REVIEW COP   review.
We would appreci___ your se___

TURNER SYNDROME

Edited by: Ron___ Rosen___
           Melvin M. Gru___

Published: 1990
552 pages, bound, illustra___

$150.00 (U.S. and Canada)
$180.00 (All other countries)
(Prices subject to change wit___   ___tice.)

marcel dekker, inc.

270 MADISON AVENUE • NEW YORK ___ 10016 • 212-696-9000

Turner Syndrome

Turner Syndrome

edited by

Ron G. Rosenfeld

Stanford University Medical Center
Stanford, California

Melvin M. Grumbach

University of California at San Francisco
San Francisco, California

Marcel Dekker, Inc.   New York and Basel

Library of Congress Cataloging-in-Publication Data

Turner syndrome / edited by Ron Rosenfeld, Melvin Grumbach.
     p.   cm.
    Based on the First International Turner Syndrome Symposium held in
San Francisco, Calif., 1988, sponsored by Genentech, Inc.
    ISBN 0-8247-8108-2 (alk. paper)
    1. Turner's syndrome--Congresses. I. Rosenfeld, Ron G.
  II. Grumbach, Melvin M. III. International Turner
Syndrome Symposium (1st : 1988 : San Francisco, Calif.)
    IV. Genentech, Inc.
    [DNLM: 1. Turner's Syndrome--congresses. QS 677 T952 1988]
RJ520.T87T87   1989
618.92'0042--dc20
DNLM/DLC
for Library of Congress   89-17131
                                                          CIP

This book is printed on acid-free paper.

MARCEL DEKKER, INC.
270 Madison Avenue, New York, New York 10016

Current printing (last digit):
10 9 8 7 6 5 4 3 2 1

PRINTED IN THE UNITED STATES OF AMERICA

Preface

Fifty-one years ago, Henry Turner described seven phenotypic females exhibiting short stature, sexual infantilism, webbing of the neck, low posterior hairline, and increased carrying angle of the elbow. Over the ensuing 5 decades, it has become apparent that the syndrome which now bears his name is a surprisingly common chromosomal disorder. Its incidence has been estimated to be between 1/2000 and 1/5000 live-born phenotypic females, and as many as 1 in 15 spontaneous abortions have karyotypes consistent with classical Turner syndrome.

Early recognition of the cardinal clinical features of Turner syndrome, combined with appropriate chromosomal analysis and thorough diagnostic evaluation, permits effective and compassionate counseling of the child and family, prompt recognition of associated disorders, and timely institution of therapy directed at promoting growth and normalizing secondary sexual development. Although the underlying pathogenesis of many of the phenotypic characteristics of Turner syndrome remains uncertain, effective clinical care of these patients requires careful integration of therapy directed toward a wide variety of primary and associated abnormalities.

On the 50th anniversary of the initial report by Henry Turner, the First International Turner Syndrome Symposium was held in San Francisco, California, under the generous sponsorship of Genentech, Inc. The six sessions were designed to explore recent developments in our understanding of: the genetics of

Turner syndrome and related abnormalities of the X and Y chromosomes, the natural history of Turner syndrome and associated abnormalities, growth hormone secretion and bone and cartilage development in Turner syndrome, endocrine therapy in Turner syndrome, intellectual and psychosocial development, and the future for women with Turner syndrome.

This volume is respectfully dedicated to all of our patients with Turner syndrome and their families. They have repeatedly instructed all of us not only about the rich phenotypic and karyotypic variability of this syndrome, but also about how one lives courageously in the face of medical adversity.

Ron G. Rosenfeld

Turner's Original Description
Reprinted from *Endocrinology*, Vol. 23, November 1938

Henry H. Turner

*From the Endocrine Clinic of the Out-Patient Department of the University
Hospital, University of Oklahoma School of Medicine,
Oklahoma City, Oklahoma*

A SYNDROME OF INFANTILISM, CONGENITAL WEBBED NECK, AND CUBITUS VALGUS

The triad, infantilism, webbing of the skin of the neck, and deformity of the elbow (cubitus valgus), occurring in the same individual is unusual, and, to my knowledge, has not been previously reported. It is sufficiently interesting to warrant this report, although the individual signs are perhaps not uncommon. Short neck, due to absence of the cervical spine, was first described by Klippel and Feil (1) in 1912. Only about 40 such cases have been reported to date, and these mostly in the French and German literature.

A similar condition (pseudo-Klippel-Feil syndrome) (2) has been reported, in which there was a numerical variation in, and more or less complete fusion of, the cervical vertebrae. Webbing of the neck was first described by Kobylinski (3) in 1882, and its relation to congenital short neck was suggested by Darchter (4) in 1922. Frawley (5) states that webbing is the most uncommon feature of congenital short neck, the most usual being the absence or fusing of the cervical vertebrae.

Sprengel's deformity (congenital elevation of the scapulae and other conditions, such as traumatic or spontaneous dislocation of the atlas on the axis

---

Read before the 22d Annual Meeting of The Association for the Study of Internal Secretions, San Francisco, California, June 13–14, 1938.

(Frissell's disease), cervical Potts disease, and sometimes torticollis) simulates congenital webbed neck. The classic objective signs of Klippel-Feil syndrome, as given by Bauman (6), are: *a*), absence or shortening of the neck; *b*), lowering of the hair-line on the back of the neck; *c*), limitation of motion. Other signs occurring in a certain percentage of cases are: *a*), torticollis, *b*), mirror movement, *c*), facial asymmetry, *d*), dorsal scoliosis, and other deformities accompanied by difficulty in breathing or swallowing and shortness of breath.

The group of patients presented in this report cannot be classified under any of the above syndromes, inasmuch as the shortening of the neck is merely apparent, due to the webbing, and not real. There is no absence or fusion of the cervical spine in any of these patients. There is some lowering of the hairline on the back of the neck, but no marked limitation of motion. Torticollis, mirror movements, facial asymmetry, and other signs and symptoms, such as difficulty in breathing or swallowing, shortness of breath, etc., are not present. There is no mental retardation. Deformity of the elbow, consisting of an increase in the carrying angle, or cubitus valgus, is constantly present.

All of my patients present osseous and sexual retardation similar to that associated with hypoantuitarism, or the Lorain-Levi type of dwarfism. Funke (7) reported a case of 'pterygium colli,' which was somewhat similar to mine, in that the patient, aged 15 years, was retarded in growth and sexual development; however, no reference was made to any osseous deformities.

CASE REPORT

Case 1. D. G., a female, aged 16 years 3 months, was first seen by me on March 28, 1932. She walked, talked, and teethed at the normal age. Her stature has always been less than that of her playmates of the same years. The patient showed somatic and sexual underdevelopment of the Lorain-Levi type. Her height was 53 in. (average 63.35 in.), and weight 78.25 lb. (average 118 lb.). There was no evidence of any secondary sex characters. Her breasts were quite masculine, and no glandular tissue was palpable.

Gynecological examination by Dr. J. B. Eskridge revealed greatly delayed development of the labia; the vagina barely admitted the index finger and was about 1.6 in. deep. The mucosa was dry and of the infantile type. The cervix was about the size of a pea, and there was an apparent congenital absence of the uterus and ovaries.

There was an internal squint of the right eye. The neck appeared very short, and there was a wing-like fold of skin extending from the mastoid region almost to the acromion. The hair-line was very low on the back of the neck. There was a marked deformity of the carrying angle of the elbow. No other abnormal physical findings were elicited.

Laboratory. The erythrocyte count showed a very moderate secondary anemia. The blood serology and chemistry gave normal reactions. The B.M.R. was +8 per cent. Roentgenograms of the skull and sella, cervical vertebrae, and

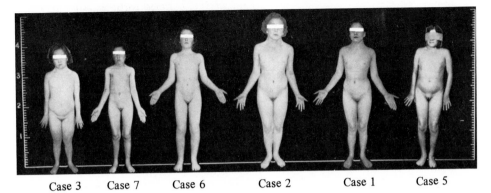

Case 3   Case 7   Case 6   Case 2   Case 1   Case 5

Figure 1 Patients illustrating the syndrome of infantilism, webbed neck, and cubitus valgus.

hips indicated normal development. A retardation of the epiphyseal union on the metacarpals and phalanges was noted. The carrying angle at the elbow measured 156° (Fig. 3).

Injections of the anterior-pituitary growth fraction, antuitrin-G, were begun, and over a period of 19 months she received 1600 cc. of this substance. Her height increased 1.75 in. (to 54.75 in.) during this period. Shortly after discontinuance of the growth hormone the patient left the city, and nothing further was heard from her until March, 1937. At that time, her height was 56.50 in. and her weight 88 lb. During the 3-year interval without treatment she had grown 1.75 in. and had gained 3 lb. There had been little, if any, change in her general appearance. The breasts and nipples continued very infantile, and there was no apparent change in her internal or external genitals. There was slightly increased hair growth over the lumbo-sacral region and over both trapezi down to the level of the scapulae. A great number of pigmented moles were noted over the trunk, with a few on the face, and there was some slight hair growth on the upper lip.

At this time, injections of 2½ cc. anterior-pituitary gonadotropic (25 U)* were administered 3 times weekly and continued for 30 days. Then, injections of 1 cc. daily were begun and continued without interruption until Oct. 11, 1937. At this time, the gynecologist reported a scant growth of hair on the mons, with rather abundant growth over the labia majora; the vagina was much larger than on the previous examination, admitting one finger very easily, and

---

*Antuitrin-G, antuitrin-gonadotropic, and theelin generously supplied by Parke, Davis & Co.; progynon-B by Schering Corp.; anterior-pituitary sex hormone, and maturity factor by Ayerst, McKenna & Harrison.

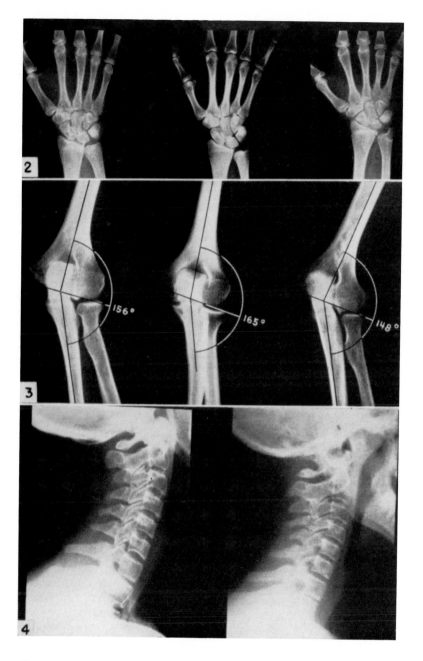

Figure 2 Case 1 (left) and case 2 (right) compared with normal of same age. Note retardation of epiphyseal union.

Figure 3 Case 1 (left) and case 2 (right) compared with normal of same age. Note increased carrying angle in both patients.

Figure 4 Case 1 (left) and case 2 (right) showing normal cervical spine.

if the vulvovaginal orifice were large enough, two fingers could be admitted. The vaginal length was 3.5 in., rugae normal and moist. The probe passed through the cervical canal to a depth of 2.2 in. With the probe in the cervix, another attempt was made to locate the uterus, but the organ or adnexa could not be palpated. It was thought the probe passed through the Müllerian duct. The cervix was 0.75 cm. in diameter, very rudimentary and short. There was no evidence of development of the nipples or breasts. It is interesting to note that there had been a definite growth in the size and depth of the vagina, to the point that it would be possible for her to marry and carry on normal marital relations.

Anterior-pituitary sex hormone (330 U maturity factor, and 75 U thyrotropic), 1 cc. daily, plus 40,000 U of theelin per week were given until Feb. 1938, at which time it was noted that the pubic hair had increased; a small uterus about the size of a pecan was palpated, and glandular tissue could be palpated in the breasts. Her weight was 94 lb., and height 57 in.

Because of the multiple injections and the fact that the buttocks were becoming quite infiltrated, it was decided to discontinue the daily injections of anterior-pituitary sex hormone but continue the 10,000 U of theelin 4 times weekly. Following the injection of a total of 170,000 U of theelin during the next four weeks, dosage was increased to 50,000 U of progynon-B 3 times weekly. Following the 6th injection, an apparently normal menstrual flow began and lasted for 3 days. She stated that the flow was moderate in amount and no pain was experienced. The injections were discontinued during this week of flow and then continued as before. Following 7 injections, or a total of 350,000 U of progynon-B, and after a rest period of 7 days, a second menstrual flow began, with an average amount of discharge for 2½ days, then scant for 3 days. No pain was encountered. Whether or not the two periods of bleeding were the true menstrual type or result of the large doses of estrin I am unable to say.

To date, she has received a total of 17 injections (850,000 U) of progynon-B. Her height is 57 in., and weight 99 lb. Pubic hair is increasing. Labia minora are still small, but showing definite evidence of development. Labia majora are small, but appear normal. The vagina easily admits one finger and is about 2.4 in. long and considered normal in size and shape for a person of this age. The cervix is about 1 inch across and much larger than on previous examination. A fundus uteri can be definitely palpated, being 1 inch across and about 1 inch thick, and approximately 2 in. long. The cervix forms about one-half of the uterus. Glandular tissue is now palpable in both breasts, and they are assuming an adolescent contour.

Case 2. O. D. L., a female, aged 18 years, was first seen on Sept. 7, 1934, because of statural underdevelopment and non-appearance of the secondary sex characters. Her height was 55 in. (average 65 in.), weight 86 lb. (average 126 lb.). There was nothing unusual in her history during infancy or childhood, with the exception that she had always been smaller than other children. She had always made excellent grades in school and at this time was taking a secretarial course. There had never been any serious illnesses. One brother, aged 15 years, and one sister, aged 25 years, father and mother, are all of average height and weight. Her general appearance was that of an anterior-pituitary dwarf of the Lorain-Levi type. There was complete absence of any secondary sexual characteristics. The breasts were flat, with no glandular tissue palpable, and the nipples were rudimentary. The neck appeared quite short, and on either side the skin appeared as a wing-like fold, extending from the mastoid almost to the acromion process. There was an abundance of black hair on the scalp, extending down the back of the neck to a point slightly below the first dorsal vertebra. The remainder of the body was devoid of hair, with the exception of very scant growth in the axillae and a few scattered over the pubis. The facial features were small, clear-cut, and there was no obvious asymmetry of the face. The eye muscles were intact. There was a marked increase of the carrying angle of the elbow.

Vaginal examination by Dr. Eskridge disclosed the labia markedly underdeveloped, and an absence of hair on the mons, with very scant growth over the labia. The vagina was too small for digital examination, and the uterus and adnexa could not be palpated. A small structure about the size of a pea was believed to be a rudimentary cervix.

Laboratory. The blood cytology, serology, and chemistry were all within normal limits. B.M.R. was +7 per cent. Chemical and microscopical examination of the urine revealed no abnormal constituents. Roentgenograms showed retardation of epiphyseal union on metacarpals and phalanges; very marked cubitus valgus; small and shallow sella; a slight osteoporosis of the spinal column; and separate ossification centers on both transverse processes of the first thoracic vertebra. The carrying angle of the elbow measured 148° (Fig. 3).

Anterior-pituitary growth hormone, 2 cc. 3 times weekly, was prescribed, and injections were continued for approximately 5 months without any appreciable increase in her height. In Oct., 1936, injections of 1 cc. maturity factor (200 U) 3 times weekly were begun and continued until April 1, 1937. Examination at this time revealed increased growth of hair on the labia and scanty growth on the mons. The labia minora were rudimentary and small. The vagina barely admitted the index finger, but the rugae were normal and moist. The cervix, about 1 cm. in diameter, did not admit a probe. The uterus and adnexa were not palpable.

Injections of antuitrin gonadotropic, 2½ cc. 3 times weekly, were then begun, and over a period of 7 months she received 70 injections, or a total of 4,375 U. At the end of the treatment period no development of the breast tissue was evident. However, the pubic hair was becoming more abundant. The vaginal canal was moist and admitted the index finger very comfortably. The uterus and ovaries still could not be palpated. At this time, her weight was 85 lb., and height 55.75 in.

Anterior-pituitary sex hormone, 2 cc. twice weekly, was begun Oct. 11, 1937, and continued to date (76 injections). At the present time her height is 56 in., and weight 91 lb. There is definite development of the labia majora. Introitus admits one finger snugly. The cervis is palpable, although still infantile, but the uterus has not yet shown signs of developing.

Case 3. V. C., a female, aged 15 years 4 months, was a normal full-term baby who had her first tooth at 9 months. She walked and talked at 13 months. Her statural development was apparently normal until the age of 9 years, but she had matured very little since then. There was no mental retardation.

The patient's general somatic development was definitely retarded, although proportional. Her height was 50 in. (average 62.27 in.), and weight 74 lb. (average 115 lb.). The upper, lower, and half-span measurements were 25 in., respectively. The neck was short and wide, and the hair-line low posteriorly. There was a moderate increase in the carrying angle of the elbow, and an internal squint of the right eye. There was no obesity. The extremities were quite acrocyanotic. The skin and hair were of normal texture. A slight hypertrichosis of the forearms was present. No breast development was evident. There were a few scattered hairs over the mons veneris. Rectal examination revealed a very infantile uterus, but no adnexa were palpated.

Laboratory. The blood count, Wassermann reaction, and chemical examinations, including serum calcium and phosphorus determinations, were all within normal limits. The urinalysis was normal. B.M.R. was +9 per cent. Roentgenograms of the wrists, shoulder, knee, skull and sella turcica, cervical spine, and elbows revealed normal osseous progress.

She received anterior-pituitary growth hormone (10 R.U.), 3 cc. subcutaneously every other day over a period of three months, with an increase in her height of 1.3 inches (theoretical normal increment 0.15 in.). Further treatment during the following 6 months, interspersed with rest periods, resulted in no further growth. In a letter received March, 1938, the mother stated that the patient's height was the same as when the growth hormone was discontinued 2½ years previously, and that sexually she remained quite infantile.

Case 4. M. B., a female, aged 16 years, consulted me first in Sept., 1934, because of dwarfism and sexual underdevelopment. Her height was 53.75 in. (average 65 in.), and weight 69 lb. (average 128 lb.). She was the second child in a family of 5, and had always been smaller than other children of her age. Examination revealed a definitely underheight and undernourished girl, with no visible evidence of secondary sex development. The neck was short and somewhat broad at the base, although there were no marked folds of skin comparable to the cases reported above. The facial features were very delicate. There was a normal amount of brown hair on the scalp, but none in the axillae or on the pubis. There was a marked increase in the carrying angle of the elbow, as observed in the other individuals of this series.

A scanty growth of hair appeared on the labia majora only. The labia minora were rudimentary, and the vagina would not admit the index finger. On rectal examination the broad ligament was found to be indistinct. There was a small mass about 0.5 in. in diameter, which was interpreted to be the cervix. The corpus uteri and ovaries were not palpable.

Roentgenograms of the skull showed an increased deposition of calcium along the coronal sutures. The sella turcia was well within normal limits, and there was no erosion of the clinoid processes. A rather marked degree of demineralization of the carpals and metacarpals, and the distal end of the ulnae and radii was demonstrated. The epiphyseal lines of the ulnae and radii and proximal ends of the metacarpals were quite visible, showing some delay in the union of the epiphyses. The cervical vertebrae were of normal number and appearance. No other laboratory procedures were recorded. No treatment.

Case 5. M. T., a female, aged 23 years, was referred to the Endocrine Clinic, University Hospital, Feb., 1935, because she was under height and had not developed sexually. She stated that she stopped growing at the age of 8 years, and was considerably disturbed because of the fact that her associates treated her as a little girl and because she feared she would never be able to marry and have a home. Her height was 52.25 in. (average 65 in.), and weight 76.75 lb. (average 130 lb.). She presented a typical picture of somatic and genital retardation with a rather oldish face. She had a very short, broad neck, with folds of skin extending from the mastoid to a point just proximally to the acromion. The hair-line extended well down the back of the neck. There was a very small amount of axillary hair, and none on the pubis. The breasts were flat with underdevelopment of the nipples, There was a marked increase in the carrying angle of the elbow.

The vaginal examination revealed very small, underdeveloped labia. The vagina admitted one finger. The uterus was about the size of that of a 6 or 7-year-old child. The ovaries could not be palpated.

Roentgenograms of the skull and sinuses revealed no apparent pathology. The epiphyses of the femurs were demonstrated. A considerable lack of calcium in the bones of the pelvis and thighs, and a demineralization in the distal end of the humerus and proximal ends of the ulna was evident, with an apparent beginning cystic degeneration in the right and left ulna. Anteroposterior and lateral views of the cervical spine revealed a spinabifida of the first cervical vertebra. The bodies of the vertebrae, however, were of normal size and position. Further laboratory investigation was refused by the patient. No treatment.

Case 6. M. A. S., a female, aged 15 years, was seen in the out-patient department of the Endocrine Clinic, University Hospital, March 1, 1937, because of her dwarfism and sexual underdevelopment. She was 51.75 in. in height (average 62.27 in.), and weighed 69 lb. (average 115 lb.). She was a normal full-term baby, and walked, talked, and teethed at the usual age, but had always grown very slowly. She was mentally alert and ahead of her class in school—an honor student.

Physical examination revealed evident infantilism, with very short neck and wing-like folds of skin extending from the mastoid region to the acromion. The hair-line was very low. There was no axillary or pubic hair. The increased carrying angle of the elbow was quite marked. Vaginal examination could not be made because of the infantile vagina. Rectal examination revealed a minute mass which was interpreted as an infantile uterus. The ovaries were not palpable.

Laboratory. The blood cytology, serology, and chemistry were all within normal limits. Roentgenograms of the cervical spine and pelvis, including both hip joints, were normal. The radial deviation of both elbows was quite prominent. The radii appeared shorter than normal, and the heads were deformed. The right wrist showed an absence of the distal epiphyses of the radius, and the carpal bones were atrophic. There was also a flattening and partial sclerosis of the epiphyses of the left ulna and radius. These observations indicated a growth disturbance; however, it was not determined whether this was of nutritional or endocrine origin. Chondrodysplasia did not seem likely. No treatment was given.

Case 7. M. B., a female, aged 16 years, was referred to the Endocrine Clinic, University Hospital, Dec. 27, 1935, because of her short stature and lack of sexual development. She was 48.50 in. in height (average 63.35 in.), and weighed 46.50 lb. (average 118 lb.). Her twin sister, who was with her, was 63 in. in height, and weighed 125 lb. The history was rather interesting, in that the patient weighed 2½ lb. at birth, while her twin weighed 5 lb. Her weight at one year was 5 lb., and that of her sister 15 lb. She had one brother and one other sister of average height and weight for their age. The parents stated that she had gained none in height or weight during the past 5 or 6 years, and that she grew very slowly before that time. She presented a rather typical picture of infantilism with congenital webbed neck and cubitus valgus. Her sister was normally developed sexually, and normal menarche was established at the age of 12 years.

Routine laboratory examinations gave essentially normal findings. Roentgenograms of the skull and sella turcica appeared normal, except for some slight demineralization. X-rays of the extremities revealed normal osseous progress, but evidence of osteoporosis. The cervical vertebrae were normal in number and appearance. No treatment was given.

SUMMARY

Infantilism with webbing of the neck and deformity of the elbow (cubitus valgus), occurring in the same individual is extremely rare, and, to the author's knowledge, has not been previously described. This unusual phenomenon was observed exclusively in seven female patients, aged 15 to 23 years. Among the characteristic signs were retardation in growth and sexual underdevelopment. Webbing of the skin of the neck was slight to marked. Absence or fusion of the cervical vertebrae was not demonstrated, and the shortening of the neck was merely apparent, due to the webbing, and not real. The posterior hair margin extended well down on the neck. Deformity of the elbow, consisting of an increase in the carrying angle, or cubitus valgus, was constantly present. Movements of the head and arms were not hindered. Fascial asymmetry, dorsal scoliosis, and other deformities, mirror movement, difficulty in breathing and swallowing, shortness of breath, or mental retardation were not present in this group of patients.

Laboratory examinations of the blood and urine showed findings that were entirely within normal limits. Roentgenograms of the skull, cervical spine, elbow, wrist, and pelvis showed no abnormalities with the exception of demineralization and evidence of delayed union of the epiphyses in 6 cases. Treatment with pituitary growth hormones has been unsatisfactory. There was definite genital development following administration of the anterior pituitary gonadotropic hormone in the two cases treated.

The author is deeply grateful to Dr. Paul C. Colonna, Department of Orthopedics; Dr. J. B. Eskridge, Department of Gynecology; Dr. Ernst Lachmann, Department of Anatomy, and Dr. A. J. Lehman, Department of Pharmacology, for their suggestions and assistance in the preparation of this report.

Addendum. Since this paper was written three additional cases have been observed making a total of ten patients to date.

REFERENCES

1. Klippel, M., and Feil, A.: Nouv. Iconogr. de la Salpetriere 25:223, 1912.
2. Roederer, C.: Bull. Soc. de Pediat. de Paris 31:255, 1933.
3. Kobylinski, O.: Arch. f. Anthrop. 14:343, 1883.
4. Drachter, R.: Klin. Wchnschr. 1:664, 1923.
5. Frawley, J. M.: Dis. Child. 29:799, 1925.
6. Bauman, G. L.: J.A.M.A. 98:129, 1932.
7. Funke: Deutsch. Ztschr. f. Chir. 63:162, 1902.

Contents

Contributors

Kersten Albertsson-Wikland, M.D., Ph.D. Associate Professor, Department of Pediatrics II and Physiology, Göteborg University, Göteborg, Sweden

David J. Baylink, M.D. Distinguished Professor of Medicine, Biochemistry and Orthopaedics, Department of Medicine, Loma Linda University School of Medicine, and Chief, Mineral Metabolism, Jerry L. Pettis Memorial Veterans' Hospital, Loma Linda, California

Jurgen R. Bierich, M.D. Professor Dr., Department of Medicine, Children's Hospital, University of Tübingen, Tübingen, Federal Republic of Germany

Robert M. Blizzard University of Virginia at Charlottesville, Charlottesville, Virginia

Nathan J. Blum, M.D.* Medical Student, Department of Pediatric Endocrinology, The Johns Hopkins University School of Medicine, Baltimore, Maryland

Werner F. Blum, M.D., Ph.D. Children's Hospital, University of Tübingen, Tübingen, Federal Republic of Germany

---

Current affiliation: Housestaff, Department of Pediatrics, The Children's Hospital of Philadelphia, Philadelphia, Pennsylvania

Patricia A. Crock, M.D. Department of Pediatrics, Monash University, Melbourne, Australia

Gordon B. Cutler, Jr., M.D. Chief, Section on Developmental Endocrinology, National Institute of Child Health and Human Development, Bethesda, Maryland

Christine M. Disteche, Ph.D. Associate Professor, Department of Pathology, University of Washington School of Medicine, Seattle, Washington

Jennifer I. Downey, M.D. Assistant Clinical Professor, Department of Psychiatry, Columbia University College of Physicians and Surgeons, and New York State Psychiatric Institute, New York, New York

Anke A. Ehrhardt, Ph.D. Professor of Clinical Psychology, Department of Psychiatry, Columbia University College of Physicians and Surgeons, New York, New York, and Research Scientist, New York State Psychiatric Institute, New York, New York

Charles J. Epstein, M.D. Professor, Department of Pediatrics and Department of Biochemistry and Biophysics, University of California at San Francisco, San Francisco, California

Harlan J. Evans, Ph.D. Senior Research Scientist, Technology Life Sciences Division, Krug International, Houston, Texas

John R. Farley, Ph.D. Research Associate Professor, Department of Biochemistry and Medicine, Loma Linda University School of Medicine, and Research Chemist, Mineral Metabolism, Jerry L. Pettis Memorial Veterans' Hospital, Loma Linda, California

Robert J. Fitzsimmons, Ph.D. Post Doctoral Fellow, Mineral Metabolism, Jerry L. Pettis Memorial Veterans' Hospital, Loma Linda, California

James W. Frane, Ph.D. Biostatistician, Department of Clinical Research, Genentech, Inc., South San Francisco, California

Frank Gasparini, Ph.D. Research Associate, Department of Chemistry, Montefiore Medical Center/Albert Einstein College of Medicine, Bronx, New York

Mitchell S. Golbus, M.D. Professor, Department of Obstetrics, Gynecology, and Reproductive Sciences and Department of Pediatrics, University of California at San Francisco, San Francisco, California

Helen E. Gruber, Ph.D. Director, Skeletal Dysplasia Morphology Lab, Medical Genetics—Birth Defects Center, Cedars-Sinai Medical Center, Los Angeles, California and Associate Researcher, Department of Pediatrics, University of California at Los Angeles School of Medicine, Los Angeles, California

Caren Grundberg, M.D.   Assistant Professor of Orthopedics, Yale University School of Medicine, New Haven, Connecticut

Judith G. Hall, M.D.   Professor, Department of Medical Genetics, University of British Columbia, Vancouver, British Columbia, Canada

Itsuro Hibi, M.D.   Director, Division of Endocrinology and Metabolism, National Children's Hospital, Tokyo, Japan

Raymond L. Hintz   Professor, Department of Pediatrics, Stanford University School of Medicine, Stanford, California

Andrew R. Hoffman, M.D.   Associate Professor, Department of Medicine, Stanford University School of Medicine, Stanford, California

William A. Horton, M.D.*   Associate Professor of Pediatrics and Medicine, Department of Pediatrics, University of Texas Medical School at Houston, Houston, Texas

Ann J. Johanson, M.D.   Associate Director, Department of Medical Affairs, Genentech, Inc., South San Francisco, California

Knud W. Kastrup, M.D.   Consultant Pediatric Endocrinologist, Department of Pediatrics, Glostrup Hospital, University of Copenhagen, Copenhagen, Denmark

John L. Kirkland, M.D.   Professor, Department of Pediatrics, Baylor College of Medicine, Houston, Texas

Rebecca Trent Kirkland, M.D.   Professor, Department of Pediatrics, Baylor College of Medicine, Houston, Texas

Ralph S. Lachman, M.D.   Professor, Radiology and Pediatrics, Harbor/University of California at Los Angeles Medical Center, Torrance, California

Yun-Fai Lau, Ph.D.   Associate Investigator and Assistant Professor, Howard Hughes Medical Institute, and Departments of Physiology and Medicine, University of California at San Francisco, San Francisco, California

Adrian D. LeBlanc, Ph.D.   Research Associate Professor, Division of Medicine, Baylor College of Medicine, Houston, Texas

Tsu-Hui Lin, M.D.   Assistant Professor, Department of Pediatrics, Baylor College of Medicine, Houston, Texas

---

Current affiliation: Professor of Pediatrics and Medicine and Director, Division of Medical Genetics, University of Texas Medical School at Houston, Houston, Texas

Susan G. Linkhart, B.S. Principal Research Assistant, Mineral Metabolism, Jerry L. Pettis Memorial Veterans' Hospital, Loma Linda, California

Thomas A. Linkhart, Ph.D. Research Associate Professor, Department of Pediatrics, Associate Professor, Department of Biochemistry, Loma Linda University School of Medicine, and Staff, Jerry L. Pettis Memorial Veterans' Hospital, Loma Linda, California

Barbara M. Lippe, M.D. Professor, Department of Pediatrics and Chief, Division of Endocrinology, University of California at Los Angeles School of Medicine, Los Angeles, California

Matthew B. Lubin, M.D. Postdoctoral Fellow, Medical Genetics—Birth Defects Center, Cedars-Sinai Medical Center, Los Angeles, California

Noel K. Maclaren, M.D. Professor and Chairman, Pathology and Laboratory Medicine, University of Florida College of Medicine, Gainesville, Florida

Frank Majewski, M.D. University of Düsseldorf, Düsseldorf, Federal Republic of Germany

Morri E. Markowitz, M.D. Associate Professor, Department of Pediatrics, Montefiore Medical Center/Albert Einstein College of Medicine, Bronx, New York

Barbara C. McGillivray, M.D. Clinical Genetics Unit, University of British Columbia, Vancouver, British Columbia, Canada

Subburaman Mohan, Ph.D. Research Associate Professor, Department of Biochemistry and Associate Professor, Department of Physiology, Loma Linda School of Medicine, Loma Linda, California

Daniel Navot, M.D. Professor, The Jones Institute for Reproductive Medicine, Department of Obstetrics and Gynecology, Eastern Virginia Medical School, Norfolk, Virginia

Johannes Nielsen, M.D. Chief of Service, Cytogenetic Laboratory, Psychiatric Hospital in Århus, Risskov, Denmark

Susumu Ohno, D.V.M., Ph.D., D.Sc. Ben Horowitz Chair of Distinguished Scientist in Reproductive Genetics, Department of Theoretical Biology, Beckman Research Institute of the City of Hope, Duarte, California

David C. Page Whitehead Institute, Cambridge, Massachusetts

Jaakko Perheentupa, M.D. Professor and Chairman, Department of Pediatrics, University of Helsinki and Director, University Children's Hospital, Helsinki, Finland

Leslie P. Plotnick, M.D. Associate Professor, Department of Pediatrics, Johns Hopkins Medical Institutions, Baltimore, Maryland

Andrea Prader Kinderspital, Zürich, Switzerland

Michael Preece, M.D. Professor of Child Health and Growth, Department of Growth and Development, Institute of Child Health, University of London, London, England

Michael B. Ranke, M.D. Professor, Department of Medicine, Children's Hospital, University of Tübingen, Tübingen, Federal Republic of Germany

David L. Rimoin, M.D., Ph.D. Director, Department of Pediatrics and The Medical Genetics Birth Defects Center, Steven Spielberg Chairman of Pediatrics, Cedars-Sinai Medical Center, and Professor of Pediatrics and Medicine, University of California at Los Angeles School of Medicine, Los Angeles, California

Arthur Robinson, M.D. Professor Emeritus, Departments of Pediatrics and Biochemistry, Biophysics, and Genetics, University of Colorado Health Sciences Center, and National Jewish Center, Denver, Colorado

Sten Rosberg, Ph.D. Professor, Department of Physiology, University of Göteborg, Göteborg, Sweden

Susan R. Rose, M.D. Adjunct Scientist, Developmental Endocrinology Branch, National Institute of Child Health and Human Development, Bethesda, Maryland

Ron G. Rosenfeld, M.D. Associate Professor, Department of Pediatrics, Stanford University School of Medicine, Stanford, California

Robert L. Rosenfield, M.D. Professor of Pediatrics and Medicine, Department of Pediatrics, The University of Chicago Pritzker School of Medicine, Chicago, Illinois

Zev Rosenwaks, M.D.* Director and Professor, The Jones Institute for Reproductive Medicine, Department of Obstetrics and Gynecology, Eastern Virginia Medical School, Norfolk, Virginia

Judith L. Ross, M.D. Associate Professor, Department of Pediatrics, Hahnemann University, Philadelphia, Pennsylvania

Karen R. Rubin, M.D. Assistant Professor, Department of Pediatrics, University of Connecticut Health Center, Farmington, Connecticut

---

Current affiliation: Director, In Vitro Fertilization, Department of Obstetrics and Gynecology, Cornell University Medical Center, The New York Hospital, New York, New York

Paul Saenger, M.D. Professor, Department of Pediatrics and Head, Division of Pediatric Endocrinology, Montefiore Medical Center/Albert Einstein College of Medicine, Bronx, New York

Desmond A. Schatz, M.D. Instructor, Department of Pediatric Endocrinology and Pathology, University of Florida College of Medicine, Gainesville, Florida

Larry J. Shapiro, M.D. Investigator, Howard Hughes Medical Institute, and Professor, Departments of Pediatrics and Biological Chemistry, University of California at Los Angeles School of Medicine, Los Angeles, California

Barry M. Sherman, M.D. Director, Department of Clinical Research, Genentech, Inc., South San Francisco, California

Kazuo Shizume, M.D. Associate Professor, Department of Medicine, Institute of Clinical Endocrinology, Tokyo Women's Medical College, Tokyo, Japan

Norman H. Silverman, M.D., D.Sc. Professor of Pediatrics and Radiology, (Cardiology), University of California at San Francisco, San Francisco, California

Joe L. Simpson, M.D. Faculty Professor and Chairman, Department of Obstetrics and Gynecology, University of Tennessee, Memphis, Memphis, Tennessee Tennessee

Annlis Söderholm, M.D. Pediatrician, Child Welfare Office, Social Service Center, Helsinki, Finland

Peter Stubbe, M.D. Professor, Department of Medicine, Children's Hospital, University of Göttingen, Göttingen, Federal Republic of Germany

Kazue Takano, M.D. Associate Professor, Department of Medicine, Institute of Clinical Endocrinology, Tokyo Women's Medical College, Tokyo, Japan

Ayako Tanae, M.D. Division of Endocrinology and Metabolism, National Children's Hospital, Tokyo, Japan

James Tanner University of Texas Health Science Center, Houston, Texas

George A. Werther, MBBS, M.Sc. (oxon), FRACP Deputy Director, Department of Endocrinology and Diabetes, Royal Children's Hospital, Melbourne, Australia

H. Norman B. Wettenhall, M.D. Consultant Endocrinologist, Department of Endocrinology, Royal Children's Hospital, Melbourne, Australia

Darrell M. Wilson, M.D. Assistant Professor, Department of Pediatrics, Stanford University School of Medicine, Stanford, California

TURNER SYMPOSIUM PARTICIPANTS

The following also participated at the First International Turner Symposium. August, Gilbert, Children's Hospital, Washington, D.C.; Becker, Dorothy, Children's Hospital, Pittsburgh, PA; Beitins, Inese, University of Michigan, Ann Arbor, MI; Bell, Jennifer, Columbia Presbyterian Medical Center, New York, NY; Bier, Dennis, St. Louis Children's Hospital, St. Louis, MO; Blethen, Sandra, Schneider Children's Hospital, New Hyde Park, NY; Brasel, Jo Anne, UCLA Medical Center, Torrance, CA; Brook, Charles, The Middlesex Hospital, London, England; Brown, David, Minneapolis Children's Health Center, Minneapolis, MN; Burstein, Stephen, University of Chicago, Chicago, IL; Butenandt, Otfrid, Universitäts-Kinderklinik, München, Germany; Cara Jr., Jose, University of Chicago, Chicago, IL; Cara Sr., Jose, Downstate Medical Center, Brooklyn, NY; Chernausek, Steven, Children's Hospital of Cincinnati, Cincinnati, OH; Conte, Felix, University of California at San Francisco, San Francisco, CA; Costin, Gertrude, Children's Hospital of Los Angeles, Los Angeles, CA; Cowell, Cristopher, The Children's Hospital, Camperdown, Sydney, Australia; Crowley, William, Massachusetts General Hospital, Boston, MA.

Elkin, Evan, Columbia University, New York, NY; Frasier, Douglas, Olive View Medical Center, Sylmar, CA; Furlanetto, Richard, Children's Hospital of Philadelphia, Philadelphia, PA; Genel, Myron, Yale University, New Haven, CT; Gertner, Joseph, New York Hospital, New York, NY; Golbus, Mitchell, University of California, San Francisco, CA; Gotlin, Ronald, University of Colorado, Denver, CO; Grumbach, Melvin, University of California, San Francisco, CA; Guidice, Linda, Stanford University, Stanford, CA; Gunnarsson, Rolf, Kabi-Vitrum, Stockholm, Sweden; Hanna, Cheryl, University of Oregon, Portland, OR; Hansen, Inger, Medical University of South Carolina, Charleston, SC; Holland, Frederick, Hospital for Sick Children, Toronto, Canada; Kaluski, Jacob, KabiVitrum, Stockholm, Sweden; Kaplan, Selna, University of California, San Francisco, CA; Klingensmith, Georgeanna, Children's Hospital of Denver, Denver, CO; Lee, Peter, Children's Hospital of Pittsburgh, Pittsburgh, PA; MacGillivray, Margaret, Children's Hospital of Buffalo, Buffalo, NY.

Mahoney, Patrick, Mason Clinic, Seattle, WA; Moore, Wayne, University of Kansas Medical Center, Kansas City, KS; Nilsson, Karl Olof, Malmo General Hospital, Malmo, Sweden; Rappaport, Raphael, Hospital des Enfants-Malades, Paris, France; Rosenthal, Stephen, University of California, San Francisco, CA; Sockalosky, Joseph, St. Paul Ramsey Medical Center, St. Paul, MN; Sotos, Juan, Children's Hospital of Columbus, Columbus, OH; Styne, Dennis, University of California, Davis, CA; Underwood, Louis, University of North Carolina, Chapel Hill, NC; Van Vliet, G., Hospital Universitaire Saint-Pierre, Bruxelles, Belgium; Van Wyk, Judson, University of North Carolina, Chapel Hill, NC; Wilton, Patrick, KabiVitrum, Stockholm, Sweden; Wyatt, David, Medical College of Wisconsin, Milwaukee, WI; Zachman, Milo, Universitäts-Kinderklinik, Zürich, Switzerland.

Part I

Genetics, Organogenesis, and Incidence

1

X and Y Chromosome Organization
The Pseudoautosomal Region

Larry J. Shapiro

*University of California at Los Angeles School of Medicine
Los Angeles, California*

This chapter provides a brief introduction to the functional anatomy and topography of the human X and Y chromosomes and describes some interests that have developed in our laboratory over the past couple of years. Together the X and the Y chromosomes make up between 5 and 8% of the haploid genome, however, there is probably no portion of the human genetic complement that we know about in more detail, at least in terms of the specific genes located in this region. More than 130 functional loci have been mapped to various portions of the X chromosome by a variety of methods over a substantial period of time (1). The map of the Y chromosome, however, is relatively barren. In addition, since the advent of recombinant DNA libraries that have been constructed from the X chromosome, it has been possible to assign more than 240 anonymous DNA segments to the X chromosome, which serve as further landmarks for genetic studies and "anatomical" dissection of this chromosome (2). A similar group of DNA markers exists for the Y chromosome. Furthermore, there are a number of human diseases that are known to be associated with mutant genes on the X chromosome. This knowledge goes back to antiquity (with several biblical references to hemophilia and its pattern of inheritance) and derives from the relative ease with which one can assign these loci to the X chromosome given a typical sex-linked pedigree. The genetic map of the Y chromosome is much more sparsely populated. For a variety of reasons, it has been difficult to identify many functional genes which map to this chromosome, although many random DNA clones have been isolated from the Y.

The questions with relevance to our interests are: (1) What are the genes on the X and the Y chromosomes that are responsible for the Turner syndrome? (2) What are the chromosomal factors that might predispose to the very high frequency of the Turner syndrome in human conceptions? and (3) Why is the Y chromosome so devoid of markers and landmarks? I would like to consider these issues from an evolutionary perspective, since that may be the easiest way to think about sex determination and the role of mammalian sex chromosomes (3). In some lower vertebrates, sex determination is not a genetic affair at all. There are a number of fishes and reptiles in which sex is determined by environmental cues. For example, in some species, sexual differentiation is established by the temperature at which eggs are incubated prior to hatching. In other animals, sexual phenotype may actually switch during the lifespan of an individual. However, somewhere in the lineage that led to modern-day humans, an absolute, programmed genetic method of sex determination developed, and it is such a system that exists in all present-day mammals. It is widely believed that the "modern-day" X and Y chromosomes evolved from a homologous chromosome pair that had most of their gene sequences and functions in common. However, a gene or a small cluster of genes that were critically involved in male sex determination became localized to the Y chromosome, and this event led to the differentiation of the ancestral Y from the ancestral X. Once this committed distinction between X and Y chromosomes was made, there was probably strong selection for a mechanism that might suppress recombination between the X and the Y, as it would not do very much good to inherit some of the male sex-determining genes without getting all of them. With some genes that might function more efficiently on the Y and others on the X, it would be disadvantageous to the organism to continue to exchange DNA between these previously homologous chromosomes. The easiest way to inhibit such recombination events at meiosis would be to grossly rearrange genes on either the X or the Y, thus preventing their pairing during spermatogenesis. However, other methods to suppress recombination may have evolved as well.

Perhaps it is easiest to contemplate the importance of genetically isolating the X and Y through consideration of situations where this mechanism has gone awry. In the sex-reversed (Sxr) mouse a Y chromosome that carries an extra male-determining gene(s) at the very distal end of the mouse Y chromosome in addition to the normal male sex-determining gene(s) residing in the proximal portion of the Y has been identified (4,5). For reasons that will be explained below, this aberrant positioning of the male sex-determining gene facilitates the transfer of such sequences to the X chromosome during meiosis, giving rise in the next generation to the individuals who are XX males. Such XX males are sterile and exemplify the disadvantageous nature of exchanging genes which are involved in male sex determination and differentiation between Y and X. Loss of fertility would represent the ultimate selection against such rearranged chromosomes. Similar problems arise in human XX males as elegantly established by Page and others (6).

Once suppression of recombination became established, several things probably happened. As the X and the Y became genetically isolated from one another and stopped exchanging information, they diverged very rapidly at a DNA sequence level. Mutations that accumulated on the Y chromosome were always covered by the presence of an X chromosome, and so with time the Y has degenerated to its present status as a much smaller chromosome than the X, with many pseudogenes, repetitive sequences, and few identifiable functional genes other than those involved in testis determination.

There are, however, several evolutionary problems created by having dimorphic, bifunctional sex chromosomes. Two of these problems are the need to establish dosage compensation between males and females who have an inequity in genetic endowment and the need to obtain proper pairing and segregation of the X and the Y chromosomes during spermatogenesis in the male. The solutions to both of these problems are probably germane to the consideration of the Turner syndrome.

Dosage compensation in mammals has, of course, been achieved by X chromosome inactivation (7). Different evolutionary solutions to this problem have been employed by other species such as *Drosophila* and *C. elegans* in which coordinate regulation of both Xs in females is effected. However, in female mammals one of the two Xs is inactivated and creates the well-known mosaicism for gene expression in females who are heterozygous for any X-linked phenotypic marker. The mechanisms by which this process is initiated remains somewhat elusive, although insight into the role of DNA methylation in the maintenance of the X inactivation has been obtained recently (8–16). In the past couple of years several laboratories have provided data regarding the molecular basis for X and Y pairing in male meiosis. There is a region of the X and the Y chromosomes in both mouse and man in which there is complete DNA sequence homology (17–21). These regions of the X and Y are identical because they undergo frequent recombination during spermatogenesis. This essentially creates a homogenization of DNA sequences in this region and keeps them identical and permits the X and Y to continue to pair with one another and recognize each other to assure proper sex chromosome alignment and segregation during meiosis. This region of X-Y homology has been termed the "pseudoautosomal segment" by Burgoyne (22) and others. This is because any genetic marker which happens to be in the pseudoautosomal region will show either partial sex linkage or no apparent sex linkage at all if subjected to pedigree analysis because alleles will recombine and keep switching back and forth between the X and the Y chromosomes.

Another point which is implicit in considerations of the region of X-Y homology is that any genes situated in this pseudoautosomal segment will be present in equivalent dosage in XX individuals as in XY individuals as distinguished from all other X- and Y-linked genes. At the present time there are only two pseudoautosomal genes of known function whose expression can be monitored, and in both instances it is of note that both are expressed from the X and Y chromosomes in males and also from both copies of the X chromosome in somatic cells in females. These genes are the steroid sulfatase gene in the mouse and a gene called *MIC2*, which encodes a cell surface antigen of unknown function but which can be readily measured in humans and is present on the human X and Y.

Peter Goodfellow's laboratory in London has shown conclusively that *MIC2* is present on the human X and on the Y (18), that both copies are expressed in males, and that the *MIC2* gene escapes inactivation and continues to be expressed from both X chromosomes in normal female somatic cells. Similarly, Stanley Gartler's laboratory in Seattle has shown that there are functional copies of the steroid sulfatase gene on the X and Y chromosomes of the mouse, that they are expressed from both X and Y in males and from both Xs in females, and also that there is recombination between the X and the Y loci (21). At the present time, there is a relative paucity of data regarding other loci in this region. While a number of anonymous DNA probes have been obtained from the pseudoautosomal regions of the mouse and human sex chromosomes, these reagents do not provide further information about expressed genes. However, for the above two described examples of STS and MIC2, it is of note that both escape from X chromosome inactivation. From a teleologic perspective, if a gene were normally expressed from both the X and Y chromosomes in males, then one might expect such a gene to be expressed equally from both Xs in females so that there would be no difference in dosage between XX females and XY males.

By electron microscopic examination, synaptonemal complexes involving the human X and Y chromosomes extend beyond what seems to be the anticipated boundaries of the pseudoautosomal region (23). Within this more proximal portion of the X and Y, there appears not to be frequent exchange between dissimilar sex chromosomes, and so strictly X-linked and strictly Y-linked sequences have developed. We have shown that the functional human STS gene is in fact located in this nonhomologous region on the X chromosome. However, similar to the situation previously described in the mouse, the human X-linked STS escapes X chromosome inactivation in females. Since there is no functional STS gene on the human Y chromosome, this ceates a curious situation in which females with two active copies of the gene express higher levels of STS in most tissues than do males with only a single active copy.

In the past few months, we have obtained data which helps to explain the differences in human and murine STS gene organization and, in the process, may provide some insight into the evolutionary history of the sex chromosomes. Based on experiments in which genomic DNA from a number of individuals was probed with a cloned STS cDNA, the presence of STS-related sequences on the long arm of the human Y chromosome was appreciated (14). To undertake a more thorough analysis of the human STS gene(s), it was necessary to clone and partially sequence both the X-encoded functional gene and these newly identified Y chromosome sequences.

The functional X-encoded gene spans approximately 150 kilobases (kb) and is organized into 10 exons. We have sequenced each of the exon-intron junctions. The first intron is the longest and spans about 40 kb. One hundred kb of the STS-like sequences from the Y chromosome long arm were cloned as well. Detailed analysis indicates that the Y locus is a pseudogene. It lacks the region which corresponds to the X-linked gene's promoter, and consequently no evidence for transcription of the Y gene has been obtained. Even if the Y gene were transcribed, there are numerous missense and nonsense mutations that would render the product nonfunctional. Both intronlike and exonlike sequences are represented in the Y-encoded locus, and so it can be characterized as a non-processed pseudogene. Direct comparison of sequencing information between the X and Y genes reveals that they are 85–92% similar, both within intronlike and exonlike segments. If one assumes that the STS gene and the STS-Y pseudogene have evolved from a common ancestor, then by the usual molecular estimates, they should have been diverging for 35 to 45 million years. It is also of interest that the extent of divergence is equivalent between intronlike and exonlike sequences suggesting that the STS-Y exon sequences have not been under any selective pressure. This indicates that the STS-Y gene probably lost its function at about the same time that the two genes began drifting apart. Based on other data including studies of STS gene organization in primates and the arrangement of other sequences on the human X and Y, it seems likely that there has been at least one pericentric inversion of the Y chromosome during primate evolution. This may explain the curious differences between the mouse and human STS gene. In an ancestor of man and mouse the STS gene was probably truly pseudoautosomal, and functional copies were present on the X and Y chromosomes. This is the situation that still pertains in the modern-day mouse genome. However, in the primate lineage, the putative pericentric inversion of the Y disrupted this X-Y homology relationship, and since the STS-X and STS-Y genes could no longer undergo recombination, they diverged. The fact that the human STS-X gene escapes inactivation is thus explained as an evolutionary remnant of its former pseudoautosomal status.

In closing, some speculation about the relationship between the pseudoautosomal region and the Turner syndrome would seem appropriate. It is tempting to attribute many of the abnormalities seen in the Turner syndrome to deficiencies of gene activity related to loci which map to the pseudoautosomal region. If X inactivation involves all genes outside the pseudoautosomal region, then there should be no dosage difference between an XO female and an XX female except at the very earliest stages of preimplantation development at loci other than those in the pseudoautosomal segment. Clearly, the identification of genes such as the human STS gene, which escape inactivation but which are not truly pseudoautosomal, would dictate an alteration of this point of view. Clinical observations, however, do not fully support this assessment of the etiology of the Turner syndrome. A number of individuals with Xp deletions involving all of the pseudoautosomal region have been reported. While some of these patients have some Turner stigmata, many do not. Thus, it would appear that simply deleting the pseudoautosomal segment is not sufficient to induce full-blown Turner syndrome. Perhaps there are other genes on the X chromosome that are not regulated by X inactivation whose expression is thus altered in the Turner syndrome as compared to normal females. This will clearly require further study. It is worth noting that XO mice have been available and studied for some time. They have some phenotypic abnormalities but lack many of the cardiovascular and lymphatic problems seen in human patients with XO karyotypes. Furthermore, XO mice are fertile although they do appear to undergo premature ovarian failure. Perhaps differences in those genes which are included in pseudoautosomal region account for some of these interspecies differences. It is likely that the pseudoautosomal region has both expanded and contracted over evolutionary time for reasons that have been described above.

A final consideration connecting the pseudoautosomal genes in the Turner syndrome relates to the etiology of this common chromosomal aneuploidy. It is well established that the Turner syndrome is among the most common cytogenetic abnormalities detectable in our species. This is particularly true if one considers early conceptions where the XO karyotype has been estimated to be found in as many as 25% of chromosomally abnormal abortuses studied (24). Why is sex chromosome aneuploidy so common? It is possible that the tenuous pairing of X and Y chromosomes which occurs during spermatogenesis may predispose to a high frequency of nondisjunction. This will have to be studied by more direct means. Consistent with this notion, however, is the observation that the remaining X chromosome in the majority of XO patients is maternally derived. This would indicate that it is the paternal sex chromosome (X or Y) that has been lost or is missing. On the other hand, the high frequency of mosaicism observed in XO individuals argues for a postzygotic event. Clearly, further research in this area is needed.

REFERENCES

1. McKusick VA. Mendelian Inheritance in Man, 8th ed. Baltimore: Johns Hopkins Press, 1988.

2. Davies KE, Mandel JL, Weissenbach J, Fellous M. Report of the committee on the genetic constitution of the X and Y chromosomes. Human Gene Mapping 9. Cytogen and Cell Genet 1987; 4611:277–315.
3. Bull JJ. Evolution of Sex Determining Mechanisms. Menlo Park, CA: Benjamin/Cummings Publishing, 1983.
4. Singh L, Jones KW. Sex reversal in the mouse (Mus musculus) is caused by a recurrent non-reciprocal crossover involving the X and an aberrant Y chromosome. Cell 1982; 28:205.
5. Evans EP, Burtenshaw MD, Cattanch BM. Meiotic crossover between the X and Y chromosomes of male mice carrying the sex-reversing (Sxr) factor. Nature 1982; 300:443.
6. Page DC. Sex reversal: deletion mapping the male-determining function of the human Y chromosome. Cold Spring Harbor Symp on Quant Biol LI 1986; 229–235.
7. Gartler SM, Riggs AD. Mammalian X-chromosome inactivation. Ann Rev Genet 1983; 17:155–190.
8. Liskay RM, Evans RJ. Inactive X chromosome DNA-mediated cell transformation for the hypoxanthine phosphoribosyl transferase gene. Proc Natl Acad Sci USA 1980; 77:4895.
9. Venolia L, Gartler SM, Wassman ER, Yen P, Mohandas T, Shapiro L. Transformation with DNA from 5-azacytidine reactivated X chromosomes. Proc Natl Acad Sci USA 1982; 79:2352.
10. Lester SC, Korn NK, Demars R. Derepression of genes on the human inactive X chromosome: Evidence for differences in locus-specific rates of derepression and rates of transfer of active and inactive genes after DNA-mediated transformation. Somatic Cell Genet 1982; 8:265.
11. Chapman VM, Kratzer PG, Siracusa LD, Quarantillo BA, Evans R, Liskay RM. Evidence for DNA modification in the maintenance of X chromosome inactivation in adult mouse tissue. Proc Natl Acad Sci USA 1982; 79:5357.
12. Kratzer PG, Chapman VM, Lambert H, Evans RE, Liskay RM. Differences in the DNA of the inactive X chromosome of fetal and extra-embryonic tissues of mice. Cell 1983; 33:38.
13. Mohandas T, Sparkes RS, Shapiro LJ. Reactivation of an inactive human X chromosome: Evidence for X-inactivation by DNA methylation. Science 1981; 211:393.
14. Yen P, Patel PI, Chinault AC, Mohandas T, Shapiro LJ. Differential methylation of HPRT genes on active and inactive X chromosomes. Proc Natl Acad Sci USA 1984; 81:1759–1763.
15. Wolf SF, Jolly DJ, Lunnen KD, Friedmann T, Migeon BR. Methylation of the hypoxanthine phosphoribosyl transferase locus on the human X chromosome: implications for X-chromosome inactivation. PNAS 1984; 81:2806–2810.
16. Keith DH, Singer-Sam J, Riggs AD. Active X chromosome DNA is unmethylated at eight CCGG sites clustered in a guanine-plus-cytosine-rich island at the 5' end of the gene for phosphoglycerate kinase. Mol Cell Biol 1986; 6:4122–4125.

17. Cooke HJ, Brown WRA, Rappold GA. Hypervariable telomeric sequences from the human sex chromosomes are pseudoautosomal. Nature 1985; 317:687–692.

18. Goodfellow PJ, Darling SM, Thomas NS, Goodfellow PN. A pseudoauto-somal gene in man. Science 1986; 234:740–743.

19. Simmler M-C, Rouyer F, Vergnaud G, Nystrom-Lahti M, Ngo KY, de la Chapelle A, Weissenbach J. Pseudoautosomal DNA sequences in the pairing region of the human sex chromosomes. Nature 1985; 317:692–697.

20. Soriano P, Keitges EA, Schorderet DF, Harbers K, Gartler SM, Jaenisch R. High rate of recombination and double crossovers in the mouse pseudo-autosomal region during male meiosis. Proc Natl Acad Sci USA 1987; 84: 7218–7220.

21. Keitges EA, Schorderet DF, Gartler SM. Linkage of the steroid sulfatase gene to the sex-reversed mutation in the mouse. Genetics 1987; 116:465–469.

22. Burgoyne PS. Genetic homology and crossing over in the X and Y chromosomes of mammals. Hum Genet 1982; 61:85–90.

23. Shapiro LJ. Steroid sulfatase deficiency and the genetics of the short arm of the human X chromosome. Adv Hum Genet 1985; 14:331–382.

24. Boue A, Boue J, Gropp A. Cytogenetics of pregnancy wastage. Adv Hum Genet 1985; 14:1–57.

DISCUSSION

DR. WILLIAM HORTON: Larry, do you have any idea how many genes ultimately will be mapped to that pseudoautosomal area?

DR. LARRY SHAPIRO: It is hard to say, Bill. It is interesting that there has been a relative dearth of expressed genes there. I mean the physical region is probably on the order of about 5 to 7 megabases, so there is room for lots of genes there, several hundred, but how many will actually be found, I don't know. More than we know of yet.

DR. ARTHUR ROBINSON: I just wondered, Larry, if anybody has looked at any of the mammals between the mouse and the human to see how this evolutionary change is coming about?

Dr. Horton is at the University of Texas, Houston, Texas. Dr. Shapiro is at the University of California at Los Angeles School of Medicine, Los Angeles, California. Dr. Robinson is at the University of Colorado, Denver, Colorado.

DR. SHAPIRO: Not yet. Clearly that is in progress. One interesting sort of observation that is slowing us down a little bit in that regard is that there has been relatively little conservation of the STS gene between mouse and man, surprisingly little compared to most other garden-variety housekeeping genes, of which this is a presumed member. And so that has slowed down our cloning efforts of actually being able to characterize the mouse gene in the detail we would like. But yet, we would obviously like to look particularly at primates to see if we can really find further evidence for this evolutionary track.

2

Mechanisms Leading to the Phenotype of Turner Syndrome

Charles J. Epstein

University of California at San Francisco
San Francisco, California

PRINCIPLES FOR ANALYZING THE EFFECTS OF ANEUPLOIDY

Why should loss of a sex chromosome, so that only a single X chromosome is present, cause the phenotype of Turner syndrome? In attempting to answer this question—or at least to suggest possible answers—I start from the same premises that apply to any other type of aneuploid condition (1). Aneuploidy (chromosome imbalance) is a disorder of gene dosage, in which the addition or loss of a chromosome or chromosome segment results in a proportionate increase or decrease in the synthesis of the products of the genes present in the region of imbalance. These gene dosage effects, which are of the order of ±50% in the synthesis of normal gene products, then lead to perturbations of structure and function which collectively constitute the phenotype. Although there may be some degree of variability among individuals with the same chromosome imbalance, the overall phenotype is nevertheless quite specific. As a result, most if not all aspects of the phenotype must be attributable to specific genes or sets of genes and not to some vague and nonspecific state of chromosome imbalance (1,2).

Sex Chromosome Aneuploidy

While the principles just stated were derived from an analysis of autosomal aneuploidy, there is no reason to believe that the situation should be any differ-

ent with sex chromosome aneuploidy. However, it is certainly more complicated, since there are two factors operative in sex chromosome imbalance
which do not enter into autosomal imbalance. The first is that there are, of
course, two different sex chromosomes—the X and the Y—which are not structurally or, for the most part, genetically homologous to one another. One of
these, the Y, carries determinants which specifically determine testicular differentiation and, as a result, masculine sexual differentiation. The second factor is
that, in individuals with two or more X chromosomes, only one X chromosome
is fully active, the other undergoing a process of inactivation. Nevertheless, the
fact that there are such disorders as Turner syndrome and the several abnormal
conditions associated with sex chromosome trisomy or higher polysomy indicates that the rules of autosomal aneuploidy must still apply.

THE PHENOTYPE OF TURNER SYNDROME

Gonadal Dysgenesis

For the purposes of discussion, the phenotype of Turner syndrome will be divided into four components: ovarian dysgenesis, major and minor congenital
malformations (or somatic stigmata), shortness of stature, and death in utero.
The first of these is the easiest to deal with and directly illustrates the point
about gene dosage just made. My basic assumption is that, as originally suggested by Ferguson-Smith (3), the problem lies in the oocytes themselves and
not in the surrounding somatic tissues. It is now known that there is a significant
period of time in oogenesis during which X-chromosome inactivation is not
operative (4). In human females, this period begins about the thirteenth or
fourteenth week of gestation, when the germ cells are about to or have just
entered meiosis, and lasts until the time in adulthood—as much as 50 years
later—when the egg is finally ovulated or becomes atretic (Fig. 1). Therefore,
the normal state of affairs is for both X chromosomes to be active during
oogenesis, and this has been shown directly in human oocytes by electrophoretic
marker techniques (5,6) and in mouse eggs by direct gene dosage measurements
(7,8). As a result, loss of a sex chromosome, so that only one X chromosome is
present, constitutes a situation of true genetic imbalance with regard to functions determined by the X chromosomes. In oocytes, then, X-chromosome
monosomy is functionally analogous to autosomal monosomy, a condition
which is highly lethal to early embryos and is known to compromise the integrity of individual monosomic cells (1).

On the basis of the considerations just outlined, it has been repeatedly suggested (1,9-13) that the monosomic state present in the germ cells and oocytes
of human female embryos lacking an X chromosome may, during the course of
gestation and infancy, lead to oocyte degeneration and secondarily to ovarian

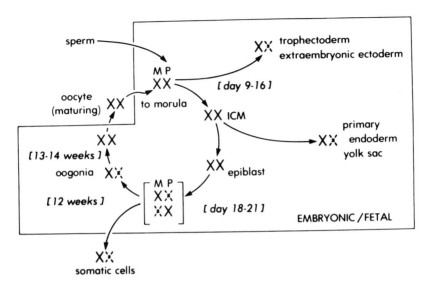

Figure 1 The cycle of X chromosome activity in the human female. All stages within the box are embryonic or fetal; those outside the box are in juvenile and adult women. M and P indicate maternally and paternally derived X chromosomes, respectively. Active X chromosomes are indicated by solid Xs, inactive chromosomes by broken Xs. 1CM, inner cell mass. (Figure redrawn and legend taken with modification from Fig. 13.1 of Ref. 1.)

dysgenesis. Although humans with monosomy X have "streak ovaries" devoid of eggs, such individuals actually do form eggs in embryonic life, which then degenerate prior to birth (14-16). In situations in which there are less complete losses of X chromosome material, such as deletions of part of the long arm (q) of the X, there may actually be a period of fertility followed by premature ovarian function. A case in point is a familial X-chromosome deletion in which the region between Xq21.3 and Xq27 was missing and in which ovarian failure occurred between 24 and 37 years of age (17). From comparisons with other similar deletions which seem to allow for normal ovarian function, it has been suggested that the "critical region" is in the vicinity of Xq26-27, as though only a single or very few loci were actually involved. This is probably not true in any absolute sense, since even deletions of the short arm of an X chromosome, Xp, can result in gonadal dysgenesis (Table 1). I would prefer to believe, therefore, that the proper genetic balance of several X-chromosomal loci is essential for normal oogenesis and maintenance of oocyte viability. However, these loci may not necessarily all be equivalent insofar as the effect of their loss is concerned. But without quantitatively examining oocyte number throughout life, it will be

Table 1 Phenotypic Features of X-Chromosome Deletions

Deleted region	Ovaries	Stature	Somatic stigmata of Turner syndrome
Short arm			
Xpter→~p21	Normal	Short	None
All of Xp	Dysgenesis	Short	Most or all
Long arm			
Xqter→~q22	Dysgenesis	Normal	None to few
Xqter→~q13	Dysgenesis	Normal[a]	None to some
All of Xq(?)	Dysgenesis	Normal[a]	Several

[a]Some cases of short stature reported
Source: Modified from Table 13.3 of Ref. 1.

difficult to define their relative importance. Nevertheless, it seems clear that given sufficient loss of X-chromosomal material, oocyte integrity is compromised and, as a consequence, overall ovarian integrity is as well.

In discussing the cases of Krauss et al. (17), Federman (18) suggested that the data indicate that the Xq26-27 "locus" is not inactivated in the normal female— i.e., that it must be present in a full double dose to preserve ovarian function. Since inactivation does not occur in oocytes, the implication is that the problem is somewhere outside of the eggs. As I have already stated, based on what is known to happen to oocytes, there is really no compelling reason to postulate the existence of such noninactivation in the distal Xq region of the X chromosome, and I do not think Federman is correct in this instance. However, as will be discussed shortly, there may be reasons to invoke the existence of noninactivated loci in other regions of the supposedly inactive X chromosome.

Somatic Abnormalities and Short Stature

When it comes to the somatic abnormalities of Turner syndrome, which include such features as lymphedema, webbed neck, widely spaced nipples, coarctation of the aorta, multiple nevi, and the like, the situation is distinctly reminiscent of autosomal aneuploidy. In the latter, the somatic abnormalities would be attributed to imbalance of loci in the aneuploid region (1), but where should we look for these loci in the case of sex chromosome aneuploidy? Contrary to first impressions, the problem is not entirely one of where on the *X chromosome* should we look. Considering that males with only one X chromosome do not have Turner syndrome, it is just as important to determine where on the *Y chromosome* are the genes we are interested in locating and what is their state of function. In a sense, then, the real answer to the question of the genesis of somatic defects may lie as much, if not more, with the Y chromosome than with the X itself.

The Role of the Y Chromosome

In approaching the problem in the manner just stated, it is assumed that the somatic abnormalities in Turner syndrome are unrelated to the gonadal dysgenesis for which a specific but somewhat special explanation has been proposed. Why then do I insist on the importance of the Y chromosome? It is because males and females are, with the exception of the particular characteristics that are sexually determined, the same insofar as somatic development is concerned. Therefore, it is my premise that whatever genes are required to balance those present on an active X chromosome, whether in a male or female cell, must be present on both X and Y chromosomes. The Y chromosome, being much smaller and devoid of any known "housekeeping genes," seems ultimately to offer the better chance for determining just what the loci are. And the way this answer is likely to come about is by examination of the structure of deleted Y chromosomes in individuals with X(del)Y or XYp-.

If the assumption about active homologous loci on both the X and Y chromosomes is not made, then it would be necessary to invoke the presence of some locus or loci on the Y which adjust the expression of certain loci on the X—a form of secondary dosage compensation—so that the net effect will be the same as is produced by an active and an inactive (actually only partially inactive) X chromosome. Although such a mechanism appears to be used in *Drosophila*, there is no evidence for it in mammals, and I find it distinctly unattractive.

A beautiful pair of cases that illustrate the point about the potential usefulness of deleted Y chromosomes are two 46,XY *females* described by Disteche et al. (19). Although normal in height, both had congenital lymphedema and one also had a short neck and widely spaced nipples. Both, who of course lacked one copy of each of a vast number of X-chromosomal loci, also had gonadal dysgenesis. By combined cytogenetic and molecular analysis, the patient with more stigmata (#2) was found to lack part of Yp, including the deletion intervals designated by Page (20) as 1, 2, and 4A (Fig. 2). The other patient (#1) lacked intervals 1, 2, and 3. These findings would suggest that the locus or loci whose absence results in lymphedema resides in intervals 1 or 2 (or the pseudoautosomal region, which is more distal on Yp) and that the locus or loci involved in the causation of the short neck (assuming that it is not really related to the presence of a cystic hygroma, also a form of congenital lymphedema) and widely spaced nipples are in interval 3. This is, of course, a very crude form of phenotypic mapping and should not be taken very seriously in the absence of further documentation. Nonetheless, these findings do compel us to consider the possibility that there are expressed genes in these regions of the Y chromosome that are essential for normal somatic development. By the same reasoning, the fact that height is normal in the two women suggests that the locus or loci required for normal stature are not in intervals 1 to 4A or that there may be other relevant loci scattered throughout Yp and perhaps even Yq.

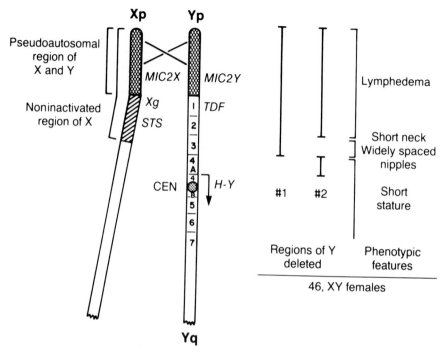

Figure 2 Genetic map of Y chromosome, showing homology with the X chromosome. The deletion intervals of Page (20) are shown within the body of the Y. On the right are shown the regions deleted in the two 46,XY cases (#1 and #2) of Disteche et al. (19) and a speculative phenotypic map based on these cases. The figures, which are based on material in Refs. 1 and 19–22, are purely schematic and not to scale.

The suggestion that there are active genes on Yp and perhaps Yq immediately raises two questions. First, what and where are these loci on the Y, and, second, where are the homologous loci on the X chromosome? With regard to the first question, certain active gene loci have been identified on the human Y chromosome and their locations specified. These include *TDF*, testis-determining factor, in interval 1 and the *H-Y* (presumably a regulatory) locus in interval 4B or in Yq (21) (Fig. 2), neither of which has a known homolog on the X chromosome. In addition, the structural locus, *MIC2Y*, for the red cell cell surface antigen recognized by monoclonal antibody 12E7 is distal to *TDF* on Yp, perhaps within 200 kilobases of it (22). *MIC2Y* is in the beginning (centromeric end) of the pseudoautosomal region of the Y and is homologous to an expressed locus, *MIC2X*, located in Xp22.32→Xpter on the distal part of the X chromosome (23)

(Fig. 2). But these loci hardly seem either sufficient or even appropriate as candidates for the loci we are seeking, although they certainly cannot be disregarded. There really ought to be many more. It would seem reasonable to look for these loci in the region of Y known to be homologous to a noninactivated region of the X chromosome, the pseudoautosomal segment telomeric to *MIC2*. A deletion of intervals 1 and 2 (as in the two cases of Disteche) would involve this pseudoautosomal region as well, but it is clear that more of the Y, and the X, must be involved.

Noninactivated Loci on the X Chromosome

Turning now to the second question, the matter of where on the X chromosome the relevant genes should be located—with the implication that these genes do not undergo inactivation—the immediate and obvious answer is once again the noninactivated and pseudoautosomal regions on distal Xp (Fig. 2) (the former including the latter but not visa versa). But this cannot really be the answer, since deletion of all of this region and more, from Xpter to ~Xp21, does not result in somatic abnormalities, although it does cause shortness of stature (see Table 1). However, somatic abnormalities occur when all of Xp is deleted and possibly when all of Xq is deleted, suggesting that regions of proximal Xp and Xq may, contrary to expectation, not be inactivated and are homologous to similar loci on proximal Yp and Yq. The most parsimonious explanation would be that there are homologous expressed loci affecting somatic morphogenesis within the pericentromeric regions of both the X and Y chromosomes. I know of no proof for this at present, and what evidence does exist indicates that anonymous sequences in Yp, if not homologous to Xp22.3 sequences, are similar to sequences in the region Xq13-q24 of the X chromosome or, in some instances, to autosomal sequences (24,25).

It is worth noting that Gartler and Riggs (26) suggested, in their review of the mechanisms of X inactivation, that it is "possible that, in an inactivated region of the X, not every piece of DNA is inactivated." Furthermore, since the genesis of the congenital defects occurs very early in gestation, the period during which the putative active genes on the Y and the inactivated X need actually express could be a relatively brief one. If such were the case, expression of these genes would not be detectable in later fetal or postnatal life.

Short Stature

The matter of short stature in Turner syndrome has already been referred to several times. The preponderance of evidence suggests that it is deletion of the distal part of Xp—the region Xp21→pter—that leads to short stature; long arm deletions do not appear to affect growth (see Table 1). These findings indicate that shortness of stature, like the somatic abnormalities, is not necessarily associated with or a consequence of gonadal dysgenesis. Although, as has already been noted, the corresponding gene or genes do not appear to be on the distal part of Yp, it is likely that relevant genes are located more proximally in Yp or in Yq. Further evidence for the presence of active genes affecting stature on the Y derives from the fact that aneuploidy involving the Y chromosome, for example 47,XXY and 47,XYY, also results in increased height.

In support of the notion that genes in distal Yp are not involved in determination of stature is de la Chapelle et al.'s conclusion (27) that translocation of part of the Y chromosome, the region encompassing intervals 1-3 and the pseudoautosomal region at most (28,29), to distal Xp to give rise to XX males does not result in increased stature. Furthermore, the fact that this translocation, which may substitute the Y sequences for equivalent X sequences in the pseudoautosomal region (30), does not result in decreased stature suggests that the stature-determining genes on Xp are not actually in the pseudoautosomal region.

Phenotypic Mapping

As was mentioned earlier, phenotypic mapping of the various features of Turner syndrome at this time is highly imperfect (see Table 1). Although I disagree with Teyssier et al.'s conclusion (31) that the actual location of the breakpoint in a deleted X chromosome might not be the major factor influencing the phenotype that results—I take it as an article of faith that it must be—I can certainly sympathize with their plight. Attempting to understand phenotypic distinctions purely on the basis of cytogenetic analyses, especially earlier analyses, is very risky. What will be required is the coupling of cytogenetic and molecular analyses using a large battery of X-chromosome probes, similar to what is being carried out for the abnormalities in which the Y chromosome is implicated. Nevertheless, despite these uncertainties, Bühler (32) has gone so far as to identify several regions on the Y which carry the loci under discussion. Two regions which act as "Turner phenotype-preventing factors," TP-1 and TP-2, have been assigned to Yq1.21 and Yp, respectively. Similarly, three regions carrying "statural determinants," STA-1, STA-2, and STA-3, have been placed in Yq11.21, Yp, and Yq21.2, respectively, with STA-1 also being associated with or even identical to a locus controlling tooth growth. For the present, these "assignments" must be considered highly speculative.

Embryonic and Fetal Death

While the phenotype of living individuals with Turner syndrome is relatively mild in comparison with what is associated with most autosomal aneuploidy, particularly when a deletion or monosomy is present, monosomy X is in fact a highly lethal condition. An estimated >95-99% of 45,X conceptuses die during gestation (33,34). The finding that early mortality is much less in 46,Xi(Xq) than in 45,X cases suggests that loss of loci on Xq may be particularly involved in the production of lethality (34). Although the period of death may extend throughout gestation, the vast majority of 45,X conceptuses die in the first trimester with a mean developmental age of 6 weeks (35).

Two general explanations for death early in gestation can be considered, and they are not dissimilar to similar arguments regarding the lethality of autosomal aneuploidy (1). One is that most 45,X embryos have such severe congenital defects that further viability is precluded. However, pathological descriptions of 45,X abortuses do not indicate any unusual degree of developmental abnormality beyond what is observed in liveborn individuals. The other explanation is that the problem is not with the 45,X embryos and fetuses themselves but, rather, with their placentas. In this event, the aneuploid state is visualized as interfering with placental growth and function so that the placenta is unable to sustain an otherwise reasonably normally functioning embryo or fetus. This interference, it has been suggested, could in turn compromise placental steroidogenesis, thereby leading to an inability to maintain an otherwise viable embryo and consequent spontaneous abortion (36).

If a placental mechanism is involved in the early lethality of 45,X, why should the placenta be abnormal at all? Once again we are forced to consider the possibility that the same type of genetic imbalance that presumably operates to produce the somatic abnormalities and growth inhibition later in life, although not necessarily the same gene(s), also acts to interfere with placental growth or function. Questions of whether X inactivation takes place on all cells of the female placenta are *not* really relevant, since the matter is not merely one of a difference between 45,X and 46,XX but equally of between 45,X and 46,XY, in which X inactivation is not an issue.

All of the above discussion of early lethality is, of course, pure conjecture, and no meaningful data, let alone a convincing explanation, yet exist. Perhaps more will be learned about the very early stages of development of 45,X embryos and their placentas as more early abortion material, both spontaneously and therapeutically derived, is examined.

Chromosomal Imprinting

Recent work in the mouse has indicated that imprinting of autosomes may occur during gametogenesis, so that these chromosomes may function differently during embryonic and fetal life depending on whether they are inherited from the father or the mother (41). Imprinting of a somewhat different nature has long been recognized with regard to the murine X chromosome, since the paternally derived X chromosome is preferentially inactivated in extraembryonic tissues (37). It is not clear whether the same occurs in the human placenta, since evidence both for (38) and against (39-40) preferential inactivation of the paternal X chromosome has been published.

Could imprinting, whether related to X inactivation or not, be involved in some way in the early lethality of 45,X? If so, and if asked to predict loss of which X chromosome would cause more difficulty, one inherited from the father or one from the mother, I would favor the paternal X, since the maternal X does perfectly well when present by itself in normal males. It is of interest, therefore, that Hassold et al. (42) found that 45,X abortuses in which the X was derived from the father, which it was about 25% of the time, did "less well" than those in which the X was maternal in origin. While consistent with some type of imprinting explanation these observations certainly cannot be construed as lending much support to a role for imprinting in the genesis of lethality.

CONCLUSIONS

The foregoing discussion, as speculative as it is, represents an attempt to demystify our understanding of the basis of the phenotypic features of Turner syndrome. While we still do not understand, at a mechanistic level, the genesis of the phenotypic features of any autosomal aneuploid state, it is quite clear that the issue is one of alterations of gene dosage and, hence, of genetic and biochemical balance. My contention in this brief review is that the same considerations apply to sex chromosome aneuploidy as well, and the arguments can be summarized as follows:

1. We should look at mechanisms of phenotypic effects of sex chromosome aneuploidy in same light as we look at autosomal aneuploidy.
2. Based on the fact that both X chromosomes function during oogenesis, 45,X results in a true monosomy, and the explanation of the gonadal dysgenesis in Turner syndrome seems therefore to be quite straightforward.
3. To explain the somatic abnormalities and effects on growth in Turner syndrome, as well as the deleterious effects of other sex chromosome aneuploidies, whether involving a Y chromosome or not, it is necessary to postulate the existence of loci on both the inactivated X chromosome of females and the Y chromosome of males, which have equivalent functions and are active at some point in development.
4. The early lethality of 45,X may result from impairment of placental functions, by mechanisms similar to those causing somatic growth impairment and congenital defects, rather than from defects of the embryo or fetus itself.
5. By molecular and cytogenetic analysis of 45,X males, 46,XX males, and 46,XY females, as well as of various 46,X(del)X females, it should be possible to develop phenotypic maps of the loci whose imbalance gives rise to the phenotype of Turner syndrome. Halting steps in this direction have already been taken.
6. Identification of the loci of interest should then permit their ultimate molecular characterization and determination of their functions and modes of expression.

Given the rapid progress in the mapping of both the X and Y chromosomes and the projected large-scale efforts to clone and sequence these chromosomes, it will hopefully be possible to arrive at the latter goals in the not too distant future.

ACKNOWLEDGMENTS

This work was supported by NIH grants HD-03132 and HD-17001.

REFERENCES

1. Epstein CJ. The Consequences of Chromosome Imbalance. Principles, Mechanisms, and Models. New York: Cambridge University Press, 1986.
2. Epstein CJ. Specificity versus nonspecificity in the pathogenesis of aneuploid phenotypes. Am J Med Genet 1988; 29:161-5.
3. Ferguson-Smith MA. Karyotype-phenotype correlations in gonadal dysgenesis and their bearing on the pathogenesis of malformations. J Med Genet 1965; 2:142-55.
4. Epstein CJ. The X chromosome in development. In Sandberg AA, ed. Cytogenetics of the Mammalian X Chromosome, Part A: Basic Mechanisms of X Chromosome Behavior. New York: AR Liss, 1983:51-65.
5. Gartler SM, Liskay RM, Campbell RK, Sparkes R, Gant N. Evidence for two functional X chromosomes in human oocytes. Cell Differ 1972; 1: 215-8.
6. Migeon BR, Jelalian K. Evidence for two active X chromosomes in germ cells of female before meiotic entry. Nature 1977; 269:242-3.
7. Epstein CJ. Mammalian oocytes: X chromosome activity. Science 1969; 163:1078-9.
8. Epstein CJ. Expression of the mammalian X chromosome before and after fertilization. Science 1972; 175:1467-8.
9. Lyon MF. Genetic activity of sex chromosomes in somatic cells of mammals. Philos Trans R Soc Lond (Biol) 1970; 259:41-52.
10. Epstein CJ. Inactivation of the X chromosome. N Engl J Med 1972; 286: 318-9.
11. Kennedy JF, Freeman MG, Benirschke K. Ovarian dysgenesis and chromosome abnormalities. Obstet Gynecol 1977; 50:13-20.
12. Burgoyne PS. The role of the sex chromosomes in mammalian germ cell differentiation. Ann Biol Anim Biochem Biophys 1978; 18(2B):317.
13. Therman E, Denniston C, Sarto GE, Ulber M. X chromosome constitution and the human female phenotype. Hum Genet 1980; 54:133-43.
14. Singh RP, Carr DH. The anatomy and histology of XO human embryos and fetuses. Anat Rec 1966; 155:369-75.
15. Carr DH, Haggar RA, Hart AG. Germ cells in the ovaries of XO female infants. Am J Clin Pathol 1968; 49:521-6.
16. Weiss L. Additional evidence of gradual loss of germ cells in the pathogenesis of streak ovaries in Turner's syndrome. J Med Genet 1971; 8:540-4.

17. Krauss CM, Turksoy RN, Atkins L, McLaughlin C, Brown LG, Page DC. Familial premature ovarian failure due to an interstitial deletion of the long arm of the X chromosome. N Engl J Med 1987;317:125-31.
18. Federman DD. Mapping of the X-chromosome. Mining its p's and q's. N Engl J Med 1987;317:161-2.
19. Disteche CM, Casanova M, Saal H, Friedman C, Sybert V, Graham J, Thuline H, Page DC, Fellous M. Small deletions of the short arm of the Y chromosome in 46,XY females. Proc Natl Acad Sci USA 1986;83:7841-4.
20. Page DC, Sex reversal: Deletion mapping the male-determining function of the human Y chromosome. Cold Spring Harbor Symp Quant Biol 1986; 51:229-35.
21. Simpson E, Chandler P, Goulmy E, Disteche CM, Ferguson-Smith MA, Page DC. Separation of the genetic loci for the H-Y antigen and for testis determination on the human Y chromosome. Nature 1987;326:876-8.
22. Pritchard CA, Goodfellow PJ, Goodfellow PN. Mapping the limits of the human pseudoautosomal region and a candidate sequence for the male-determining gene. Nature 1987;328:273-5.
23. Goodfellow PJ, Darling SM, Thomas NS, Goodfellow PN. A pseudoautosomal gene in man. Science 1986;234:740-3.
24. Goodfellow PN, Davies KE, Roper H-H. Report of the committee on the genetic constitution of the X and Y chromosomes. Eighth International Workshop on Human Gene Mapping. Cytogenet Cell Genet 1985;40:296-352.
25. Affara NA, Florentin L, Morrison N, Kwok K, Mitchell M, Cook A, Jamieson D, Glasgow L, Meredith L, Boyd E, Ferguson-Smith MA. Regional assignment of Y-linked probes by deletion mapping and their homology with X-chromosome and autosomal sequences. Nucleic Acids Res 1986; 14:5353-73.
26. Gartler SM, Riggs AD. Mammalian X-chromosome inactivation. Annu Rev Genet 1983;17:155-90.
27. de la Chapelle A, Savikurti H, Herva R, Tippett PA, Knutar F, Gröhn P, Siponen H, Huovinen K, Korhonen T. Aetiological studies in males with the karyotype 46,XX. In San Román C, McDermott A, eds. Aspects of Human Genetics with Special Reference to X-linked Disorders. Basel: Karger, 1984:125-42.
28. Page DC, de la Chapelle A, Weissenbach J. Chromosome Y-specific DNA in related human XX males. Nature 1985;315:224-6.
29. Vergnaud G, Page DC, Simmler M-C, Brown L, Rouyer F, Noel B, Botstein D, de la Chapelle A, Weissenbach J. A deletion map of the human Y chromosome based on DNA hybridization. Am J Hum Genet 1986; 38: 109-24.
30. Page DC, Brown LG, de la Chapelle A. Exchange of terminal portions of X- and Y-chromosomal short arms in human XX males. Nature 1987; 328:437-40.
31. Teyssier JR, Bajolle F, Caron J. Complete deletion of long arm of X chromosome in woman without Turner syndrome. Lancet 1981;1:1158-9.

32. Bühler EM. Clinical and cytologic impact of X-chromosome abnormalities. In: Sandberg AA, ed. The Y Chromosome, Part B: Clinical Aspect of Y Chromosome Abnormalities. New York: AR Liss, 1985:61–93.
33. Simpson JL. Disorders of Sexual Differentiation. New York: Academic Press, 1976.
34. Hook EB, Warburton D. The distribution of chromosomal genotypes associated with Turner's syndrome: Livebirth prevalence rates and evidence for diminished fetal mortality and severity in genotypes associated with structural X abnormalities or mosaicism. Hum Genet 1983; 64:24–7.
35. Boué J, Phillippe E, Giroud A, Boué A. Phenotypic expression of lethal chromosome anomalies in human abortuses. Teratology 1976; 14:3–20.
36. Burgoyne PS, Tam PPL, Evans EP. Retarded development of XO conceptus during early pregnancy in the mouse. J Reprod Fert 1983; 68:387–93.
37. Harper MJ, Foster M, Mark M. Preferential paternal X inactivation in extraembryonic tissues in early mouse embryos. J Embryol Exp Morphol 1982; 67:127–35.
38. Harrison KB, Warburton D. Preferential X-chromosome activity in human female placental tissues. Cytogenet Cell Genet 1986; 41:163–8.
39. Migeon BR, Wolf SF, Axelman J, Kaslow DC, Schmidt M. Incomplete X chromosome dosage compensation in chorionic villi of human placenta. Proc Natl Acad Sci USA 1985; 82:3390–4.
40. Mohandas T, Passage MB, Williams J III, Sparkes RS, Yen PH, Shapiro LJ. X-chromosome inactivation in cultured cells from human chorionic villi. Am J Hum Genet 1987; 41:A151.
41. Searle AG, Beechey CV. Noncomplementation phenomena and their bearing on nondisjunctional effects. In Dellarco VL, Voytek PE, Hollaender PE, eds. Aneuploidy. Etiology and Mechanisms. New York: Plenum, 1985: 363–76.
42. Hassold T, Benham F, Kobryn C, Leppert M, Whittington E. Cytogenetic and molecular studies of sex chromosome monosomy. Am J Hum Genet 1987; 41:A121.

DISCUSSION

DR. JOE LEIGH SIMPSON: It seems to me that there is another potential possibility with respect to the lethality being due to 45 X placental abnormalities. One possibility is that we have over estimated the lethality of 45X. We certainly know from chorionic villi studies of sampling, both the direct and the long-term culture, that not infrequently we detect a monosomy X line that particularly if present in a mosaic state we do not act upon and rather wait until amniocentesis at 16 weeks and if not infrequently we detect a normal chromosomal compliment without the monosomy X at 16 weeks. So it seems to me that that would be a point against the hypothesis that placental abnormalities of 45 X would cause the lethality. In addition, if you remember that most of the studies giving rise to the percentages of intrauterine lethality are derived from abortive studies that show that about 25 percent of all spontaneous abortuses that are abnormal of 45 X, remember that most of those are not from studies of the embryonic tissue per se, but rather from membranes or villi. Perhaps we have a spuriously overestimate of the frequency of the 45 X in early abortuses and hence a spurious overestimate of the lethality of 45 X.

DR. CHARLES EPSTEIN: That may be the case, but I think that in any aneuploid situation there is a high intrauterine lethality whether human or mouse and in most instances you are hard put to explain why the fetus dies at all. And I think in many of these the explanation may reside in the placenta no matter what the actual numbers turn out to be one way or the other. The fact that the abortus materials often show a 45,X placenta, whatever the fetus turns out to be, might suggest that the 45,X placenta in many instances does not support a fetus through gestation.

DR. GORDON CUTLER: Is it known how many genes might be involved in the short stature, and is it possible there could be a single gene that might be amenable some day to gene therapy apart from the other problems?

DR. EPSTEIN: I do not know the answer to that question. I do not know how many genes are involved. I think you would have to look at the karyotypic/ phenotypic kind of correlations in that to get an idea of how many loci might be

Dr. Simpson is at the University of Tennessee, Memphis, Tennessee. Dr. Epstein is at the University of California at San Francisco, San Francisco, California. Dr. Cutler is at the National Institutes of Health, Bethesda, Maryland. Dr. Shapiro is at the University of California at Los Angeles School of Medicine, Los Angeles, California. Dr. Hall is at the University of British Columbia, Vancouver, Canada.

involved. Probably more than one locus would be involved, but it could very well be relatively few. I think the answer is: nobody knows.

DR. LARRY SHAPIRO: XOs have been well studied in the mouse. Can you make any inferences since the mice, although they develop gonadal dysgenesis, look relatively normal phenotypically and you are a better mouse dysmorphologist than I. Can one make any inferences about what might be different between the mouse sex chromosomes and human sex chromosomes that would permit mouse XOs to do so well?

UNIDENTIFIED: This is a critical question because we have been talking about the mouse and the human as if they have homologous genes and so forth and yet the striking feature of the XO mouse is really almost restricted to, well there are a few other things too, gonadal difference, and that has always troubled me.

DR. EPSTEIN: Well, mice are mice and people are people. I wish I knew the explanation. The gonadal situation in the mouse is interesting in that the XO mouse is actually fertile, but their period of fertility gives out relatively early. So I think the inference from that is their eggs cannot survive too long, but of course, between the period of conception and the period at which the end of fertility occurs is about nine or ten months which is not much different from what it is in the human during intrauterine ooogenesis actually, but they do maintain that problem with the eggs. They do not have the somatic problem and I think my inference would be the same as yours: that whatever the somatic genes that seem to be still operative either on the inactivated X chromosome or on the Y chromosome if that is in fact what is going on for one reason or another are not working any more in the mouse situation in that the mouse is much better compensated than we are. That is a circular answer to a question which says that I do not know the answer.

UNIDENTIFIED: One thing about the gonad too, is that it has always struck me having looked at a number of these and having looked at some of our fetuses with XO gonadal dysgenesis and then following through, these gonads have trouble undergoing myosis and when the start, when the go from the oogonial to the "oogonial" which is no different than a spermatogonia, to the oocyte phase they fall apart and you may have ordinarily a few persisting, but very few. And that is why when you look at these gonads, they really are not ovaries, they are an arrest in maturation and then yes, a few of the oogonial become oocytes and some of them may become perhaps as in the vole as Dr. Ohno might mentioned from myototic nondisjunction even, we do not know. But even if some of them remained, where even the OO may persist, it is sort of almost an arrest in gonadal organoogenesis with a few persisting and escaping and perhaps it is the same in the mouse.

DR. EPSTEIN: Well I think the arrest in the human situation is due to the fact that the oocytes are no good and that they cannot survive. There are many situations in the mouse where, if the migrating germ cells do not make it to the gonadal ridges, you end up with a streak ovary or with ovarian dysgenesis. The problem is not a somatic problem; the problem is intrinsic in the oocyte itself.

UNIDENTIFIED: So in that sense perhaps the mouse and the human may not be that different, in terms of the oocyte.

DR. EPSTEIN: I do not think they are different at all. I think it is just that the mouse comes and goes so fast that it does not have enough time for its oocytes to degenerate. But they do live less long.

DR. JUDITH HALL: My question is pretty much along the same line and that is is it really the oocyte or is it the supporting cells that crump? It seems to me that the supporting cells may just as much need that extra material on the other X or on the Y to be able to function and in fact when it is Y material they do bad things. So my question is, is there evidence that it is really the absence of the X or is it really the supporting tissue that goes to pot?

DR. EPSTEIN: As I have just said, I cannot give you absolute evidence, but the precedent is again going back to the mouse where we know experimentally is that there are many mutations which affect the migration of the germ cells into the ovary and that if the germ cell does not get to the ovary from the gonadal ridge, you do not get an ovary. So you cannot form an ovary without the germ cell. The other part of it is an inference and that is that every situation that I know of, and we have worked with this experimentally a lot, in which you have a monosom, monosomic cell populations just do not do well. You may not want to call them cell lethals, but nonetheless they do not proliferate well, they do not survive well. So it seems to me quite reasonable to postulate that the germ cell, with only one X chromosome when it ought to have two, is just as monosomic as any other autosomal monosomic cell would be and does extremely poorly as a result of that.

3

The Genetic Basis of Gonadal Sex Determination

Barbara C. McGillivray

University of British Columbia
Vancouver, British Columbia, Canada

David C. Page

Whitehead Institute, Cambridge, Massachusetts

Whether a human fetus becomes a phonopypic male or female has been the subject of both scientific and nonscientific speculation for as long as we know. Environmental factors were first thought important, but in this century the chromosomal constitution was recognized as the initiating factor. In insects, sex was recognized to be determined by the number of X chromosomes, and to have nothing to do with the presence or absence of a Y chromosome (1). Therefore, it was assumed that sex in mammals was determined by the number of X chromosomes. In 1959, clinical observations of both mice and humans with abnormal sex constitutions revealed that the Y chromosome were always female regardless of the number of X chromosomes, and those with a Y chromosome were always male regardless of the number of Xs (2,3,4).

Although the presence of the Y chromosome was obviously important as a switch mechanism in the decision of male versus female development, we also know that development of the internal and external genitalia are directly influenced by hormonal output *and* that many X-linked or autosomal genes contribute to the development of one particular sex. We also know from observations in humans and other animals, that the innate tendency, or the default pathway, is female (5). The question then has been: how does the Y chromosome divert from this ovarian pathway?

In diversion to the testicular pathway, the Y chromosome, or genes on the Y chromosome, are thought to act on the four components of the gonad. These include the supporting cell precursors, the primordial germ cells, the steroid cell precursors, and the blood vessels and connective tissues. The prevailing model dictates that the Y chromosomal genes encode a testis determining molecule of some type, and that this molecule then diffuses and affects all four components of the gonad (6).

As has been the case in other normal pathways, initial clinical observations involving individuals differing from the norm have allowed the detection of an abnormality, and go on to define that normal pathway. This has also been true in the pathway involving normal sexual differentiation. The initial clinical observation was sex reversal.

Similarly, such patients with sex reversal without adrenal hyperplasia or androgen insensitivity have aided in the delineation of the Y-linked gene involved in testis determination. These patients fall into two main categories: the XX males without obvious Y chromosomal material, and the XY females not fitting the androgen insensitivity groups and generally normal appearing Y chromosome (7,8).

The XX males usually come to attention with Klinefelter-like features. They are distinguished by their XX karyotype and a male gonad without dysgenetic features but with hyalinization. XX males are uncommon with an incidence of about 1/20,000 in Europe and North America, usually sporadic within a family and sterile very much like Klinefelter syndrome.

Some cytogenetic observations first pointed to the possible mechanisms explaining the XX males. In 1976, some of the males were noted to have one X chromosome slightly larger than the other (9). In 1980, Ellen Magenis described such a male with a larger X chromosome and felt that a portion of the short arm of the Y chromosome had been translocated to the X (10). In 1986 Ferguson-Smith, who had studied a number of XX males, observed that while a small proportion of the males did have the larger X chromosome, the majority had no such difference (11).

Page suggested that the fathers of those males had had an aberrant or nonmatching XY interchange, and felt that a small portion of the Y chromosome had therefore been translocated to the X (12). That portion of the Y chromosome was then postulated to contain the male determining factor.

The reverse clinical situation, the XY females, were a heterogeneous group (13,14). Many were found to have streak gonads and often presented with features of Turner syndrome. While some were familial, others were sporadic within families, and some of these females showed small Y chromosome deletions or rearrangements. It was suggestive that this might be the reverse situation to that seen in XX males. Therefore, we and other groups England and Europe postulated that both XX males and XY females resulted from an XY interchange, and that it was the presence or absence of this factor that resulted in the sex reversal.

The Y chromosome has been a difficult one to map as there are few genes known to be linked to the chromosome, but there are three strategies important for mapping. The goal for many investigators has been to isolate probes which have a complimentary DNA sequence to only the Y chromosome. These specific sequence probes may then be used to analyze regions of the Y chromosome. Using these kinds of techniques, various investigators began to isolate specific Y sequences. One of the first was isolated by Page (15). This probe mapped to the short arm and is called DXY S-1 meaning that it maps to sections of both the Y and the Xq chromosome. Goodfellow, shortly after that, using different techniques, localized a gene MIC2 which makes an antigen 12E7 to both the short arms of the X and Y chromosomes (16).

The next step was to use the patients, both the XX males and the XY females, to map the most likely region for the testis determining factor (TDF). With a whole series of probes identifying small areas on both the long and short arm of the Y chromosome, the investigators hoped to find one area of the Y chromosome in common to all XX males and a similar area deleted in the XY females.

With 135 probes outlining 155 distinct loci, the Y chromosome was divided into twenty intervals. Specific probes were used on DNA from XX males, and the males were then divided according to the length of the Y fragment found. All of the XX males with demonstrated Y chromosomal material have in common the intervals 1A1 and 1A2 (17).

A particularly valuable female presenting with an abdominal mass determined to be a gonadoblastoma, and later identified to have an apparently balanced translocation involving her Y and chromosome 22 (18). When the same set of probes were used, she was found to have a deletion of only two intervals of the Y, and the deletion overlapped one of the intervals (1A2) seen in common with all the XX males. This interval was then most likely to contain the TDF sequence.

From then on, his laboratory used overlapping human inserts from recombinant phages, a technique where the space is gradually filled in, and the region was cloned (19).

What are the characteristics of the sequence identified? The portion cloned thus far appears to be one long segment free of any nucleotide sequences suggesting stops. This suggests the segment is actually transcribed or is an exon. The sequence had zinc fingers, a repetitive array of structural elements, similar to a described transcription factor. The particular sequence was thought to allow a tetrahedral shape to enclose a zinc molecule and project into the grooves of either DNA or RNA. The protein is thought to be regulatory in nature, acting in the nuclei of cells, without the characteristics of either a hormone or a cell surface protein.

A similar coding sequence, labeled TDX, was found on the X chromosome. The location appears not to be in the pseudoautosomal region (i.e. the region normally interchanging with the Y chromosome), but appears to be in a central portion of the X short arm.

As the sequence was postulated to be the TDF, homologous sequence were sought on the X and Y chromosomes of other mammals. The sequence was found to be highly conserved in all mammals examined, and detected a fragment in both males and females. Therefore, this area on the Y chromosome appears to be highly conserved, with a similar locus on the X chromosome.

Possible explanations for the existence of an X-linked gene include the possibility that the TDX gene is similar but unrelated to the TDY, or that TDX and TDY encode different subunits of one protein, that the products are similar but competitive, or that the two genes are interchangeable, and that the dosage is the important thing. As the location of the X-linked gene is in an area of the X normally inactivated in a female, the dosage would be half in a normal female.

Still unexplained is where the gene acts, and therefore what is the immediate next step of the pathway. There are still unexplained clinical situations such as the XX true hermaphrodites where no evidence of Y-linked material has yet been found. A third question is whether the mechanism works for other, as yet untested, animal species.

In summary, the work to date indicates that interval 1A2 of the Y chromosome is male determining, and that all individuals having a Y chromosome or this interval will make testes regardless of the number of X chromosomes present. In contrast, all individuals having only X chromosomes or lacking the interval will make ovaries. The discovery is exciting, and the wait to understand the mode of action of this newly identified protein will be an anxious one.

REFERENCES

1. Bridges, CB. Non disjunction as proof of the chromosome theory of heredity. Genetics 1 1916; 1-51:107-163.
2. Jacobs, PA, Strong, JA. A case of human intersexuality having a possible XX sex-determining mechanism. Nature 1959; 83:302-303.
3. Ford, CE, Miller, OJ, Polani, PE, de Almeida, JC, Briggs, JH. A sex-chromosome anomaly in a case of gonadal dysgenesis (Turner's syndrome). Lancet 1959; 1:711.
4. Welshcins, WJ, Russell, LB. The Y chromosome as the bearer of male determining factors in the mouse. Proc. Natl. Acad. Sci. USA 1959; 45:560-566.
5. Jost, A. Problems of fetal endocrinology, the gonadal and hypophyseal hormones. Rec. Pogr. Horm. Res. 1983; 8:379-418.
6. Wachtel, SS, Ohno, S, Koo, gC, Boyse, EA. Possible role for H-Y antigen in the primary determination of sex. Nature 1975; 257:235-236.

7. Guellaen, G, Casanova, M, Bishop, C, Geldwerth, D, Andre, G, Fellous, M, Weissenbach, J. Human XX males with Y single-copy DNA fragments. Nature 1984;307:172–173.
8. Disteche, CM, Casanova, M, Saal, H, Friedman, C, Sybert, V, Graham, J, Thuline, H, Page, DC, Fellous, M. Small deletions of the short arm of the Y chromosome in 46,XY females. Proc. Natl. Acad. Sci. USA 1986; 83: 7841–7844.
9. Kunkel, LM, Smith, KD, Boyer, SH. Human Y-chromosome-specific re-iterated DNA. Science 1976; 191:1189–1190.
10. Magenis, RE, Casanova, M, Fellous, M, Olson, S, Sheehy, R. Further cyto-logic evidence for Xp-Yp translocation in XX males using in situ hybridiza-tion with Y-derived probe. Hum. Genet. 1987; 75:228–233.
11. Affara, NA, Ferguson-Smith, MA, Tolmie, J, Kwok, K, Mitchell, M, Jame-son, D, Cooke, A, Florentin, L. Variable transfer of Y specific sequences in XX males. Nucl. Acids Res. 1986; 14:5375–5387. Altaba, AR, Perry-O'Keefe, H, Melton, DS. Xfin: an embryonic gene encoding a multifingered protein in Xenopus. EMBO J 1987;6:3065–3070.
12. Page, DC, Brown, LG, de la Chapelle, A. Exchange of terminal portions of X- and Y-chromosomal short arms in human XX males. Nature 1987;328: 437–440.
13. German, J. Gonadal dimorphism explained as a dosage effect of a locus on the sex chromosomes the Gonad-Differentiation Locus (GDL). Am. J. Hum. Genet. 1988; in press.
14. Berstein, R, Koo, GC, Wachtel, SS. Abnormality of the X chromosome in human 46,XY female siblings with dysgenetic ovaries. Science 1980; 207: 768–769.
15. Page, DC, Harper, ME, Love, J, Botstein, D. Occurrence of a transposition from the X-chromosome long arm to the Y-chromosome short arm during human evolution. Nature 1984;311:119–123.
16. Goodfellow, PJ, Darling, SM, Thomas, NS, Goodfellow, PN. A pseudo-aurosomal gene in man. Science 1986; 243:740–743.
17. Page, DC. Sex reversal deletion mapping the maldetermining function of the human Y chromosome. Cold Spring Harbor Symp. Quant. 1986; Biol. 51:229–235.
18. Page, DC. Hypothesis: a Y-chromosomal gene causes gonadoblastoma in dysgenetic gonads. Development 1987; in press.
19. Page, DC, Mosher, R, Simpson, EM, Fisher, MC, Mardon, G, Pollack, J, McGillivray, B, de la Chapelle, A, Brown, LG. (1987). The Sex-Determining Region of the Human Y-Chromosome Encodes a Finer Protein. Cell 1987; 51:1091–1104.

DISCUSSION

DR. PAUL SAENGER: Weissenbach and his group published in the June 1987 issue of *Cell* a bunch of XX males that did not have any of the TDF material, at least according to their probes. Any speculation of how that came about?

DR. DAVID C. PAGE: In the past we could look at these XX hermaphrodites and the unexplained XX males with a collection of Y DNA probes, but we were always left with the out that, "Oh, well they have a smaller portion of the Y." But now we can say rather definitively that there are XX males and there are XX hermaphrodites who do not have TDF. They likely constitute mutations on the X chromosome or on autosomes in genes that function together with or down-stream in TDF in a pathway. Let us say for instance, if the sex determining gene is a transcriptional regulatory factor, you could for instance have a mutation, perhaps it regulates a gene that is on an autosome that is present in both males and females, chromosomal males and females, that if you had a mutation in the site, in the gene which is regulated by that transcriptional factor, you could have sort of a constitutive male mutation that would circumvent the need for the Y chromosomal factor.

DR. MELVIN M. GRUMBACH: Is there anything, David, that is inconsistent in your hypothesis because of a lot of other evidences that the TDF Y that you call this factor on the Y may be a regulatory rather than a constitutive, regulating the HY, something, another factor?

DR. PAGE: It certainly is going to be clear, it *is* clear that this gene has to control the activity of a number of other genes. The terminology can be a bit confusing because structural and regulatory genes have had different meanings to different audiences and basically we would say that this is a structural gene in the sense that it encodes a protein. But it is probably a regulatory gene in the sense that it influences the activity of other genes downstream.

UNIDENTIFIED: There are a variety of rare autosomal recessive conditions which regularly have sex reversal. Have you had a chance to look at those syndromes to see if they have missing areas on the Y or whether they are potentially the area that then gets acted on by this gene?

Dr. Saenger is at Montefiore Medical Center/Albert Einstein College of Medicine in Bronx, New York. Dr. Page is at the Whitehead Institute, Cambridge, Massachusetts. Drs. Grumbach and Lau are at the University of California at San Francisco, San Francisco, California. Dr. Simpson is at the University of Tennessee at Memphis, Memphis, Tennessee, Dr. Shapiro is at the University of California at Los Angeles School of Medicine, Los Angeles, California.

Dr. PAGE: We really have not had a chance to look at that yet.

DR. CHRIS LAU: I just want to ask you whether you have any evidence that the X chromosome is inactive, that the sequences are on the X chromosome.

DR. PAGE: We do not know yet if the X locus is subject to inactivation.

DR. LAU: What I mean is do you know if the sequence on the X chromosome is a pseudogene or is it an active gene, I mean is it a functional gene?

DR. PAGE: We do not have any functional assay to answer that question. However, the X chromosomal locus is extremely highly conserved during mammalian evolution which I think is a strong argument that it is a real functional gene.

DR. JOE L. SIMPSON: My question, David is similar. On the portions of the region in which you are attempting to localize TDF you have a material that is also present on the X. Is it conceivable that the material on the X that you have is active as is the Y, in which case you would have the same gene present, only X and the Y, and you might need to postulate something like X inactivation as a method to control the amount of gene product. That would be similar to a males hypothesis about regulatory locus.

DR. PAGE: I think that the locus on the X is an active gene. Whether the model building as to the relationship of the X and the Y loci is, in our minds at least, already extremely complex, whether the X and the Y genes are functionally equivalent or whether they differ subtly would be crucial to any kind of model building of that sort. It is possible, as you suggest, that the X and the Y genes are functionally interchangeable, functionally equivalent, and that X inactivation is sex determining.

DR. LARRY J. SHAPIRO: Dave, where are they expressed? What tissues?

DR. PAGE: Well we have not been able to detect any significant levels of expression of . . . well, I should say at this point, we cannot distinguish the X from the Y loci, let us say on Northerns or what have you, and in fact we cannot see either locus on a Northern. We have just detected rare transcripts in various CDNA libraries.

DR. GRUMBACH: One of the issues David, that does come up is really the location of whatever this factor is on the Y and the evidence has suggested in the past that it is in the pericentric region probably on the short-arm side. Now, looking at gross deletion maps when we are talking about structural chromosome abnormalities (not your beautiful probe analyses), it did seem that you could have some terminal deletions of the Y, as small as they may be, without getting into trouble and I think that led some people to believe this. Now there are a variety of things that could have happened—inversions and so forth—and the questions is as you walk the chromosome, there is no question in your mind where 1A is.

DR. PAGE: The deletion map is strong simply by virtue of reinforcement. I showed you the slides of the 20-interval deletion map. That is really a summary of about 90 patients and it is quite unambiguous as far as we are concerned. The TDF is quite distal in the short arm of the Y despite all the previous suggestions that it was near the centrum area or perhaps on both the long and the short arms.

4

Use of DNA Probes to Characterize Sex Chromosome Anomalies

Christine M. Disteche

University of Washington School of Medicine, Seattle, Washington

INTRODUCTION

In 1959, Ford et al. (1) reported that female individuals with Turner syndrome were 45,X, and Jacobs and Strong (2) reported that male individuals with Klinefelter syndrome were 47,XXY. This established that the presence of a Y chromosome and not the absence of an X chromosome determines male sex in humans. The study of additional sex chromosome anomalies resulted in the assignment of different loci playing a role in gonadal development to specific regions of the sex chromosomes. Until recently phenotype-genotype correlations related to sex differentiation were based mainly on classical cytogenetic studies. These studies can now be expanded by using DNA probes located on the X and Y chromosomes. These DNA probes are either cloned, functional genes or anonymous DNA sequences mapping to the sex chromosomes. Many of these DNA sequences originated from chromosome-specific libraries (e.g., 3-9).

Some of the DNA sequences isolated exhibit restriction fragment length polymorphisms (RFLPs) providing genetic markers that can be mapped along the chromosomes by following their recombination and segregation in families. Linkage analysis is complemented by physical mapping of the DNA sequences. Physical mapping methods include: (1) the analysis of somatic cell hybrids containing different portions of chromosome, (2) in situ hybridization of the DNA sequences directly to metaphase chromosomes, and (3) pulse-field electrophoresis for the separation of large DNA fragments. Detailed maps of the X chromosome have been established with genetic markers separated by a few centimorgans (10,11). In contrast to the X chromosome, most of the Y chromosome cannot be mapped by family studies since it does not recombine with the X chromosome, with the exception of a small region at the tip of the short arm. This region pairs and recombines at male meiosis and thus exhibits pseudoautosomal, as opposed to sex-linked, inheritance (12-14). Mapping of the remainder of the Y chromosome relied on physical mapping methods and the analysis of individuals with cytogenetically defined sex chromosome abnormalities.

The first Y chromosome–specific DNA of human origin was detected by Cooke (15), who compared HaeIII-digested DNA from male and female individuals, and by Kunkel et al. (16), who did subtraction hybridization of male and female DNA. Subsets of this repetitive DNA were cloned and located to the distal bright Q-band of the Y chromosome (17-19). These repeated DNA sequences are now being used as markers for the presence of the heterochromatic region of the Y chromosome (e.g., 20). Another tandem repeat located on the Y chromosome is a subset of the centromeric alphoid family that can be distinguished from the X-linked alphoid repeat (21-23).

Single-copy or low-copy Y chromosome DNA probes have also been isolated and sublocalized on the Y chromosome. A series of DNA probes were ordered along the short arm of the Y chromosome by the analysis of (1) 46,XX male individuals retaining portions of the short arm; (2) 46,XY females with deletions of the short arm; and (3) individuals with other rearrangements involving the short arm (24-26). Similarly, deletions of the long arm of the Y chromosome have been used to order DNA probes on the long arm. A map of the Y chromosome dividing it into seven regions (or deletion intervals) recognized by specific DNA probes was constructed by Vergnaud et al. (24) and has been recently refined (see Chapter 3). As the Y chromosome map is filled with additional genetic markers, other methods of mapping (e.g., cosmid cloning or pulse-field electrophoresis) can be used to order the loci at the molecular level (27).

Several of the Y chromosome DNA probes isolated share homologous DNA sequences with the X chromosome or with autosomes (6,7,28-30). Large regions of the X and Y chromosomes appear to carry homologous sequences that may have evolved from an ancestral, homologous sex chromosome pair (31). In addition, transfer of material from the X to the Y chromosome has occurred recently, when the human lineage diverged from that of the apes (32,33). Strictly Y-linked DNA fragments are useful for clinical studies because they allow the detection of specific regions of the Y chromosome by dot blot analysis. Rapid prenatal sex determination has been achieved by hybridization of a repeated Y chromosome DNA probe to very small amounts of amniotic fluid (19,34). We have recently isolated a series of DNA fragments from different regions of the Y chromosome by extensive hybridization of purified Y chromosome DNA to DNA from patients with partial deletions of the Y chromosome (M. A. Cantrell and C. M. Disteche, unpublished work) using a phenol-enhanced reassociation technique (35). This method enriches for DNA sequences that are strictly Y-linked and are located in specific regions of the Y chromosome.

Among the Y-linked DNA sequences that have been reported in the literature, some are low repeats with copies located in different regions of the Y chromosome. Thus, on a Southern blot hybridized with a single probe, one can visualize bands characterizing different regions of the Y chromosome (e.g., 6,24). The presence of homologous sequences on the short and long arm of the Y chromosome indicates that inversions may have occurred often in the evolution of the Y chromosome.

The abundance of X and Y chromosome DNA sequences available has only begun to aid our understanding of the pathogenesis of gonadal dysgenesis. The following section illustrates use of the complementary molecular cytogenetic techniques of Southern blot and in situ hybridization of X and Y chromosome-specific DNA probes in the analysis of human sex chromosome anomalies. Anomalies involving the Y chromosome are emphasized, although anomalies of the X chromosome have been studied with DNA probes as well.

THE X CHROMOSOME

A striking example of the ability of molecular cytogenetic techniques to extend the cytogenetic analysis of human sex chromosome disorders is the reevaluation of a long-arm deletion of the X chromosome in a family of patients with premature ovarian failure recently reported by Krauss et al. (36) using X chromosome probes. What appeared to be a terminal deletion by cytogenetic studies was shown to be an interstitial deletion by DNA analysis. The authors' interpretation of the anomaly suggests that a region of the X chromosome between bands q26 and q28 may be important for ovarian function. Careful analysis at the DNA level of additional breakpoints in X chromosome anomalies may help identify regions of the X chromosome that play a role in producing different features of Turner syndrome.

Another application of X chromosome RFLP analysis is the determination of the parental origin of the chromosome abnormality. Hassold et al. (37) recently used such a method to determine the origin of the X chromosome in Turner syndrome abortuses and newborns.

THE Y CHROMOSOME AND SEX REVERSAL

Anomalies of the Y chromosome have been extensively studied with DNA probes. In particular, the study of individuals with sex reversal (46,XX males and 46,XY females) and 45,X males has greatly advanced our understanding of sex determination in humans (38) (see Chapter 3).

46,XX Males

The phenotype of 46,XX males resembles that of Klinefelter patients (47,XXY), with the exceptions of short stature and an absence of mental retardation (39). The testes are very small with abnormal tubules and few, if any, spermatogenic elements. It was postulated that 46,XX males may carry Y chromosome material due to an exchange between the X and Y chromosomes at meiosis (40). Indeed, in 1984, de la Chapelle et al. (41) and Guellaen et al. (42) showed that 46,XX males carried Y chromosome genetic markers. Subsequent studies by in situ hybridization showed that the Y chromosome material is located at the tip of the short arm of the X chromosome (43,44).

By following the inheritance of paternal pseudoautosomal markers, Petit et al. (45) showed that an abnormal X-Y interchange causes XX maleness. Because the abnormal interchange can occur at different points on the sex chromosomes, a variable amount of Y chromosome material is translocated to the X chromosome in different patients (24,26,46,47). However, this Y chromosome material always includes region 1 of the Y chromosome (Fig. 1, Table 1) (24). Region 1 contains the testis-determining factor (*TDF*) gene that is accidentally translocated to the X chromosome at paternal meiosis and causes male gonadal differentiation in the 46,XX patient (38) (see Chapter 3).

Males with a 46,XX karyotype who do not appear to contain any Y chromosome material have also been described. In these individuals, sex reversal is likely to have resulted from mutations in other genes (sex-linked or autosomal) involved at other steps in the chain of events leading to gonadal differentiation. Waibel et al. (48) reported that 46,XX true hermaphrodites did not show Y chromosome DNA, indicating that the etiology of true hermaphroditism is different from that of 46,XX male syndrome.

46,XY Females

In 1979, Rosenfeld et al. (49) described a female infant with Turner-like features who had a deletion of the short arm of the Y chromosome. Patients with a similar Y chromosome anomaly have been diagnosed by cytogenetic and/or DNA analysis (46,47,50,51). Three Y chromosome deletions that we have studied appear similar by cytogenetic analysis, but differ at the molecular level (Figs. 1 and 2; 51). All three patients are missing region 1 and 2 of the Y chromosome; in addition, patients 1 and 3 are missing region 3, while patient 2 lacks region 4A due to an inversion of the paternal Y chromosome (Fig. 1, Table 1; 51).

Phenotypic features characterizing our three patients include streak gonads in each patient, with the variable occurrence of lymphodema at birth, wide-spaced nipples, and short neck. Two of the patients (patients 2 and 3) developed gonadoblastoma, a tumor that frequently occurs in females with a Y chromosome (52). This would indicate that a locus conferring susceptibility to gonado-

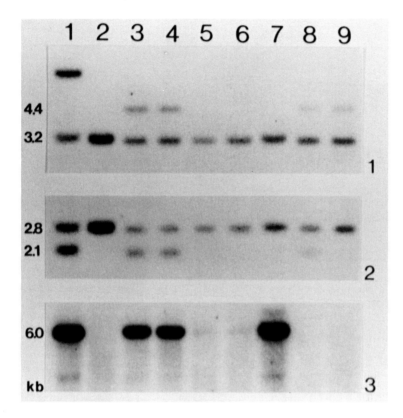

Figure 1 Southern blot hybridization of three Y chromosome probes: (1) pDP132 for region 1, (2) pDP61 for region 2, and (3) MC23 for region 3 to DNA from a normal male (lane 1), a normal female (lanes 2), two 46,XY females (lanes 3 and 4), 46,X,Yp- female patient 3 (lane 5), 46,X,Yp- female patient 1 (lane 6), 46,X,Yp- female patient 2 (lane 7), 46,XX male patient 1 (lane 8), and 46,XX male patient 2 (lane 9). Probe pDP132 recognizes a 3.2 kb (or RFLP 5.7 kb) X-linked band and a 4.4 kb (or RFLP 5.7 kb) Y-linked band (24); probe pDP61 recognizes a 2.8 kb X-linked band and a 2.1 kb Y-linked band (74), and probe MC23 recognizes a 6.0 kb Y-specific band (M.A. Cantrell and C.M. Disteche, unpublished work). The two 46,XX male patients (lanes 8 and 9) show positive hybridization of the region 1 probe and patient 1 (lane 8) of the region 2 probe. The three 46,X,Yp- females (lanes 4, 5, and 6) show deletion of DNA sequences homologous to the probes for regions 1, 2, and 3, except patient 2 (lane 7), who shows positive hybridization of a probe for region 3. The two 46,XY females (lane 3 and 4) show positive hybridization of all three probes with no evidence of deletion of the Y chromosome. DNA was digested with TaqI and hybridized with ^{32}P-labeled probes as described in Disteche et al. (51).

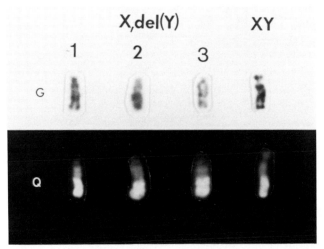

Figure 2 Examples of deleted Y chromosomes in 46,X,Yp- patients 1, 2 and 3. A normal Y chromosome is shown at the right. The prometaphase chromosomes obtained from methotrexate-synchronized lymphocyte cultures are stained with G-banding (G) and Q-banding (Q) as described in Disteche et al. (51).

Table 1 Hybridization Data on Patients with Sex Reversal

		\multicolumn{7}{c}{Y chromosome region[a]}						
		1	2	3	4	5	6	7
46,XX ♂	1:	+	+	−	−	ND	−	ND
	2:	+	−	−	−	ND	−	ND
45,X ♂	1:	+	+	+	+	+	−	−
46,X,Yp- ♀	1:	−	−	−	+	+	+	ND
	2:	−	−	+	−	+	+	ND
	3:	−	−	−	+	ND	+	ND
46,XY ♀	1:	+	+	+	+	ND	+	ND
	2:	+	+	+	+	ND	+	ND

[a]Region 1 was identified by probe pDP132 (24); region 2, by probe pDP61 (74); region 3, by probe MC23 (M. A. Cantrell and C. M. Disteche, unpublished work); region 4, by probe pD34 (28); region 5, by probe 12f (6); region 6, by probe pDP105 (D. C. Page, unpublished work); region 7, by probe pY3.4 (19).

blastoma might be located in the proximal portion of region 4, or in the long arm of the Y chromosome. The patients that we studied and that Magenis et al. (50) reported were not short and may even be tall for females. Thus, a gene for stature, postulated to reside on the Y chromosome (review in 53), could also reside in the proximal short arm or in the long arm. The same region of the Y chromosome may also carry a gene (or a controlling gene) for the cytotoxic HY antigen that tested positive in patients 1 and 2 (54).

The phenotypic sex of 46,X,Yp- females can be explained by a deletion of region 1 where the *TDF* is located (38). Occasionally a female carries Y chromosome material in the form of a translocation to an autosome or to the X chromosome, rather than as a free Y chromosome. These patients also lack region 1 of the Y chromosome (24,38,55). However, there are 46,XY females with gonadal dysgenesis who appear to carry a normal Y chromosome, do not show evidence of Y-chromosome mosaicism, and have no detectable deletion by cytogenetic or DNA analysis (Fig. 1, Table 1; 38,47). These individuals may result from other mutations in the *TDF* gene or in other genes involved in sex differentiation.

45,X Males

The 45,X males are much rarer than 46,XX males or 46,XY females. Individuals with this karyotype may or may not have phenotypic abnormalities. We have studied a 45,X male who was retarded, although his developmental delay may have resulted from asphyxia at birth rather than from his chromosome constitution (56). The patient's chromosomes appeared cytogenetically normal. However, hybridization of a series of Y chromosome DNA probes to DNA from this individual showed that the patient's genome contained regions 1 to 5 of the Y chromosome (Table 1). By in situ hybridization to a moderately repeated DNA probe (pDP105) that recognizes regions 3 and 6 of the Y chromosome (D. C. Page, unpublished work), we showed that this individual had a translocation between the Y chromosome and chromosome 15 (Fig. 3). The chromosome 15 breakpoint appeared to be located in the proximal portion of the long arm, with the centromere of the derivative chromosome being of Y-chromosomal origin, although we could not exclude that the derivative chromosome was dicentric (56).

Other 45,X males have been shown to result from Y autosome translocations by DNA analysis (57–60). The autosomes involved in the translocations were chromosomes 5 (2 cases), 15 (2 cases) and 18 (1 case). In one 45,X male, no Y chromosome DNA was detected, while another 45,X male was shown to be a hidden 45,X/46,XY mosaic (61; see below).

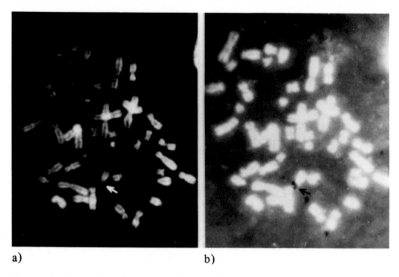

a)   b)

Figure 3 Example of a metaphase cell from a 45,X male patient hybridized with probe pDP105 that recognizes regions 3 and 6 of the Y chromosome (D.C. Page, unpublished work). a) Chromosome identification by Q-banding and b) grain localization to the short arm of one chromosome 15 (arrow). Forty-one percent of the sites of hybridization on a total of 53 metaphases were on the short arm of one chromosome 15 indicating that this chromosome carries a Y chromosome translocation. In situ hybridization was performed with a ^{3}H-labeled probe as described in Disteche et al. (56).

SEX CHROMOSOME MOSAICISM

45,X/46,XY and 45,X/46,XX

Sex chromosome-specific DNA probes are useful to detect hidden mosaicism in 45,X individuals, as exemplified by the case of de la Chapelle et al. (61) mentioned above. In a fibroblast culture from this individual, the 46,XY cells were estimated to represent 1-3% of the cells. A 46,XX/69,XXY mosaic with a rare occurrence (1-3%) of 69,XXY cells has also been detected by using a repeated Y chromosome DNA probe (62). Polymorphic X chromosome DNA probes can also be useful to detect hidden mosaicism. RFLP analysis of an X-linked sequence revealed polymorphic bands from the mother and the father of an individual who was a hidden 45,X/46,XX mosaic (37). The advantage of using DNA probes to detect mosaicism is that the material examined can be nondividing tissue, while cytogenetic studies require actively dividing cells.

Most Turner fetuses die between conception and birth and it has been postulated that most of the surviving 45,X individuals are in fact hidden mosaics (63).

Burns et al. (64) have examined this question by cytogenetic studies of different tissues and found no clear evidence of mosaicism. It may be of interest to re-examine this question using DNA probes. Clinically, it is also important to detect a 46,XY cell line in a 45,X individual as this would place the individual at higher risk of developing gonadoblastoma (52).

Mosaicism can be quantified by using DNA probes (65). We have hybridized DNA from control males and from mosaic patients to probe pDP34 that recognizes X-linked and Y-linked loci (28). Densitometric measurements of the intensity of the X- and Y-linked bands were compared to calculate the percentage of cells with a Y chromosome in 45,X/46,XY mosaic individuals. Such measurements showed a good correlation with the cytogenetic estimates (65).

45,X/45,XYnf

The presence of an abnormal Y chromosome called a nonfluorescent (nf) Y chromosome can be associated with a male or female phenotype. Although some patients appear to be nonmosaic, most cases are mosaic 45,X/45,XYnf with their phenotypic sex dependent on the predominant cell line. Nonfluorescent Y chromosomes are of normal length, though appear to lack the bright (Yq12) Q-band. Magenis and Donlon (66) showed that the abnormal chromosome is in fact a dicentric Y chromosome with two copies of the short arm and proximal long arm. Figure 4 shows an example of Ynf found in 88% of cells from a female indi-

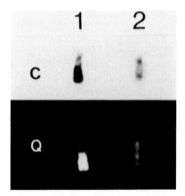

Figure 4 Examples of a normal Y chromosome (1) and a Ynf chromosome (2) stained with C-banding (C) and with Q-banding (Q). The Ynf shows two positive centromeric C-bands and absence of the bright Q-band (or dark C-band) q12 indicating that the Ynf is a dicentric chromosome with two copies of the short arm and proximal long arm of the Y chromosome. Preparation and staining of chromosome is as described in Disteche et al. (65).

vidual with short stature, wide-spaced nipples, and bilateral gonadoblastoma. Hybridization of a region 7 probe (pY3.4) that recognizes the 3.4 kb HaeIII male repeat (19) to DNA from this patient was positive, although very faint (65; Fig. 5). This indicates that the breakpoint in the long arm of the Ynf chromosome is likely to be in region 7 very close to the junction of region 6 and 7. When a probe for region 3 was hybridized to DNA from the Ynf patient, a hybridization intensity greater than that observed with normal male DNA was observed, confirming the presence of two copies of the short arm in the Ynf (65). Similar findings were reported in three cases of 45,X/46,XYnf by Gänshirt-Ahlert et al. (67), although these authors found no evidence of the 3.4 and 2.1 kb HaeIII male repeats in their patients. Thus, there appears to be heterogeneity in the long-arm breakpoint of Ynf chromosomes.

The phenotype of individuals carrying a Ynf chromosome includes mixed gonadal dysgenesis and variable features of Turner syndrome. Interpretation of

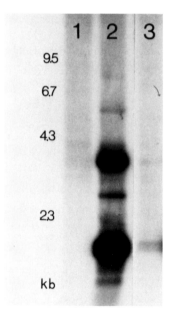

Figure 5 Southern blot hybridization of repeated probe pY3.4 that recognizes region 7 of the Y chromosome (19) to DNA from a normal female (lane 1), a normal male (lane 2), and a female patient with a Ynf chromosome (shown in Fig. 4). The two prominent Y chromosome–specific bands seen in the normal male at about 2.0 and 3.5 kb are very faint in the patient indicating deletion of most of region 7 in the Ynf. DNA was digested with MboI and hybridized with the ^{32}P-labeled probe as described in Disteche et al. (65).

phenotype-genotype relationships is difficult in these patients due to mosaicism. The frequent finding of a 45,X cell line in these individuals may result from the mitotic instability of the dicentric Y chromosome. Female individuals with a Ynf chromosome usually do not develop gonadoblastoma (68), although the patient that we reported had bilateral gonadoblastoma (65). Lukusa et al. (68) argued that the absence of the Q-band bright region 7 was correlated with the absence of gonadoblastoma in female individuals carrying a Ynf chromosome. The presence of residual DNA sequences homologous to a probe for region 7 in our patient would suggest that, unless probe pY3.4 cross-hybridizes to sequences located elsewhere on the Y chromosome, a gene for gonadoblastoma may be located in the distal portion of region 6 or the proximal portion of region 7. This would agree with our study of 46,X,Yp- females, which located the gonadoblastoma locus to the long arm or proximal short arm of the Y chromosome (see above; 69). More refined analysis of the breakpoints involved in the formation of Ynf chromosomes and other Y chromosome deletions in patients with and without gonadoblastoma will be necessary to map the locus of susceptibility to gonadoblastoma. Evaluating the association of cytogenetic or molecular genetic abnormalities and the subsequent development of gonadoblastoma will be difficult, however, as these patients' gonads are often removed at an early age to prevent the subsequent development of the tumor.

SMALL MARKER SEX CHROMOSOMES

Small marker sex chromosomes are difficult to analyze using classical cytogenetic techniques. Individuals who are 46,X,del(?) or 46,Xr(?) may be of male or female sex depending on the origin of the small marker chromosome. In prenatal diagnosis when the sex of the fetus is unknown, it is even more difficult and critical to determine the origin of a small marker sex chromosome. Magenis and Donlon (66) showed that with G11 staining, the centromere of the X and Y chromosome could be distinguished, and thus the origin of markers identified. Alternatively, one can use probes for the X and Y chromosomes to characterize the marker. Even in cases where cytogenetic studies appear sufficient to identify the origin of the small sex chromosome, DNA probes can be used to confirm the cytogenetic results or to further delineate the deletion. For example, in one case described by Gemmill et al. (70), DNA analysis showed the presence of Y chromosome sequences in a G11 negative chromosome.

The two cases described below are examples of small marker sex chromosomes that we found in prenatal diagnosis. Case 1 was a fetus with a small Y chromosome, while the paternal Y chromosome was of normal length (71). Hybridization of a DNA probe for region 7 (ps4, K. K. Smith, unpublished work) to DNA from the fetus revealed that about 20% of region 7 remained on the short Y chromosome. This indicated that the infant was likely to be a normal male with a variant Y chromosome, which was confirmed at birth. Case 2 had a small marker sex chromosome that appeared as a ring chromosome in about 20% of amniotic fluid cells. The rest of cells were 45,X. In situ hybridization with Y chromosome probe pDP105 that recognizes regions 3 and 6 (D. C. Page, unpublished work) was performed. A control male individual was analyzed by the same in situ hybridization protocol (Figs. 6a and b). Although the control showed positive hybridization in 60% of the cells, the small marker chromosome was negative in all cells examined. The fetus was stillborn at 39 weeks of gestation and appeared as a female with Turner syndrome. No further material could be obtained to confirm the suspected X chromosome origin of the small ring chromosome.

Müller et al. (72) used a Y chromosome DNA fragment Y-190 that recognizes repeated DNA sequences located on the short arm to confirm the Y chromosome origin of two small marker chromosomes. Another probe for the short arm of the Y chromosome was used by Münke et al. (73) to characterize a marker present in two male patients, one with azoospermia and the other with short stature. Further studies of small deleted Y chromosomes or ring Y chromosomes in patients with specific phenotypic features will aid the construction of the de-

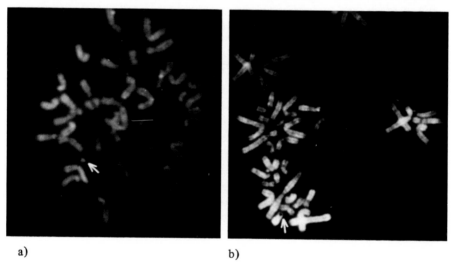

a)   b)

Figure 6 In situ hybridization of probe pDP105 that recognizes regions 3 and 6 of the Y chromosome (D. C. Page, unpublished work): a) to a 46,X,r(?) metaphase cell and b) to a control normal male metaphase cell from amniotic fluid cultures. Positive hybridization is indicated on the normal male cell by a grain on the Y chromosome (arrow), while the r(?) appears negative (arrow). The cells are stained with Q-banding. In situ hybridization was performed with ^{3}H-labeled probe pDP105 as described in Disteche et al. (56).

letion map of the Y chromosome and correlation of the presence of specific Y chromosome sequences with specific phenotypic features.

CONCLUSION

DNA analysis using X- and Y-linked DNA probes has greatly advanced our understanding of sex chromosome anomalies. Sex reversal—46,XX and 45,X males and 46,XY females—can be explained in many cases by the presence or the absence of region 1 of the Y chromosome that contains the TDF gene. Sex chromosome mosaicism can be detected and quantified by hybridization of X- and Y-specific DNA probes to patient DNA. Finally, more complex sex chromosome rearrangement including dicentric and small marker sex chromosomes can be identified and further delineated by using DNA analysis. Accurate determination of chromosomal breakpoints at the molecular level in patients with abnormal sex chromosomes will lead to the identification of specific genes on the sex chromosomes that affect specific phenotypic features.

ACKNOWLEDGMENTS

We thank Drs. M. A. Cantrell, J. Bicknell, D. A. Adler, and J. M. Garr (Department of Pathology, University of Washington, Seattle, WA) for their help. We thank Dr. Y-F. Lau (University of California, San Francisco, CA), Dr. D. C. Page (Whitehead Institute, Cambridge, MA), Dr. K. K. Smith (Johns Hopkins, Baltimore), and Drs. J. Weissenbach and M. Fellous (Institut Pasteur, Paris), for DNA probes. We thank Dr. J. Graham (Dartmouth Medical School, Hanover, NH), Drs. R. A. Pagon and V. P. Sybert (University of Washington, Seattle, WA), Dr. H. Saal (Children's Hospital, Washington, DC), Dr. H. C. Thuline (Genetics Program, Department of Social and Health Sciences, Seattle, WA), and Dr. A. Zinn (Case Western University, Cleveland, OH) for referring patients to us. We thank the patients and their families for their participation. This work was supported by a March of Dimes grant 1-1019 and an American Cancer Society grant CD305.

REFERENCES

1. Ford CE, Jones KW, Polani PE, de Almeida JC, Briggs JH. A sex-chromosome anomaly in a case of gonadal dysgenesis (Turner's syndrome). Lancet 1959;i:711–713.
2. Jacobs PA, Strong JA. A case of human intersexuality having a possible XXY sex-determining mechanism. Nature 1959;183:302–303.
3. Davies KE, Young BD, Elles RG, Hill M, Williamson R. Cloning of a representative genomic library of the human X chromosome after sorting by flow cytometry. Nature 1981;293:374–376.

4. Kunkel LM, Tantravahi U, Eisenhard M, Latt SA. Regional localization on the human X of DNA segments cloned from flow sorted chromosomes. Nucl Acids Res 1982; 10:1557–1578.
5. Müller CR, Davies KE, Cremer C, Rappold G, Gray JW, Ropers HH. Cloning of genomic sequences from the human Y chromosome after purification by dual beam flow sorting. Hum Genet 1983; 64:110–115.
6. Bishop C, Guellaen G, Geldwerth D, Fellous M, Weissenbach J. Extensive sequence homologies between Y and other human chromosomes. J Mol Biol 1984; 173:403–417.
7. Wolfe J, Erickson RP, Rigby PWJ, Goodfellow PN. Regional localization of 3 Y-derived sequences on the human X and Y chromosomes. Ann Hum Genet 1984; 48:253–259.
8. Hofker MH, Wapenaar MC, Goor N, Bakker E, van Ommen G-JB, Pearson PL. Isolation of probes detecting restriction fragment length polymorphisms from X chromosome-specific libraries: potential use for diagnosis of Duchenne muscular dystrophy. Hum Genet 1985; 70:148–156.
9. Affara NA, Florentin L, Morrison N, Kwok K, Mitchell M, Cook A, Jamieson D, Glasgow L, Meredith L, Boyd E, Ferguson-Smith MA. Regional assignment of Y-linked DNA probes by deletion mapping and their homology with X-chromosome and autosomal sequences. Nucl Acids Res 1986; 14:5353–5373.
10. Drayna D, White R. The genetic linkage map of the human X chromosome. Science 1985; 230:753–758.
11. Donis-Keller H, Green P, Helms C, Cartinhour S, Weissenbach B, Stephens K, Keith TP, Bowden DW, Smith DR, Lander ES et al. A genetic linkage map of the human genome. Cell 1987; 51:319–337.
12. Cooke HJ, Brown WRA, Rappold GA. Hypervariable telomeric sequences from the human sex chromosomes are pseudoautosomal. Nature 1985; 317:687–692.
13. Simmler M-C, Rouyer F, Vergnaud G, Nyström-Lahti M, Ngo KY, de la Chapelle A, Weissenbach J. Pseudoautosomal DNA sequences in the pairing region of the human sex chromosomes. Nature 1985; 317:692–697.
14. Rouyer F, Simmler M-C, Johnsson C, Vergnaud G, Cooke HJ, Weissenbach J. A gradient of sex linkage in the pseudoautosomal region of the human sex chromosomes. Nature 1986; 319:291–295.
15. Cooke HJ. Repeated sequence specific to human males. Nature 1976; 262:182–186.
16. Kunkel LM, Smith KD, Boyer SH. Human Y-chromosome-specific reiterated DNA. Science 1976; 191:1189–1190.
17. McKay RDG, Borrow M, Cooke HJ. The identification of a repeated DNA sequence involved in the karyotype polymorphism of the human Y chromosome. Cytogenet. Cell Genet 1978; 21:19–32.
18. Schmidtke J, and Schmid M. Regional assignment of a 2.1 kb repetitive sequence to the distal part of the human Y heterochromatin. Hum Genet 1980; 55:255–257.

19. Lau Y-F, Huang JC, Dozy AM, Kan YW. A rapid screening test for antenatal sex determination. Lancet 1984; i:14–16.
20. Lau Y-F. Detection of Y-specific repeat sequences in normal and variant human chromosomes using in situ hybridization with biotinylated probes. Cytogenet Cell Genet 1985; 39:184–187.
21. Willard HF, Smith KD, Sutherland J. Isolation and characterization of a major tandem repeat family from the human X chromosome. Nucl Acids Res 1983; 11:2017–2033.
22. Wolfe J, Darling SM, Erickson RP, Craig IW, Buckle VJ, Rigby PWJ, Willard HF, Goodfellow PN. Isolation and characterization of an alphoid centromeric repeat family from the human Y chromosome. J Mol Biol 1985; 182:477–485.
23. Tyler-Smith C, Brown WRA. Structure of the major block of alphoid satellite DNA on the human Y chromosome. J Mol Biol 1987; 195:457–470.
24. Vergnaud G, Page DC, Simmler M-C, Brown L, Rouyer F, Noel B, Botstein D, de la Chapelle A, Weissenbach J. A deletion map of the human Y chromosome based on DNA hybridization. Am J Hum Genet 1986; 38: 109–124.
25. Page DC. Sex reversal: Deletion mapping the male-determining function of the human Y chromosome. Cold Spring Harbor Symposia on Quantitative Biology 1986; 51:229–235.
26. Affara NA, Ferguson-Smith MA, Tolmie J, Kwok K, Mitchell M, Jamieson D, Cooke A, Florentin L. Variable transfer of Y-specific sequences in XX males. Nucl Acids Res 1986; 14:5375–5387.
27. Pritchard CA, Goodfellow PJ, Goodfellow PN. Mapping the limits of the human pseudoautosomal region and a candidate sequence for the male-determining gene. Nature 1987; 328:273–275.
28. Page D, de Martinville B, Barker D, Wyman A, White R, Francke U, Botstein D. Single-copy sequence hybridizes to polymorphic and homologous loci on human X and Y chromosomes. Proc Natl Acad Sci USA 1982; 79: 5352–5356.
29. Cooke HJ, Brown WRA, Rappold GA. Closely related sequences on human X and Y chromosomes outside the pairing region. Nature 1984; 311:259–261.
30. Koenig M, Moisan JP, Heilig R, Mandel JL. Homologies between X and Y chromosomes detected by DNA probes: localisation and evolution. Nucl Acids Res 1985; 13:5485–5501.
31. Ohno S. *Sex Chromosomes and Sex-linked Genes*. New York: Springer-Verlag, 1967:1–23.
32. Page DC, Harper ME, Love J, Botstein D. Occurrence of a transposition from the X-chromosome long arm to the Y-chromosome short arm during human evolution. Nature 1984; 311:119–123.
33. Bickmore WA, Cooke HJ. Evolution of homologous sequences on the human X and Y chromosomes, outside of the meiotic pairing segment. Nucl Acids Res 1987; 15:6261–6271.

34. Gosden JR, Gosden CM, Christie S, Cooke HJ, Morsman JM, Rodeck CH. The use of cloned Y chromosome-specific DNA probes for fetal sex determination in first trimester prenatal diagnosis. Hum Genet 1984; 66: 347–351.

35. Kunkel LM, Monaco AP, Middlesworth W, Ochs HD, Latt SA. Specific cloning of DNA fragments absent from the DNA of a male patient with an X chromosome deletion. Proc Natl Acad Sci USA 1985; 82:4778–4782.

36. Krauss CM, Turksoy N, Atkins L, McLaughlin C, Brown LG, Page DC. Familial premature ovarian failure due to an interstitial deletion of the long arm of the X chromosome. N Engl J Med 1987; 317:125–131.

37. Hassold T, Benham F, Kobryn C, Leppert M, Whittington E. Cytogenetic and molecular studies of sex chromosome monosomy. Am J Hum Genet 1987; 41(3 Suppl):A121.

38. Page DC, Mosher R, Simpson EM, Fisher EMC, Mardon G, Pollack J, McGillivray B, de la Chapelle A, Brown LG. The sex-determining region of the human Y chromosome encodes a finger protein. Cell 1987; 51:1091–1104.

39. de la Chapelle A. The etiology of maleness in XX men. Hum Genet 1981; 58:105–116.

40. Ferguson-Smith MA. X-Y chromosomal interchange in the aetiology of true hermaphroditism and of XX Klinefelter's syndrome. Lancet 1966; ii:475–476.

41. de la Chapelle A, Tippett PA, Wetterstrand G, Page D. Genetic evidence of X-Y interchange in a human XX male. Nature 1984; 307:169–173.

42. Guellaen G, Casanova M, Bishop C, Geldwerth D, Andre G, Fellous M, Weissenbach J. Human XX males with Y single-copy DNA fragments. Nature 1984; 307:172–173.

43. Andersson M, Page DC, de la Chapelle A. Chromosome Y-specific DNA is transferred to the short arm of X chromosome in human XX males. Science 1986; 233:786–788.

44. Magenis RE, Casanova M, Fellous M, Olson S, Sheehy R. Further cytologic evidence for Xp-Yp translocation in XX males using in situ hybridization with Y-derived probe. Hum Genet 1987; 75:228–233.

45. Petit C, de la Chapelle A, Levilliers J, Castillo S, Noël B, Weissenbach J. An abnormal terminal X-Y interchange accounts for most but not all cases of human XX maleness. Cell 1987; 49:595–602.

46. Müller U, Lalande M, Donlon T, Latt SA. Moderately repeated DNA sequences specific for the short arm of the human Y chromosome are present in XX males and reduced in copy number in an XY female. Nucl Acids Res 1986; 14:1325–1340.

47. Affara NA, Ferguson-Smith MA, Magenis RE, Tolmie JL, Boyd E, Cooke A, Jamieson D, Kwok K, Mitchell M, Snadden L. Mapping the testis determinants by an analysis of Y-specific sequences in males with apparent XX and XO karyotypes and females with XY karyotypes. Nucl Acids Res 1987; 15:7325–7342.

48. Waibel F, Scherer G, Fraccaro M, Hustinx TWJ, Weissenbach J, Wieland J, Mayerova A, Back E, and Wolf U. Absence of Y-specific DNA sequences in

human 46,XX true hermaphrodites and in 45,X mixed gonadal dysgenesis. Hum Genet 1987; 76:332–336.

49. Rosenfeld RG, Luzzatti L, Hintz RL, Miller OJ, Koo GC, Wachtel SS. Sexual and somatic determinants of the human Y chromosome: Studies in a 46,XYp-phenotypic female. Am J Hum Genet 1979; 31:458–468.

50. Magenis RE, Tochen ML, Holahan KP, Carey T, Allen L, Brown MG. Turner syndrome resulting from partial deletion of Y chromosome short arm: Localization of male determinants. J Pediatr 1984; 105:916–919.

51. Disteche CM, Casanova M, Saal H, Friedman C, Sybert V, Graham J, Thuline H, Page DC, Fellous M. Small deletions of the short arm of the Y chromosome in 46,XY females. Proc Natl Acad Sci USA 1986; 83:7841–7844.

52. Scully RE. Gonadoblastoma: A review of 74 cases. Cancer 1970; 25:1340–1356.

53. Bühler EM. A synopsis of the human Y chromosome. Hum Genet 1980; 55:145–175.

54. Simpson E, Chandler P, Goulmy E, Disteche CM, Ferguson-Smith MA, Page DC. Separation of the genetic loci for the H-Y antigen and for testis determination on human Y chromosome. Nature 1987; 326:876–878.

55. Bernstein R, Rosendorff J, Ramsay M, Pinto MR, Page DC. A unique dicentric X;Y translocation with Xq and Xp breakpoints: Cytogenetic and molecular studies. Am J Hum Genet 1987; 41:145–156.

56. Disteche CM, Brown L, Saal H, Friedman C, Thuline HC, Hoar DI, Pagon RA, Page DC. Molecular detection of a translocation (Y;15) in a 45,X male. Hum Genet 1986; 74:372–377.

57. Maserati E, Waibel F, Weber B, Fraccaro M, Gal A, Pasquali F, Schempp W, Scherer G, Vaccaro R, Weissenbach J, Wolf U. A 45,X male with a Yp/18 translocation. Hum Genet 1986; 74:126–132.

58. Gal A, Weber B, Neri G, Serra A, Müller U, Schempp W, Page DC. A 45,X male with Y-specific DNA translocated onto chromosome 15. Am J Hum Genet 1987; 40:477–488.

59. Weber B, Schempp W, Orth U, Seidel H, Gal A. A Y/5 translocation in a 45,X male with cri du chat syndrome. Hum Genet 1987; 77:145–150.

60. Sheehy RR, Brown MG, Warren RJ, Schwartzman M, Magenis RE. Y-derived sequences detected in a 45,X male by in situ hybridization. Am J Med Genet 1987; 27:831–839.

61. de la Chapelle A, Page DC, Brown L, Kaski U, Parvinen T, Tippett PA. The origin of 45,X males. Am J Hum Genet 1986; 38:330–340.

62. Tantravahi U, Bianchi DW, Haley C, Destrempes MM, Ricker AT, Korf BR, Latt SA. Use of Y chromosome specific probes to detect low level sex chromosome mosaicism. Clin Genet 1986; 29:445–448.

63. Hecht F, MacFarlane JP. Mosaicism in Turner's syndrome reflects the lethality of XO. Lancet 1969; i:1197–1198.

64. Burns JL, Hall JG, Powers E, Callis JB, Hoehn H. No evidence for chromosomal mosaicism in multiple tissues of 10 patients with 45,XO Turner syndrome. Clin Genet 1979; 15:22–28.

65. Disteche CM, Saal H, Friedman C, Sybert V, Thuline H. Quantitative analy-
     sis of sex-chromosome mosaicism with X-Y DNA probes. Am J Hum Genet
     1986; 38:751–758.
66. Magenis E, Donlon T. Nonfluorescent Y chromosomes. Cytologic evidence
     of origin. Hum Genet 1982; 60:133–138.
67. Gänshirt-Ahlert D, Pawlowitzki IH, Gal A. Three cases of 45,X/46,XYnf
     mosaicism: Molecular analysis revealed heterogeneity of the nonfluorescent
     Y chromosome. Hum Genet 1987; 76:153–156.
68. Lukusa T, Fryns JP, van den Berghe H. Gonadoblastoma and Y-chromo-
     some fluorescence. Clin Genet 1986; 29:311–316.
69. Page DC. Hypothesis: a Y-chromosomal gene causes gonadoblastoma in
     dysgenetic gonads. Development 1987; in press.
70. Gemmill RM, Pearce-Birge L, Bixenman H, Hecht BK, Allanson JE. Y
     chromosome-specific DNA sequences in Turner-syndrome mosaicism. Am
     J Hum Genet 1987; 41:157–167.
71. Disteche C, Luthy D, Haslam DB, Hoar D. Prenatal identification of a de-
     leted Y chromosome by cytogenetics and a Y-specific repetitive DNA
     probe. Hum Genet 1984; 67:222–224.
72. Müller U, Donlon TA, Kunkel SM, Lalande M, Latt SA. Y-190, a DNA
     probe for the sensitive detection of Y-derived marker chromosomes and
     mosaicism. Hum Genet 1987; 75:109–113.
73. Münke M, de Martinville B, Lieber E, Francke U. Minute chromosomes re-
     placing the Y chromosome carry Y-specific sequences by restriction frag-
     ment analysis and in situ hybridization. Am J Med Genet 1985; 22:361–
     374.
74. Geldwerth D, Bishop C, Guellaön G, Koenig M, Vergnaud G, Mandel J-L,
     Weissenbach J. Extensive DNA sequence homologies between the human
     Y and the long arm of the X chromosome. EMBO J 1985; 4:1739–1743.

DISCUSSION

DR. DAVID PAGE: Have you done in situ hybridization on any of those nonfluorescent Y chromosomes with the interval 7 probes?

DR. CHRISTINE M. DISTECHE: No, I haven't done that.

DR. DARRELL WILSON: Is it known which area of the Y, or are there any
probes for that area, that confer the risk for the gonadoblastoma?

Dr. Page is at the Whitehead Institute, Cambridge, Massachusetts. Dr. Disteche is at the
University of Washington School of Medicine, Seattle, Washington. Drs. Wilson and Rosenfeld are at Stanford University, Stanford, California. Dr. Cutler is at the National Institutes of Health, Bethesda, Maryland. Dr. Grumbach is at the University of California at
San Francisco, San Francisco, California.

DR. DISTECHE: No, it is not known. From these female patients that we have that have deletion, it appears to be in all the rest of the Y chromosome.

DR. WILSON: It is possible that it may be related to the dysorganogenesis of whatever testicular tissue you have rather than the specific.

DR. DISTECHE: Rather than have a specific gene that confers the tumor, yes.

DR. GORDON B. CUTLER: Do you have any comments about how closely the areas conferring shortness on the Turner's syndrome patients can be localized?

DR. DISTECHE: No, again all that we know from the deleted patients is that it is outside the region that is deleted, but from classical cytogenetic studies people have put regions that are important in growth both on the proximal short arm and on the long arm of the Y chromosome.

DR. CUTLER: You mentioned that some of the 1, 2, 3, Y-deleted patients were not short. Of course there is always the possibility that there are extra enhancers on the Y chromosome that also increase height in males, say relative to females, but do you think that the whole short arm is necessary for normal height? Or is there anything more than that?

DR. DISTECHE: No, these patients that have deletion of a large region of the short arm are not short so that it would be located elsewhere than the region that is deleted.

DR. CUTLER: Okay, and that is between 4 and the centromere, or?

DR. DISTECHE: It will include the long arm also. These patients do have the long-arm region.

DR. MELVIN M. GRUMBACH: Some of the patients with a dicentric that looks like it is two short arms with some extra material around it, or two centromeres, have not been short.

DR. RON G. ROSENFELD: I think you have to be a little bit careful about how you evaluate stature in the deletions of the Y chromosome because remember they are actually males, and while they may not be short for females, they are short relative to what their parenteral heights are, at least the cases we have seen are. We should remember to evaluate them as genetic males, and while they are not as short as a Turner patient would be, they are short for males.

5

Overview and Summary of Y Chromosome/ XY Antigen/Organogenesis

Susumu Ohno

Beckman Research Institute of The City of Hope, Duarte, California

The testis and the ovary are comprised of homologous elements; male versus female germ cells, Sertoli versus granulosa cells, and Leydig versus theca cells. A difference between these two organs can't be as great as that between, say, liver and kidney. They are more like sebaceous glands and sweat glands of the skin or, better still, mesonephros and metanephros in embryonic development. This extreme similarity explains the ready transformation of the testis to the ovary or vice versa in asynchronously hermaphroditic species commonly found among advanced teleosts. It follows that the protein responsible for testicular organogenesis must necessarily be very similar to that for ovarian organogenesis. This readily explains evolutionary interchangeability between the male heterogamety of XY/XX type and the female heterogamety of ZZ/ZW type during the course of vertebrate evolution. Plasma membrane proteins involved in organogenesis came to be known as both CAM (cell adhesion molecule) proteins and cadherins by different groups of investigators. The first among them apparently arose when multicellular organisms first emerged on this earth. They are extremely hydrophobic proteins rich in Leu, Ile, Val, and Phe, made partially hydrophilic by glycosylation. Such proteins should normally be forming α-helices, instead they form β-pleated sheet structures because of the relative abundance of Thr, Ser, and Pro. β_2-microglobulin-like domains from which all components of the adaptive immune system sprung first arose in some of these proteins. Human testis-organizing antigen with the subunit molecular weight of 18,000 that we previously identified clearly belongs to this family of proteins. Inasmuch as the first sex as we understand it arose in unicellular eukaryotes, such as baker's yeast, it is of interest to note that the ultimate ancestor of this family of proteins also arose in the protozoa. The coding sequence for the sex factor glycoprotein of *Volvox carteri*, which is effective at the astoundingly low concentration of 10^{-17} *M*, is tetrameric repeats; the most prominent tetramer is T G C A, with T A T C being the second. Thus, we come back to the sex-specific repeats that Singh and Jones originally found on the W-chromosome of certain poisonous snake species and subsequently found in the functionally pertinent portion (*Sxr*) of the mouse Y-chromosome, for their transcripts, too, are tetrameric repeats of T A T C and T G T C.

INTRODUCTION

First, I'd like to emphasize two facts of life which are rather obvious, but for that very reason, often overlooked: (1) The chromosomal sex-determining mechanism as it applies to mammals and probably to all other organisms concerns itself only with the question of whether to organize an ovary or a testis. Accordingly, it is a matter involving organogenesis and nothing else. (2) As with all events in this universe, the initial stage was the most innovative stage in evolution of life on this earth. Accordingly, the ultimate ancestor of every family of proteins as we understand them arose at the very beginning of life on this earth, usually before the division of eukaryotes from prokaryotes.

Mammals are, as a rule, extremely sexually dimorphic species; larger males look very different from females. This fact tends to give us an illusion of great genetic differences between the two sexes. However, it is well to remember that all symbols of masculine supremacy are mere androgen-induced traits and that XX cells and XY cells in corresponding organs are equally responsive to androgens.

As to the initial innovativeness, one of the more versatile families of proteins is the rhodopsin family of proteins equipped with seven transmembrane α-helices. Among mammals, this family is represented not only by retinal rhodopsin, but also by β-adrenergic receptor as well as muscarinic acetylcholine receptor of neuronal organs. The presence of bacterial rhodopsin reveals that this family indeed arose before the division of eukaryotes from prokaryotes and that its relevance to the sex was established in baker's yeast, for mating factor receptor of this unicellular organism is a representative of this family. Keeping the above in our minds, let us first consider the question of ovary versus testis strictly as a matter of organogenesis.

OVARY VS. TESTIS

The ovary and the testis cannot be as different as liver and kidney but more like sebaceous glands and sweat glands. Although there are multitudes of proteins, the number of families to which they belong is rather small indeed. Similarly, there appear to be a rather small number of organ types. The type consisting mainly of ducts is represented by a variety of organs called glands. Pancreas, kidney, and seminal vesicles, among others, should also be included. Then there is the type consisting mainly of strands of cells. Liver and adrenal cortex are of this type. It would be realized that there are only a few other types left; the central nervous system, built of layers of cells, constitutes one unique type.

As to the question of the ovary versus the testis, the two are comprised entirely of homologous cell types: (1) First of all, there are germ cells. Although oogonia and spermatogonia follow very different pathways of differentiation, both are, nevertheless, germ cells. (2) Testicular Sertoli cells and ovarian granulosa cells are apparently homologous, for both synthesize anti-mullerian factor although in different ontogenic sequences, and both are rich in aromatase, which converts androstenedione to estrone and testosterone to estradiol. The only reason that aromatase of testicular Sertoli cells is not normally utilized is that Sertoli cells are sequestered from Leydig cells by the basement membrane of the seminiferous tubules. Once this barrier is broken, as occurs in Sertoli cell tumors of the dog, the testis become an estradiol producer. (3) Similarly, testicular Leydig cells are homologous with ovarian theca cells. Although synthetic pathway by theca cells stops at androstenedione, not proceeding to testosterone, this must be considered as an evolutionary quirk, for aromatase converts testosterone to estradiol as readily as it converts androstenedione to estrone.

From the above, it would appear that the ovary and the testis are not two entirely different organs but, rather, merely represent two sides of the same coin. Indeed, among advanced teleost fish, there are numerous asynchronously hermaphroditic species of both protogynous and protoandrous types. Ready interconvertibility between the ovary and the testis with age seen in these species can only be understood by the realization of the two being homologous organs. The most notable in this regard are tropical coral dwellers represented by *Anthias squaminipinnis* (1). In this species, the removal of a solitary male from each breeding unit causes the conversion of a dominant female to a male. It would thus appear that a difference between the testis and the ovary is far less than that between, say, liver and kidney, but rather more like that between sebaceous glands and sweat glands of the skin. I would even go so far as to say the difference is more like that between fetal mesonephros and metanephros, which is to replace the former. It follows then that the testis-organizing protein, if there is such an independent entity, must necessarily be exceedingly similar to the ovary-organizing protein. One should even entertain the possibility of the two being one and the same, the organ fate being determined by dosage effect. If the mammalian X and Y carry the homologous locus for gonadal organogenesis, and if the X-linked locus is subjected to X inactivation in females, for example, the male would receive two active doses and the female only a single dose of this gene.

THE FAMILY CHARACTERISTIC OF CAM
(CADHERIN) PLASMA MEMBRANE PROTEINS
FOR ORGANOGENESIS

Since the classical experiment by Moscona in 1957 (2), it was realized that organogenesis is primarily the function of like cells aggregating with each other. Plasma membrane proteins responsible for such like cell aggregation have been recognized and studied by independent groups. They have been defined as CAM proteins by one (3) and as cadherins by another group (4). A β_2-microglobulin-like domain 90 to 100 residues long is comprised of a series of β-sheet loops held together by one intrachain disulfide bridge. This disulfide bridge formation is a latecomer in evolution of CAM, first identified in chicken N-CAM (5). Thus, it cannot be included in the family characteristics of CAM proteins. The ancestry of the CAM family has thus far been traced back to the slime mold, *Dictyostelium discoideum*, who lives as amoeboid unicellular organisms in a favorable environment but undergoes organogenesis to become a multicellular slug and then a miniature mushroom with a stalk and a fruiting body (6). This again confirms the initial innovativeness in evolution of life on this earth. The nature of amino acid sequence homology that unite all CAMs on the one hand and components of the adaptive immune system on the other (7) is as follows: They are all extremely hydrophobic polypeptide chains rich in Ala, Val, Leu, Ile, and Phe. Were it not for invariable glycosylation, they might not be able to protrude above the plasma membrane. Normally, such proteins expected to form α-helices for four of the five resides noted above have S' values greater than 1 (8). Instead, they form β-pleated sheet structures only because of frequent inclusion of Thr, Ser, and Pro; all three having low S' values. Recently, the ancestry of the CAM family has been pushed back further to protozoa, at the same time establishing the connection with sex determination. The sexual inducer of *Volvox carteri f. nagariensis* is glycoprotein, synthesized and released by sexual males, and it is fully effective in converting asexually growing organisms to males and females at the concentration of $10^{-17} M$. The coding sequence for this protein rich in Ala, Val, Leu, Phe, Met, but also in Cys, Thr, Pro, His, is essentially tetrameric repeats (9). While the primordial tetramer of this coding sequence is T G C A, three consecutive copies of which giving the Cys-Met-His-Ala tetrapeptidic periodicity to this polypeptide chain, there is no shortage of another tetramer, T A T C, which gives another tetrapeptidic periodicity Tyr-Leu-Ser-Ile, as shown in Figure 1. Thus, we come back to the sex-specific repeats of Singh and Jones (10). This family of tetrameric sex-specific repeats was first found on the W chromosome of certain poisonous snake species, and subsequently found to be included in the functionally critical *Sxr* region of the mouse Y chromosome (11). While such sequence today probably has nothing to do with either organogenesis in general or gonadal organogenesis in particular, I regard this to be the

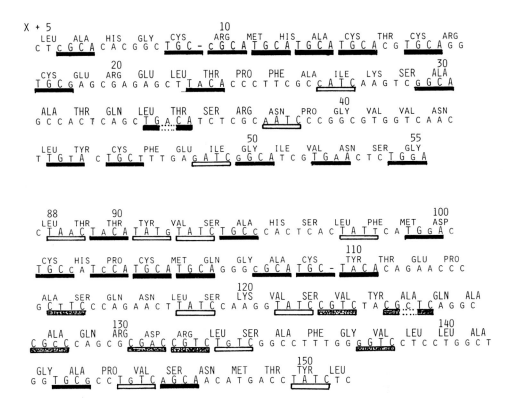

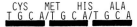 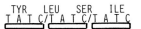

Figure 1 Two coding sequence fragments accompanied by corresponding amino acid residues of the sexual inducer of *Volvox carteri* (9). Amino acid sequence fragments that matched tryptic digests of the purified protein are shown in large capital letters. One specific primordial tetramer T G C A and its single-base-substituted copies are underlined by solid bars of two different widths. The other primordial tetramer T A T C and its single-base-substituted copies are underlined by open bars. Locally prominent C G T C and its single-base-substituted copies are identified only in the second fragment, underlined by shaded bars. At the bottom the tetrapeptidic periodicity of Cys-Met-His-Ala encoded by three consecutive copies of T G C A tetramer is shown on the left, while Tyr-Leu-Ser-Ile periodicity encoded by three copies of T A T C tetramer is shown on the right.

ultimately ancestral sequence of all CAM genes, therefore, genes for components of the adaptive immune system. Their transcript comprised of T A T C and T G T C and each ones' derivatives give two tetrapeptidic periodicities, Tyr-Leu-Ser-Ile and Cys-Leu-Ser-Val, to a polypeptide chain translated from it (12). We have previously identified human testis-organizing protein excreted by β_2-microglobulin (-), HLA (-) Daudi male Burkitt lymphoma cells by its binding affinity to the plasma membrane of bovine fetal ovarian cells as comprised of 18,000 dalton subunit (13). Its amino acid composition readily qualifies it as a member of CAM family. Soon the long-sought-after testis-determining gene on the Y shall be identified either through XX^{Sxr} male mice or XX human males. It would be no surprise if the testis-determining gene encodes one of the CAM proteins.

WHAT IF THERE IS A MORPHOGEN FOR GONADAL ORGANOGENESIS?

CAM protein for gonadal organogenesis, on the other hand, might be encoded exclusively either by an X-linked gene or by an autosomal gene. If that is the case, one should recall the frequent presence of morphogens directing the onset of organogenesis. Such morphogens are, as a rule, small molecular weight compounds. Indeed, a morphogen of the aforementioned slime mold has recently been identified as 1-(3,5-dichloro-2,6-dihydroxyl-4-methoxyphenyl)-1 hexanone (14). Since the classical experiment by Grobstein in 1955 (15), it has been well established that the fate of an organ is more often than not determined by underlying mesenchymal cells rather than by epithelial elements. It is thus possible that the Y-linked testis-determining gene encodes a key enzyme for testis-organizing morphogen to be secreted by mesenchymal cells of indifferent gonads. Its receptor, however, is likely to be a member of the rhodopsin family with seven transmembrane helices (16). It would be recalled that the sex-factor receptor of baker's yeast belongs to this family.

REFERENCES

1. Shapiro DY. Sequence of coloration changes during sex reversal in the tropical marine fish *Anthias squaminipinnis* (Peters). Bull Marine Science 1981; 31:383–398.
2. Moscona A. The development *in vitro* of chimaeric aggregates of dissociated embryonic chick and mouse cells. Proc Natl Acad Sci USA 1957; 43:184–189.
3. Edelman GM. Evolution and morphogenesis: The regulator hypothesis. In: Gustafson JP, Stebbins GL, Ayala FJ, eds. Genetics, Development and Evolution, 17th Stadler Genetics Symposium. New York-London: Plenum Press, 1986.
4. Takeichi M. Cadherins: a molecular family essential for selective cell-cell adhesion and animal morphogenesis. Trends in Genetics 1987; 3:213–217.

5. Hemperly JJ, Murray BA, Edelman GM, Cunningham BA. Sequence of a cDNA clone encoding the polysialic acid-rich and cytoplasmic domains of the neural cell adhesion molecule N-CAM. Proc Natl Acad Sci USA 1986; 83:3037–3041.
6. Noegel A, Gerisch G, Stadler J, Westphal M. Complete sequence and transcript regulation of a cell adhesion protein from aggregating *Dictyostelium* cells. EMBO J 1986; 5:1473–1476.
7. Matsunaga T, Mori N. The origin of the immune system: The possibility that immunoglobulin superfamily molecules and cell adhesion molecules of chicken and slime mold are all related. Scandinavian J Immunol 1987; 25:485–495.
8. Vasquez M, Pincus MR, Sheraga HA. Helix-coil transition theory including long-range electrostatic interactions: Application to globular proteins. Biopolymers 1987; 26:351–371.
9. Tschochner H, Lottspeich F, Sumper M. The sexual inducer of *Volvex carteli*: Purification, chemical characterization and identification of its gene. EMBO J 1987; 6:2203–2207.
10. Singh L, Purdom IF, Jones KW. Sex chromosome associated satellite DNA: Evolution and conservation. Chromosoma (Berl) 1980; 79:137–157.
11. Singh L, Phillips C, Jones KW. The conserved nucleotide sequences of Bkm, which define *Sxr* in the mouse are transcribed. Cell 1984; 36:111–120.
12. Ohno S, Epplen J. The primitive code and repeats of base oligomers as the primordial protein-encoding sequence. Proc Natl Acad Sci USA 1983; 80:3391–3395.
13. Nagai Y, Ciccarese S, Ohno S. The identification of human H-Y antigen and testicular transformation induced by its interaction with the receptor site of bovine fetal ovarian cells. Differentiation 1979; 13:155–164.
14. Morris HR, Taylor GW, Masento MS, Jermyn KA, Kay RR. Chemical structure of the morphogen differentiation inducing factor from *Dictyostelium discoideum*. Nature 1987; 328:811–814.
15. Grobstein C. Inductive interaction in the development of the mouse metanephros. J Exptl Zool 1955; 130:319–340.
16. Kubo T, Fukuda K, Mikami A, Maeda A, Takahashi H, Mishina M, Haga T, Haga K, Ichiyama A, Kojima M, Matsuo H, Hirose T, Numa S. Cloning, sequencing and expression of complementary DNA encoding the muscarinic acetylcholine receptor. Nature 1986; 323:411–416.

6

Localizing Ovarian Determinants Through Phenotypic-Karotypic Deductions
Progress and Pitfalls

Joe L. Simpson

University of Tennessee, Memphis, Memphis, Tennessee

Correlating the phenotype of abnormal individuals with their chromosomal status (phenotypic-karyotypic correlations) has served as a useful initial step in localizing genes to chromosomes. The hope is that information gained through such deductions can be used to facilitate the localization of gonadal determinants, whose gene products can eventually be synthesized. Indeed, recent molecular advances presage the ability to achieve the above with respect to ovarian determinants.

Unlike autosomal loci or even Y-linked testicular determinants, however, there are reasons to suspect that progress will continue to be slow in elucidating ovarian determinants. Certain cytogenetic pitfalls remain a constant problem, and the nature of gonadal gene products may be more difficult to elucidate than sometimes presumed. For these reasons, it is appropriate at this symposium to review available information derived from phenotypic-karyotypic correlations, in particular noting potential pitfalls and identifying regions of the genome that appear integral for ovarian development.

PITFALLS IN PHENOTYPIC-KARYOTYPIC CORRELATIONS

A problem in both phenotypic-karyotypic correlations and molecular analysis is that certain pitfalls are inevitable. Thus, certain cytogenetic caveats should be restated.

First, correlations should be restricted to well-studied individuals, preferably those with either simple terminal deletions or (the rare) interstitial deletions verified by DNA studies. Mosaicism should be reasonably excluded (at least 25–50 cells per tissue) and chromosomal composition unequivocally determined utilizing modern banding techniques. Second, modes of ascertainment and biases of reporting should be addressed. Detecting a cytogenetic abnormality in a clinically abnormal individual does not necessarily imply cause and effect between the two phenomena. Unusual cases are more likely to be prepared for publication and accepted. Thus, pooling available literature does not necessarily provide truly representative samples. Unfortunately, these biases are unavoidable because prospective cohort studies cannot be performed. No X deletions have been identified among 50,000 consecutively born neonates.

OVARIAN DEVELOPMENT AS EMBRYOLOGICALLY CONSTITUTIVE

In the absence of the Y chromosome, the indifferent gonad develops into an embryonic ovary. As evidence, germ cells clearly exist in 45,X fetuses (1). In 39,X mice, oocytes are also present, albeit fewer in number than in normal XX mice (2). We can thus deduce that human 45,X oocytes undergo attrition more rapidly than 46,XX oocytes. If two intact X chromosomes are not present, ovarian follicles degenerate by birth.

It follows that the X ovarian determinants that we shall below attempt to localize must be responsible for *oocyte maintenance*, rather than *oocyte differentiation*. Further supporting constitutive ovarian development are observations that oocyte differentiation may occur in mammals with a Y chromosome. Ovaries (oocytes) exist in human XY gonadal dysgenesis (3), in several other XY human syndromes (e.g., genito-palato-cardiac syndrome) (4), and in mice with a Y chromosome (5).

The clinical significance of 45,X embryos and 45,X neonates having germ cells, albeit destined for accelerated attrition, is that 45,X individuals would sometimes be expected to menstruate spontaneously (6). Indeed, fertile 45,X individuals have been reported (7).

OVARIAN MAINTENANCE DETERMINANTS ON THE X SHORT ARM (Xp)

By the early 1970s, a scientific consensus had developed that ovarian determinants existed on both Xp and Xq. Each arm was considered essential for ovarian maintenance (8). Such deductions were based upon observations that del(Xp) and del(Xq) individuals usually manifested streak gonads indistinguishable from those in 45,X individuals. More recently, the question of whether some del(Xp) deletions may be innocuous has arisen.

Among 24 reported del(X)(p11.2→11.4) cases, 11 (45.8%) had primary amenorrhea (9). Thirteen (13) (54.2%) menstruated spontaneously (Fig. 1); however, menstruation was rarely normal, often leading to secondary amenorrhea and infertility. One tempting explanation for some, yet not other, del(X)(p11.2) individuals showing primary amenorrhea is that break points in those individuals were proximal (centromeric) to ovarian maintenance determinants, whereas break points in menstruating individuals are distal (telo-

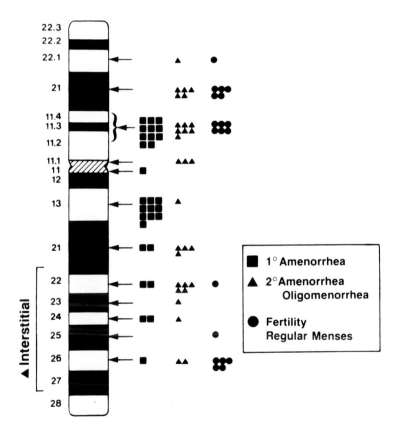

Figure 1 Schematic diagnosis of X chromosome showing degree of ovarian function in individuals with various terminal deletions of the X chromosome, as reported in literature and studied personally. The bracket signifies the region involved in the interstitial deletion of Krauss et al. (13).

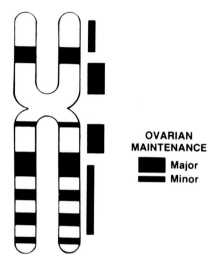

Figure 2 Schematic drawing of X chromosome illustrating relative importance of various region for ovarian maintenance. Wider bar connotes more important regions. Limits of regions are mere approximations.

meric) to those determinants. Against such a hypothesis, however, are observations that all three reported telocentric X individuals showed secondary (not primary) amenorrhea. Of course, discrepant cases can also be explained by invoking undetected 45,X or 46,XX lines; however, no data support existence of such lines.

Concerning more telomeric deletions, all 10 reported del(X)(p21) subjects menstruated spontaneously (Fig. 1) (9). However, 5 of the 10 proved infertile, manifesting secondary amenorrhea (9). Thus, region Xpter→Xp21 seems more important for ovarian development than originally proposed by Fraccaro et al. (10). Presumably the integral region lies centromeric to the pseudoautosomal region.

That deletion of Xp21→pter is not being associated with primary amenorrhea favors existence of two Xp regions (loci), influencing ovarian maintenance (Fig. 2). We shall see that a similar arrangement probably exists for the X long arm.

OVARIAN MAINTENANCE DETERMINANTS ON THE
X LONG ARM (Xq)

With respect to X long arm deletions, terminal deletions originating at Xq13 are usually (10/11 reported cases) associated with primary amenorrhea and complete ovarian failure (9). Region Xq13 would thus seem to be the single most important region for ovarian maintenance, deletions leading to complete ovarian failure more often than other X deletions. The key region might actually lie in proximal Xq21, but it would not appear to be more distal because del(X)(p22 or 24) individuals menstruate far more often. That is, menstruating del(X)(q21) women (Fig. 1) might have terminal deletions just distal to an ovarian maintenance locus, whereas del(X)(q13 or 21) women with primary amenorrhea might have terminal deletions proximal to an ovarian maintenance locus. The denouement awaits reports utilizing more refined cytogenetic analysis.

In more distal deletions (Xq25→27), the deleterious effect seems restricted to premature ovarian failure (POF). Thus, Krauss et al. (11) observed POF in a mother and two daughters having an interstial deletion [Xpter→q21.3::q27→ qter] involving Xq26. Our group has observed premature ovarian failure in a woman with an apparent terminal deletion at Xq25; the women transmitted the deletion to her daughter (12). Familial del(X)(q26) producing premature ovarian failure was also observed in two daughters by Fitch et al. (13). In fact, among 8 reported terminal del(X)(q26) cases there are a total of 5 fertile females, 2 menstruating but infertile females, and only 1 female with primary amenorrhea (9) (Fig. 1).

If a locus on distal Xq protects against POF, it follows that two or more regions on Xq must play roles in ovarian maintenance. The regions must also differ in importance, perhaps analogous to the situation postulated above for Xp. Proximal Xq13 or proximal Xq21 is of greatest importance, whereas distal Xq(Xq25 or 26) is of secondary importance.

AUTOSOMAL FACTORS IN OVARIAN DEVELOPMENT

That autosomal loci are essential for ovarian differentiation in humans can be deduced readily on the basis of autosomal recessive mutations causing gonadal dysgenesis in 46,XX individuals (XX gonadal dysgenesis). The gonadal dysgenesis observed in 46,XX individuals is histologically similar to that detected in individuals with an abnormal sex chromosomal complement (14,15).

External genitalia and streak gonads of affected individuals are indistinguishable from those of individuals who have gonadal dysgenesis and an abnormal chromosomal complement. Likewise, the characteristic endocrine findings (e.g., elevated FSH and LH) and the lack of secondary sexual development do not differ from those of other individuals with streak gonads. Most individuals with XX gonadal dysgenesis are normal in stature (mean height 165 cm) (14), and somatic features of the Turner stigmata are usually absent.

In many families more than one sib has had XX gonadal dysgenesis, and in several instances parents are consanguineous. Available data are thus consistent with autosomal recessive inheritance. Of special note are the few families in which one affected sib had streak gonads, whereas another had primary amenorrhea and extreme ovarian hypoplasia (i.e., a few ova were detected) (16,17). Such families suggest that the mutant gene responsible for XX gonadal dysgenesis can exert a more variable effect than previously supposed. It follows that the gene may be responsible for some sporadic cases of premature ovarian failure.

In several other entities XX gonadal dysgenesis coexists with distinctive patterns of somatic anomalies. The combination of XX gonadal dysgenesis and neurosensory deafness (Perrault syndrome) has been observed in affected sibs (18-20). The mutation is presumably due to a different gene or allele than that causing XX gonadal dysgenesis alone. Other syndromes due to distinct genes include XX gonadal dysgenesis and myopathy (21); XX gonadal dysgenesis and cerebellar ataxis (22); and XX gonadal dysgenesis, microcephaly, arachnodactyly, and skeletal anomalies (23).

Gonadal dysgenesis in 46,XX individuals may also result from nongenetic causes (phenocopies). Plausible causes include infections (e.g., mumps), infarctions, infiltrative processes (e.g., tuberculosis, tumors), and autoimmune phenomena (24).

GERM CELL FAILURE IN BOTH SEXES

In each of five sibships, both male and female sibs have shown germinal cell failure. Affected females showed streak gonads, whereas affected males showed germ cell aplasia (Sertoli-cell only syndrome or del Castillo phenotype). In several of these families parents were consanguineous, suggesting autosomal recessive inheritance. In two families somatic anomalies did not coexist (25,26). In three other families distinctive patterns of somatic anomalies coexisted, indicating distinct entities. Hamet et al. (27) observed coexisting somatic features of hypertension and deafness; Al-Awadi et al. (28) observed alopecia; Mikati et al. (29) observed microcephaly, short stature, and various minor anomalies.

These families demonstrate that several different autosomal genes are capable of affecting XX and XY germ cells. Presumably pathogenesis involves steps common for germ cell development in both males and females. Elucidation of such genes could have profound implications for normal developmental processes.

RELATIONSHIP OF OVARIAN AND TESTICULAR DETERMINATION

As cytogenetic and molecular techniques are increasingly used in concert, investigators will be able to focus upon three interrelated questions: (1) What mechanisms (loci?) are responsible for X-Y pairing? (2) What is the relationship between the X-Y pairing regions and gonadal determinants? (3) What is the relationship between X-Y homologies and control of sex differentiation?

X-Y Pairing

We now know that distal Xp contain several genes that could facilitate X-Y pairing: MIC2X and MIC2Y (loci-defining antigen 12E7), and DNA sequences like DXYS14, DXYS15, and DXYS17 (30,31). The pairing region of Xp escapes X inactivation, assuring that its loci act in pseudoautosomal fashion. Of relevance to the present symposium, I still remain intrigued with our old hypothesis that statural determinants are integral for pairing (32). The attractiveness of that hypothesis is that when recombination inevitably occurs, it might actually be favorable by providing a mechanism assuring that the two sexes remain approximately equal in height. Nevertheless, we can envision a logical topographical scheme by which gonadal determinants on both the X and the Y are located relatively near the centromere and relatively further from the telomeric pairing regions (Xp-Yp).

Homologies and Sex Determination

We have noted that the most important region for ovarian maintenance is Xq13 or proximal Xq21. Elsewhere (9) we discuss that the testes-determining factor (*TDF*) localized to Yp11.2 (see Chapter 3). Do homologies exist between these and other regions on the X and Y? If so, what do they mean? Given pseudoautosomal pairing, homologies between Xp and Yp are already accepted (31,32). However, a surprisingly common site of homology involves Yp and Xq (13→22) (33). A logical deduction is that Yp evolved from Xq as result of transposition during speciation. In fact, in hominoid apes, DXYS1 is present on Xq but not concurrently on the Y, as it is in humans and other primates (33). Thus, the Xq to Yp transposition presumably occurred after man diverged from the hominoid ape.

Do the above discoveries alter basic assumptions concerning genetic control of sex determination? Prevailing assumptions dictate that sex differentiation is controlled by a few loci (one?) that direct the indifferent gonad toward male differentiation. We further assume that these loci are governed by the same rules as other genes. Is there reason to alter these assumptions, specifically in view of X-Y homologies vis-à-vis gonadal localizations?

Two disparate thoughts arise. First, the "classical" genetic assumptions could indeed remain correct. On the other hand, an argument might be pursued as follows. If the key gonadal determinants are localized to Yp and Xq, could they be identical? Specifically, could both the Y and X gonadal determinants be regulatory? Structural gonadal loci would then exist on autosomes. If true, one potential mechanism to maintain sexual dimorphism might be X inactivation. Inactivation of X chromosomes in excess of one would produce less gene product in XX than in XY individuals, for the Y is not inactivated. Indeed, X inactivation as a method to govern sex determination was suggested by Chandra (34) for reasons other than those proposed by me (9,12) and by German (35). Chandra's hypothesis (34) was derived from two observations: (1) Sex determination in mealy bugs is governed by X inactivation of an entire haploid set, producing males in this lecanoid species. (2) Not the expected male but, rather, female phenotypes are observed in *Sxr* T16H/mice in which the translocation (T16H) chromosome is inactivated.

Compatible with this postulate are otherwise enigmatic observations by Mittwoch (36), who observed that gonadal growth occurs more rapidly in (XY) embryos destined to develop testes than in (XX) embryos destined to develop ovaries. That testicular development occurs earlier in embryogenesis than does ovarian development would be expected if males had more gonadal gene product than females.

Another potentially compatible set of observations concerns localization of the X inactivation center (XCE), which if discrete may be used to locate region Xq13. One expects a spreading effect originating at XCE. X inactivation might thus be expected to be more complete in that area most important to inhibit, namely ovarian (gonadal) determinants postulated here to lie on Xq13 or proximal Xq21.

Of course, many questions arise before one could accept the hypothesis that X inactivation directs sex determination in humans. As an obvious example, explaining abnormalities in 45,X individuals would require one to hypothesize synthesis of at least some gene product by X chromosomes in excess of one, i.e., less than complete X inactivation. The amount of gene product might be 2X in normal males, 1.5X in normal females, and 1X in monosomy X females.

Nonetheless, the possibility that X inactivation evolved not solely for dosage compensation but for sex determination as well deserves thought. Even if such a mechanism were no longer extant, it could have been important in evolution.

STATURAL DETERMINANTS ON THE X CHROMOSOME

Elsewhere in this volume the somatic anomalies of monosomy X are considered in detail. The short stature and various somatic anomalies (termed Turner stigmata by this author) characteristic of 45,X individuals are well known. The expected adult height is considered in particular by Frane in Chapter 33.

Of relevance in the present context is whether only certain portions of the X chromosome must remain intact for normal somatic growth. Initially, it appeared that statural determinants were present on the X short arm but not on the X long arm. Later analysis revealed decreased statural growth in del(Xq) individuals as well (37). (The original erroneous conclusion may have resulted from unbanded 46,XY gonadal dysgenesis patients having been misclassified as 46,X,del(X)(q13), an understandable error if an unbanded Y were mounted upside-down.) Of note is that some del(X)(p21) individuals may be short yet still fertile (10). Thus, regions on Xp responsible for ovarian and statural determinants were distinct (10).

Analysis of cases reported since our 1981 publication (37) have not fundamentally altered conclusions. Figure 3 suggests that distal Xq deletions may be less deleterious than proximal deletions; however, data are still limited. Also of special interest, however, are several familial deletions, one studied by our group (Table 1). The advantage of studying familial cases is that undetected 45,X lines are much less likely to exist recognized than in sporadic cases. Familial data (11–13) further indicate that Xq is necessary for growth and, perhaps, protection

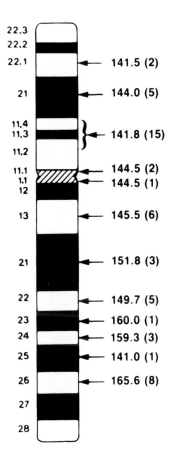

Figure 3 Heights in adults reported to have terminal deletions at various regions of the X. Sample restricted to adult cases (>15 years) in which mosaicism excluded.

Table 1 Familial Deletions of Xq

	Age (yr)	Height (cm)
Fitch et al[a]		
Daughter	40	160
Daughter Xq26	37	155
Simpson[b]		
Mother	38	141
Daughter Xq25	10	138.5
Krauss et al, 1987[c]		
Mother	55	≃153
Daughter Xq21.3 27	31	152.5
Daughter	27	155

[a]*Source*: Ref. 13.
[b]*Source*: Ref. 12.
[c]*Source*: Ref. 11.

against other somatic anomalies of the Turner stigmata, some of which were observed in these familial cases. Some authors still favor these somatic anomalies being associated only with short-arm deletions (38).

Further localization of statural determinants has proved elusive. On Xp a statural determinant can be localized to Xp21→Xpter; del(X)(p21) women are short even if displaying normal ovarian functions. Unlike the situation with respect to ovarian maintenance, deletions throughout Xq seem equally likely to produce short stature, even if to a lesser extent than observed with complete monosomy X. One possible explanation for the failure to localize statural determinants is that terminal Xq deletions are actually interstitial; a common region might actually be missing in ostensibly different deletions. If so, the essential region probably involves Xq13 or a more proximal region. Alternatively, the region could be distal Xq, but not the telomere.

The cellular explanation for short stature is considered by others in this symposium and will not be discussed in detail here. Suffice to acknowledge our observation that cell generation time (CGT) is increased in 45,X;46,X,del(X)(p11); 46,X,del(X)(q13); and 46,X,del(X)(q22) fibroblasts (37). Increased CGT could explain not only short stature but other related phenomena-intrauterine growth retardation, anomalies (the end result of decreased cell number in a given anlage), and embryonic lethality. Consistent with this hypothesis are our more recent experiments involving co-cultivation of 45,X or 46,XX cells (39). The former proved at selective disadvantage. We are now applying flow cytometry techniques for cell cycle analysis.

On the other hand, other studies (40–43) have not only failed to confirm our findings of increased CGT but actually observed decreased CGT! Discrepancies between these results and those we observed are not only difficult to reconcile, but teleologically puzzling to this author.

If CGT is indeed characteristic of monosomy X, its significance with respect to therapeutic intervention could be significant. End organ response might never allow normal growth, even if amelioration were possible. Further investigation is thus obviously necessary.

REFERENCES

1. Jirasek J. Principles of reproductive embryology. In Simpson JL, ed. Disorders of Sexual Differentiation: Etiology and Clinical Delineation. New York; Academic Press, 1976:51–110.

2. Burgoyne PS, Baker TG. Perinatal oocyte loss in XO mice and its implication for the etiology of gonadal dysgenes in XO women. J Reprod Fertil 1988; 75:633–45.

3. Cussen LK, MacMahon RA. Germ cells and ova in dysgenetic gonads of a 46,XY female dizygotic twin. Arch Dis Child 1979; 133:373–75.

4. Greenberg F, Gresik MW, Carpenter RJ, Law SW, Hoffman LP, Ledbetter DH. The Gardner-Silengo-Wachtel or genito-palato-cardiac syndrome: Male pseudohermaphroditism with micrognathia, cleft palate, and conotruncal cardiac defect. Am J Med Genet 1987; 26:59–64.

5. Evans EP, Ford CE, Lyon MF. Direct evidence of the capacity of the XY germ cell in the mouse to become an oocyte. Nature 1977; 267:430.

6. Simpson JL. Gonadal dysgenesis and abnormalities of the human sex chromosomes: Current status of phenotypic-karyotypic correlations. Birth Defects. Orig Artic Ser 1975; 11(4):23–59.

7. Simpson JL. Pregnancies in women with chromosomal abnormalities. In Genetic Diseases in Pregnancy. Schulman JD and Simpson JL, eds. New York: Academic Press, 1981: 439–71.

8. Ferguson-Smith MA. Karyotype-phenotype correlations in gonadal dysgenesis and their bearing on the pathogenesiasal malformations. J Med Genet 1965; 2:142–53.

9. Simpson JL. Phenotypic-karyotypic correlations of gonadal determinants: Current status and relationship to molecular studies. In Sperling K and Vogel F, eds. Human Genetics: Proceedings 7th International Congress (Berlin, 1986.) Heidelberg, Berlin, 1987:224–32.

10. Fraccaro M, Maraschio P, Pasquali F, Scappaticci S. Women heterozygous for deficiency of the (Xpter→Xp21) region of the X chromosome are fertile. Hum Genet 1977; 39:283–92.

11. Krauss CM, Turksoy RN, Atkins L, McLaughlin C, Brown LG, Page DC. Familial premature ovarian failure due to an interstitial deletion of the long arm of the X chromosome. N Engl J Med 1987; 317:125–31.

12. Simpson JL. Genetic control of sexual development. In Ratnam SS, ed. Proceedings 12th World Congress on Fertility and Sterility. Lancaster, UK: Parthenon Press, 1987:165–73.

13. Fitch N, de Saint Victor J, Richer CL, Pinsky L, Sitahal S. Premature menopause due to small deletion in the long arm of the X chromosome: A report of three cases and a review. Am J Obstet Gynecol 1982; 142: 968–72.

14. Simpson JL, Christakos AC, Horwith M, Silverman F. Gonadal dysgenesis associated with apparently normal chromosomal complements. Birth Defects. Orig Artic Ser 1971; 7(6):215–18.

15. Simpson JL. Disorders of sexual development. New York: Academic Press, 1976.

16. Boczkowski K. Pure gonadal dysgenesis and ovarian dysplasia in sisters. Am J Obstet Gynecol 1971; 106:626.

17. Simpson JL. Unpublished data.

18. Christakas AC, Simpson JL, Younger JB, Christian CD. Gonadal dysgenesis as an autosomal recessive condition. Am J Obstet Gynecol 1969; 104:1027.

19. Pallister PD, Opitz JM. The Perrault syndrome: Autosomal recessive ovarian dysgenesis with facultative, non-sex-limited sensorineural deafness. Am J Med Genet 1979; 4:239–46.

20. McCarthy DJ, Opitz JM. Perrault syndrome in sisters. Am J Med Genet 1985; 22:629–31.

21. Lundberg PO. Hereditary myopathy, oliogophrenia, cataracts, skeletal abnormalities and hypergonadotrophic hypogonadism: A new syndrome. Europ Neural 1973; 10:261–80.

22. Skre H, Bassoe HH, Berg K, Frovis AG. Cerebellar ataxia and hypergonadism in two kindreds. Chance concurrence, pleiotropism or linkage? Clin Genet 1976; 9:234–44.

23. Maximillian G, Ionescu B, Becur A. Deux soers avec dysgenesie majeure, hypotrophic staturale, microephalie, arachnodactylie et caryotype 46,XX. J Genet Hum 1970; 18:365–78.

24. Verp MS. Environmental causes of ovarian failure. Semin Reprod Endocrinol 1983; 1:101–12.

25. Smith A, Fraser IS, Noel M. Three siblings with premature gonadal failure. Fertil Steril 1979; 32:528–30.

26. Granat M, Amar A, Moy-Yosef S, Brautbar C, Schenker JG. Familial gonadal germinative failure: Endocrine and human leukocyte antigen studies. Fertil Steril 1983; 40:215–19.

27. Hamet P, Kuchel O, Nowacynski JM, Rojo-Ortega C, Sask C, Genest J. Hypertension with adrenal, genital, renal defects, and deafness. Arch Intern Med 1973; 131:563–69.

28. Al-Awadi SA, Farag TI, Teebi AS, Naguib K, Elkhalifa MY, Ketani Y, AlAnsari A, Schimke RN. Primary hypogonadism and partial alopecia in three sibs with Mullerian hypoplasia in the affected females. Am J Med Genet 1985; 22:619–22.

29. Mikati MA, Samir SN, Sahli IF, Melhem RE, Mansour S, Kaloustian VM. Microcephaly, hypergonadotropic hypogonadism, short stature, and minor anomalies: a new syndrome. Am J Med Genet 1985; 22:599-608.

30. Cooke HJ, Brown WRA, Rappold GA. Hypervariable telomeric sequences from the human sex chromosomes are pseudoautosomal. Nature 1985; 317:687-92.

31. Simmler MC, Rougher F, Vergnaud G. Pseudoautosomal DNA sequences in the pairing region of the human sex chromosomes. Nature 1985; 317:692-97.

32. German J, Simpson JL, McLemore G. Abnormalities of human sex chromosomes. I. Abnormal human Y chromosome 46,XYr. Ann Genet 1973; 16:225-31.

33. Page DC, Harper ME, Love J, Botstein D. Occurrence of a transposition from the X chromosome long arm to the Y chromosome short arm during human evolution. Nature 1984; 311:119-23.

34. Chandra HS. Is human X chromosome inactivation a sex-determining device? Proc Natl Acad Sci 1985; 82:6947-949.

35. German J. Gonadal dimorphism explained as a dosage effect of a locus on the sex chromosomes, the Gonadal-Differential Locus (GDL). Am J Hum Genet 1988; 42:414-21.

36. Mittwoch A. Males, females and hermaphrodites. Ann Hum Genet 1986; 50:103-21.

37. Simpson JL, LeBeau MM. Gonadal and statural determinants on the X chromosome and their relationship to in vitro studies showing prolonged cell cycles in 45,X;46,X del(X)(p11); 46,X del(X)(q13) and q(22) fibroblasts. Am J Obstet Gynecol 1981; 141:930-39.

38. Shapiro LR. Phenotypic expression of numeric and structural X-chromosome abnormalities. In A.A. Sandberg, ed. Cytogenetics of the Mammalian X Chromosome, Part B: X Chromosomes Anomalies and Their Clinical Manifestations. New York: Alan R. Liss, 1983:321-39.

39. Verp MS, Rosinsky B, LeBeau MM, Martin AO, Kaplan R, Wallemark CB, Olano L. Growth disadvantages of 45,X and 46,X del(X)(pii) fibroblasts. Clin Genet 1988; 33:277-85.

40. Barlow P. The influence of inactive chromosomes on human development. Humangenetik 1973; 17:105-36.

41. Curé S, Boué J, Boué A. Growth characteristics of human embryonic cell lines with chromosomal anomalies. Biomedicine 1974; 21:233-36.

42. Kukharenko VI, Grinberg, KN, Kuliev AM. Mitotic cycles in human cell strains with sex chromosomes aneuploidy. Hum Genet 1978; 42:157-62.

43. Frias S, Carnevale A. Cell cycle in normal individuals and in patients with Down, Cri-du-chat and Turner syndromes. Ann Genet 1983; 26:60-2.

7

The Function of H-Y Antigen
Yes, No, and Maybe

Yun-Fai Lau

*Howard Hughes Medical Institute and University of California
at San Francisco, San Francisco, California*

INTRODUCTION

In recent years, there have been several scientific debates regarding the function of the male-specific histocompatibility-Y antigen, known as the H-Y antigen (1-10). Two major hypotheses invoke the H-Y antigen. The first, put forward in 1975 by Wachtel, Ohno, and associates, postulated that the H-Y antigen is the inducer molecule for mammalian testis differentiation (1). The second hypothesis, by Burgoyne and colleagues in 1986, postulated that the H-Y antigen is an essential factor for normal spermatogenesis in mammals (2). At present there is no conclusive evidence to support either of these two hypotheses. In fact, despite the recent advances and applications of the recombinant DNA technology in many biomedical disciplines, molecular studies of the H-Y antigen have been lacking. This chapter will comment on the merits of these two hypotheses and discuss recent studies designed to identify the candidate gene for the H-Y antigen and to elucidate its function.

TWO HYPOTHESES AND TWO ANTIGENS?

The controversy regarding the function of the H-Y antigen arose partly from the operational definitions of the molecule itself (6,10,11). This antigen was first demonstrated in 1955 by skin transplantation experiments among inbred strains of mice in which male to female grafts showed rejection, while male-male, female-male, and female-female combinations did not (12). This difference was attributed to a minor histocompatibility antigen encoded by the Y chromosome (13). Subsequently, two other immunological methods, the cell-mediated cytotoxicity and serology tests, were developed to demonstrate the presence of this male-specific antigen (14,15). However, it is still uncertain whether these immunological methods detect the same or a different but related antigen (16).

Experimental evidence for the sex-determining role of the H-Y antigen was obtained mainly from studies using serological methods. Three lines of data support the hypothesis of the serological H-Y antigen as the inducer molecule for primary testicular differentiation. The first group of experiments showed that the serological H-Y antigen was phylogenetically conserved as demonstrated by cross-immunoreactive binding of mouse antibodies to cells from other mammalian species (10,11). The antigen was invariably detected in individuals who developed testicular tissues, irrespective of their sex chromosome constitution (10,11). The second group of studies involved the technique of dissociation and reaggregation of gonad tissues (10,17-19). In these experiments, the dissociated gonad cells assembled into testicular structures in vitro in the presence of either testicular or other male cell extracts which presumably contained the H-Y antigen. When the H-Y antigen was removed by immunoprecipitation, ovarian structures were reorganized. Since total tissue or cellular extracts were used in these studies, the role of the H-Y antigen in the assembly of testicular architecture could be implied but not confirmed. The third type of study demonstrated by immunofluorescence methods that preimplantation male embryos expressed the serological H-Y antigen on their cell surface as early as the 8-cell stage (20,21). These results stimulated considerable interests among researchers in the field of embryo sexing using H-Y antisera in domestic animals (22,23). Even though the function of the serological H-Y antigen is unclear, its association with male embryos suggests it may play an important role in male development.

Despite supporting evidence derived from these studies, most antisera and monoclonal antibodies against the H-Y antigen react weakly to the antigen and vary among different laboratories (6,24,25). Very often its male-specific reaction cannot be demonstrated unambiguously. This technical deficiency not only makes purification of the antigen difficult, but has sparked controversy regarding the value of its role in sex determination (1-10). The terms serologically detected male antigen (SDM antigen) (4) and serologically detected male predominant antigen (SDMP antigen) (25) have been proposed for the H-Y antigen demonstrated by serological methods to distinguish it from the H-Y antigen demonstrated by the transplantation and cytotoxicity assays. The original hypothesis was modified by other investigators to account for the detection of the serological H-Y antigen in female cells (26-28). The modified versions suggest that the structural gene encoding the H-Y antigen is not located on the Y chromosome, but is on an autosome or even the X chromosome. A regulatory gene present on the Y chromosome is expressed during gonadogenesis, and its product(s), either directly or indirectly, stimulates the transcription of the H-Y structural gene and leads to the biosynthesis of the H-Y antigen. This antigen then induces the indifferent gonads to differentiate into embryonic testes. These modifications are compatible with the recent findings (see Chapter 3) that the human testis-determining factor (TDF) mapped on the short arm of the Y chromosome is a DNA-binding factor likely to be involved in the regulation of transcription of other genes.

Experimental evidence supporting the role of the H-Y antigen as a spermatogenic factor has been derived from studies using both transplantation and cell-mediated cytotoxicity assays. In a series of studies involving a special strain of mice carrying a sex-reversal factor (*Sxr*), which causes XX individuals to develop as males, McLaren and coworkers produced evidence that the H-Y antigen is not involved in primary sex determination, but rather may be involved in spermatogenesis (29). Subsequently, Singh and Jones demonstrated that XX^{Sxr} carriers harbor a variant Y chromosome that contains a duplication of the segment containing the testis-determining gene, *Tdy* (29). This duplicated segment is located on the telomere of the Y chromosome. XX sex-reversal occurs when this segment is transferred to the paternal X chromosome by unequal crossing-overs during meiosis of these XY^{Sxr} carriers. The XX^{Sxr} mice were typed H-Y antigen-positive by serology and cell-mediated cytotoxicity assays. However, McLaren and associates further identified a second sex-reversal mutation, $XX^{Sxr'}$, in individuals who harbored the *Tdy* gene but lost the H-Y antigenicity (30,31). These observations, hence, separate the locus for *Tdy* from that of H-Y antigen. Histological studies of the gonads from the sex-reversed mice revealed an association between spermatogenic failure and the lack of H-Y antigen in male mice. Based on the above studies, Burgoyne and McLaren suggested that the H-Y antigen is a spermatogenic factor in mammals (2). More recent studies by Simpson on H-Y antigen expression in cells of human XX male and XY female sex-reversed patients also showed that the H-Y locus may be separate from the testis-determining locus, *TDF*, in man (32). Since in these experiments, the H-Y typings were performed with the cell-mediated cytotoxicity and transplantation assays, the status of the serologically defined H-Y, or SDM, antigen in these sex-reversed individuals is not clear.

ISOLATION OF A CANDIDATE GENE FOR THE H-Y ANTIGEN

For the past few years our laboratory has been interested in the molecular genetics of mammalian sex determination. As a first step to ascertain the function of the H-Y antigen, we initiated recombinant DNA experiments to isolate candidate genes for this antigen. Even though both transplantation and cell-mediated cytotoxicity assays seem to detect accurately the H-Y antigen, they cannot be used to identify the protein in molecular terms. On the other hand, despite its weak reactivity, the serologic test presumably involves the biosynthesis of specific antibodies which can be used to recognize the molecule in antibody-antigen reactions. We used the prokaryotic expression system (lambda gt11) to isolate the complementary DNA (cDNA) of the H-Y antigen. In this recombinant DNA cloning system, the target DNAs are inserted in the middle of a bacterial gene to generate hybrid genes which are transcribed and translated in the bacterial hosts. The resulting hybrid proteins can be detected by antibody reactions (33). Using antisera against the H-Y antigen from immunized female mice (antisera kindly provided by Dr. Ellen Goldberg of the University of New Mexico), we screened a mouse testicular cDNA library constructed in lambda gt11. Several cDNA clones representing one particular mRNA were consistently isolated in the immunoscreening procedure. Since the H-Y antigen has never been purified to homogeneity for protein analysis, we cannot at present conclusively identify the isolated gene as that for the H-Y antigen. In view of past difficulties in H-Y antigen studies, we have termed this candidate gene the male-enhanced antigen (MEA) gene. Detailed molecular isolation and characterization of the MEA gene have been reported elsewhere (28,34,35). In order to discuss further the candidacy of the MEA gene for the serological H-Y antigen, its molecular characteristics are summarized (Table 1) and compared to those attributed to the H-Y antigen as defined by serological methods (9-11). Striking

Table 1 Similar Properties of Serological H-Y Antigen and Male-Enhanced Antigen

Serological H-Y antigen[a]	Male-enhanced antigen[b]
1. Male-specific glycoprotein	1. Male-enhanced transcription
2. Molecular weight about 18–20 KD	2. Molecular weight about 18.6–20 KD
3. Phylogenetically conserved, immunological	3. Phylogenetically conserved, genomic
4. Detected in mammalian testes	4. Expressed in mammalian testes
5. Expressed in Sertoli cells	5. Transcribed in Sertoli cells
6. Sperms contain the most amount	6. Spermatids transcribe most abundantly
7. Located on autosome or X chromosome (?)	7. Located on human chromosome 6 and mouse chromosome 17

[a]Results from immunological and biochemical studies (from References 6,9,10,11).
[b]Results from molecular analyses (from References 28,34,35 and Lau et al., 1989 in preparation).

similarities between the properties of the MEA gene and the serological H-Y antigen can be noted. It may be premature to equate these genes without further characterizations of both molecules, however, the isolation of the MEA gene will provide a means of testing this candidate gene for the postulated function of the H-Y antigen.

WHAT IS THE FUNCTION OF THE MALE-ENHANCED GENE?

Although the MEA gene is a strong candidate gene for the serological H-Y antigen, it is important to recognize its molecular properties as those of a gene that may be critical for the normal development and function of the mammalian testis. Further molecular studies of the MEA gene have identified two other linked genes which showed similar genetic conservation and expression pattern in mammals. The identification of an MEA gene family suggests that other linked genes may also play an important role in these processes. Its location on chromosome 17 of the mouse is especially noteworthy, since several interesting loci such as *Hye, Tas*, the T/t and major histocompatibility (H-2) complexes, have been mapped to this chromosome. The *Hye* locus has been mapped between the T and H-2 complexes and is related to the regulation of H-Y antigen expression (36). The *Tas* is a dominant autosomal sex-determining locus associated with a partial deletion of chromosome 17 in the t^{hp} haplotype of the t complex. The XY individuals carrying this mutation develop sex-reversals and form either ovaries and/or ovotestes in their gonads (37). Whether or not the MEA gene and the H-Y antigen are the same or different entities, the MEA gene family is certainly located in the portion of the mouse genome that is important for sex determination, spermatogenesis, and cell-cell recognition.

It is reasonable to assume that for any gene to play a positive role in either sex determination or spermatogenesis, as postulated for the H-Y antigen, it must be expressed at the time when these developmental processes are in progress. Molecular studies on the expression of the MEA and related genes have demonstrated that they are abundantly transcribed in all mammalian testes examined. Significantly, the MEA transcriptional activity seems to be associated with specific stages of spermatogenesis in the mouse, and is at its highest level in the round spermatids (Lau et al., unpublished observations). Such expression pattern suggests that MEA may be involved in the sperm cell differentiation, and hence may be an essential factor for this process. However, MEA-specific transcripts have also been detected in RNA derived from the testes of fetal mice at 12th day of gestation when primordial germ cells have migrated to the genital ridge and gonadogenesis is in progress (Fig. 1). Even though the level of transcription is much lower in the fetal testis than in the adult testis and its expression in other

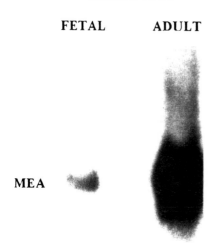

TESTIS RNA

FETAL   ADULT

MEA

Figure 1 Northern hybridization of total RNA derived from fetal and adult mouse testes. Fetal testes were dissected from mouse embryos at 12.5 days of gestation. Total RNA from both fetal and adult tissues were isolated, size-fractionated by agarose gel electrophoresis, and blotted onto a Biodyne membrane filter according to standard procedures. The filter was hybridized with a ^{32}P-labeled cDNA probe for the mouse MEA gene. The autoradiogram represents hybridization signals from about 10 μg of total RNA derived from each sample.

fetal tissues is now known, the possible involvement of MEA in gonadogenesis cannot be completely ruled out. Further studies are needed to elucidate its exact role and mechanism of action in these two differentiation processes.

ACKNOWLEDGMENTS

I thank Mr. K. Chan and Dr. C. Nagamine for technical assistance. This work is partly supported by grant HD24384 from the National Institutes of Health.

REFERENCES

1. Wachtel SS, Ohno S, Koo GC, Boyse EA. Possible role for H-Y antigen in the primary determination of sex. Nature 1975; 257:235–236.

2. Burgoyne PS, Levy ER, McLaren A. Spermatogenic failure in male mice lacking H-Y antigen. Nature 1986; 320:170–172.

3. Goodfellow PN, Andrews PW. Sexual differentiation and H-Y antigen. Nature 1982; 295:11–13.

4. Silvers WK, Gasser DL, Eicher EM. H-Y antigen, serologically detectable male antigen and sex determination. Cell 1982; 28:439–440.

5. Simpson E. The H-Y antigen and sex reversal. Cell 1986; 44:813–814.

6. Wiberg U. Facts and considerations about sex-specific antigens. Hum Genet 1987; 76:207–219.

7. Goodfellow PN. The case of the missing H-Y antigen. Trends Genet 1986; 2:87.

8. McLaren A. Testis determination and the H-Y antigen hypothesis. Cur Top Devel Biol 1987; 23:163–183.

9. Andrews PW. The male-specific antigen (H-Y) and sexual differentiation. In P Goodfellow, ed. Genetic Analysis of the Cell Surface. London: Chapman and Hall, 1984:159–190.

10. Wachtel SS. H-Y Antigen and the Biology of Sex Determination. New York: Grune and Stratton, 1983.

11. Muller U. The H-Y antigen identification, functions, and role in sexuality. In A A Sandberg, ed. The Y Chromosome, Part A: Basic Characteristics of the Y Chromosome. New York: Alan R. Liss, 1985:63–80.

12. Eichwald EJ, Silmser CR. Untitled communication. Transplant Bull 1955; 2:148–149.

13. Billingham RE, Silvers WK. Studies on tolerance of the Y chromosome antigen in mice. J Immunol 1960; 85:14–16.

14. Goldberg EH, Boyse EA, Bennett D, Scheid M, Carswell EA. Serological demonstration of H-Y (male) antigen on the mouse sperm. Nature 1971; 232:478–480.

15. Goldberg EH, Shen F, Tokuda S. Detection of H-Y (male) antigen on mouse lymph node cells by the cell to cell cytotoxicity test. Transplantation 1973; 15:334–336.

16. Simpson E, McLaren A, Chandler P. Evidence for two male antigens in mice. Immunogenet 1982; 15:609–614.

17. Zenzes MT, Wolf U, Engel W. Organization in vitro of ovarian cells into testicular structures. Hum Genet 1978; 44:333–338.

18. Nagai Y, Ciccarese S, Ohno S. The identification of human H-Y antigen and testicular transformation induced by its interaction with the receptor site of bovine fetal ovarian cells. Differentiation 1979; 13:155–164.

19. Muller U, Singh L, Grund S, Jones KW. Ovarian cells participate in the formation of tubular structures in mouse/rat heterosexual gonadal co-cultures: A direct demonstration by in situ hybridization. Differentiation 1982; 22:136–138.

20. Krco CJ, Goldberg EH. Detection of H-Y (male) antigen on 8-cell mouse embryos. Science 1976; 193:1134–1135.

21. Epstein CJ, Smith S, Travis B. Expression of H-Y antigen on preimplantation mouse embryos. Tissue Antigens 1980; 15:63–67.

22. Wachtel SS. H-Y antigen in the study of sex determination and control of sex ratio. Theriogenology 1984; 21:18–28.

23. Anderson GB. Manipulation of the mammalian embryo. J An Sci 1985; 61, Suppl.3:1–13.

24. Sharpiro M, Erickson RP. Genetic effects on quantitative variation in serologically detected H-Y antigen. J Reprod Immunol 1984; 6:197–210.

25. Zenzes MT, Reed TE. Variability in serologically detected male antigen titer and some resulting problems: a critical review. Hum Genet 1984; 66: 103–109.

26. Wolf U, Fraccaro M, Mayerova A, Hecht T, Maraschio P, Hameister H. A gene controlling H-Y antigen on the X chromosome. Hum Genet 1980; 54:149–154.

27. Polani PE, Adinolfi M. The H-Y antigen and its functions: A review and a hypothesis. J Immunogenet 1983; 10:85–102.

28. Lau Y-F, Chan K, Kan YW, Goldberg E. Male-enhanced expression and genetic conservation of a gene isolated with an anti-H-Y antibody. Trans Ass Am Phys 1987; 100:45–53.

29. Singh L, Jones KW. Sex reversal in the mouse (Mus musculus) is caused by a recurrent nonreciprocal crossover involving the X and an aberrant Y chromosome. Cell 1982; 28:205–216.

30. McLaren A, Simpson E, Tomonari K, Chandler P, Hogg H. Male sexual differentiation in mice lacking H-Y antigen. Nature 1984; 312:552–555.

31. Simpson E, Chandler P, Hunt R, Hogg H, Tomonari K, McLaren A. H-Y status of X/XSxr$'$ male mice: in vivo tests. Immunology 1986; 57:345–349.

32. Simpson E, Chandler P, Goulmy E, Page DC, Disteche C, Ferguson-Smith MA. Separation of the genetic loci for the H-Y antigen and testis determination on human Y chromosome. Nature 1987; 326:876–878.

33. Young RA, Davis RW. Efficient isolation of genes by using antibody probes. Proc Natl Acad Sci USA 1983; 80:1194–1198.

34. Lau Y-F, Chan K, Kan YW, Goldberg E. Isolation of a male-specific and conserved gene using an anti-H-Y antibody. Am J Hum Genet 1986; 39(suppl):142A.

35. Lau Y-F. Localization of a gene for the male enhanced antigen on human and mouse chromosomes. In FP Haseltine, ME McClure, and EH Goldberg, eds. *Genetic Markers of Sex Differentiation* New York: Plenum Press, 1987:161–167.

36. Kralova J, Lengerova A. H-Y antigen: Genetic control of the expression as detected by host-versus-graft popliteal lymp node enlargement assay maps between the T and H-2 complexes. J Immunogenet 1979; 6:429–438.

37. Washburn LL, Eicher EM. Sex reversal in XY mice caused by dominant mutation on chromosome 17. Nature 1983; 303:338–340.

Summary of Part I

Barbara C. McGillivray

University of British Columbia
Vancouver, British Columbia, Canada

Dr. Shapiro opened by commenting that the X and Y chromosome make up 5-8% of the human genome, but while many loci have been assigned to the X chromosome, little assignment has been made to the Y. The X and Y chromosomes were thought to be initially homologous, but at some point a gene or genes involved in male sex determination distinguished the Y from the X. A potential problem would be exchange between the nonhomologous regions of the chromosomes. Dosage compensation and segregation of the X and Y chromosomes during spermatogenesis became important as well.

The pseudo autosomal region of the X and Y chromosome allows frequent recombination during spermatogenesis. Genes in this region would be expected to behave as autosomal genes. Two such genes have been identified, steroid sufatase and MIC2. Both escape inactivation, are present on both the X and the Y, and are expressed from both X chromosomes in the normal female.

Dr. Shapiro went on to discuss the STS gene locus in humans, and commented that the situation differed from most in that the gene was situated on the Y chromosome in an area not having sequence homology with the X, and although the gene escapes X chromosome inactivation, because there is not a homologous functional locus on the Y chromosome there is a dosage inequity. Using CDNA probes with genomic blocks from individuals with varying numbers of X or Y chromosomes, dosage can be shown with increasing numbers of X chromosomes.

Analysis of the X and Y locuses for the STS gene have shown a high degree of homology, but inactivation of the gene on the Y chromosome. Dr. Shapiro postulated that a percentric inversion involving the Y chromosome could explain its location on YP.

Two questions brought up by Dr. Shapiro: 1. Which areas must be deleted to give the clinical features of Turner's syndrome and 2. Why is there such a high frequency of X chromosome aneuploidy in humans?

Dr. Epstein reviewed the four important elements in the Turner phenotype; namely, the ovarian dysgenesis, the major and minor congenital malformations, the short stature, and the intrauterine lethality. In the normal ovary, both X chromosomes are active from 13–14 weeks of gestation until menopause. Therefore, in the 45,X Turner's syndrome female a true monosomy will exist in the ovary, and will probably lead to cell death. The critical region for maintenance of ovarian integrity appears to be XQ 26 but there may well be multiple areas required.

Dr. Epstein made the important point that deletions of the Y chromosome in a 46,XY individual can also give features of Turner's syndrome (without the short stature). He suggested that loss of Y chromosomal material near interval 1 and 2 (or a homologous area on the X) could give rise to the lymphedema and shield chest. XP, but not XQ, deletions give rise to short stature, as well as most of the other Turner's syndrome stigmata.

While it is clear that the vast majority of Turner's syndrome conceptuses result in spontaneous losses, and most of these at about 6 weeks gestation, the etiology of the losses is not clear. Possible reasons are abnormal placental function (perhaps because both X chromosomes are normally active), chromosomal imprinting (that is whether the single X chromosome is maternally or paternally derived), or perhaps that our impression of frequent early loss of a 45,X conceptus comes from studies of the membranes rather than of the embryo itself.

Dr. Disteche reviewed the clinical use of the Y chromosome probes especially with XX males, and those XY females having deletions of the YP region. Dr. Disteche reemphasized that the XY females with the YP deletions had some Turner's syndrome features including lymphoedema at birth and streak gonads. Unfortunately, these women are at increased risk for gonadoblastoma and therefore require surgical removal of the gonads.

The use of the Y chromosome probes has also demonstrated that 45,X males are usually the result of Y autosomal translocations, especially involving chromosome 15. As these individuals also have small deletions of autosomal material, they are also present with somatic abnormalities and mental retardation.

In males having particularly small Y chromosome the use of probes can allow determination of which areas have been deleted. This can be used in a predictive way with prenatal diagnosis, or at a later stage to predict fertility.

Comments made in the discussion included a careful consideration of height in the XY females with deletions. It was pointed out that one needed to remember that such individuals may be short for the expected *male* height.

Dr. Ohno emphasized the similarity between the testis and the ovary. The seminiferous tubule has a similar structure in the ovary (the folliculus), the Leydig and theca cells are homologous cell types, and in some animal species the gonad can change from ovary to testis when there are insufficient numbers of males.

Dr. Ohno pointed out the very similar characteristics of all proteins involved in organogenesis, all having a $beta_2$ microglobulin-like domain.

Dr. Ohno has identified a protein he believes responsible for testicular organogenesis, and with this protein can convert bovine ovarian tissue to a miniature testis (very much like the Freemartin gonad). This protein, the testis organizing antigen, is also known as the HY antigen. There was no attempt to correlate these findings with those of David Page's.

Dr. Simpson warned us of potential pitfalls in correlating the phenotype of individuals having sex chromosome abnormalities with the view to localizing genes. Individuals with well studied deletions, and without mosaicism are most useful, and one must consider the bias of ascertainment. Two possible areas on the short arm, and probably two areas on the long arm of the X chromosome are associated with amenorrhea. Proximal XXq13, or Xq21 are important in ovarian maintenance, with Xq25 or 26 of lesser importance.

Autosomal loci were also discussed, as there are autosomal recessive syndromes giving rise to gonadal dysgenesis. Germ cell failure in both sexes may be genetic, with most families suggesting autosomal recessive inheritance. The association of other abnormalities in specific families suggests that more than one gene is involved.

Dr. Simpson also reviewed the areas of the X chromosome potentially involved in stature. From limited data, proximal Xq deletions are thought to be more important than those of the distal Xq. Those families with deletions indicate that Xq is necessary for growth and some somatic features of Turner's syndrome.

The information now accumulated was a result of careful observation of clinical cases with subsequent delineation of sex chromosome abnormalities and now the addition of the Y and X specific probes are beginning to delineate gene functions. The exciting work of David Page with the testis determining gene or genes has posed several questions: How to explain the similar gene on the X chromosome, whether to invoke problems with inactivation, and of course how to consider the subsequent steps in testis determination.

Similar work is needed to sort out the gene locations for the various Turner's syndrome features. Here, we may be looking at a much more complex situation.

It seems very likely that several areas on the X chromosome (and perhaps on the Y) are important not only for ovarian maintenance, but also stature. This volume underscores the importance of close working relationships between clinicians who ascertain the patients, and the basic scientists who can then help correlate the clinical findings with identification of specific genes.

Part II

Natural History and Assorted Abnormalities

8

Demography and Prevalence of Turner Syndrome

Arthur Robinson

*University of Colorado Health Sciences Center and National Jewish Center
Denver, Colorado*

INTRODUCTION

Most of the data concerning Turner syndrome stems from cytogenetic surveys of a variety of populations. In addition, Turner syndrome is both clinically and cytogenetically heterogeneous. For purposes of this chapter, Turner syndrome may be considered ovarian dysgenesis with short stature and a variety of other somatic anomalies in a liveborn female who has total or partial monosomy X. The diagnosis in spontaneous abortions (SABs), however, will be cytogenetic and not clinical. This definition does also omit mosaics who do not fit the clinical description but who still are partially X-monosomic.

No one would have predicted in 1956 (1), when the first report of the normal human karyotype appeared, that at least 5% of 5-week-old conceptuses are chromosomally abnormal (2) and that greater than 60% of abortuses of a developmental age less than 12 weeks have chromosome abnormalities (3). Hamerton (4) collected six studies of chromosome anomalies among spontaneous abortions, in which 4813 spontaneous abortions were successfully karyotyped. Forty-six percent were abnormal as follows:

45,X	19%
Autosomal trisomy	51%
Polyploid	23%
Structural	4%
Mosaics	3%

45,X is the commonest individual chromosomal anomaly in this group. More than 99% of 45,X conceptions are eliminated before birth (5). Obviously, there is strong intrauterine selection against 45,X zygotes. If roughly 15% of all known pregnancies (not those diagnosed in the first 2 weeks after conception) end as SABs and 50% of these are chromosomally abnormal, with 20% of them being 45,X, then we must conclude that at least 1.5% of all known conceptuses are 45,X. The reason for the lethality of 45,X is unknown. One wonders if recent data on chromosomal imprinting in the mouse, showing that the parental origin of a chromosome can influence the phenotype of the offspring (6), might have any relevance. Hassold et al. (7) suggest that spontaneous abortions in which the paternally derived X is present (X^P) fare less well than X^M abortions.

An older maternal age is not present in 45,X SABs as in trisomics. In fact, a New York study (8) claims just the reverse, namely an association between the incidence of SABs and *young* maternal age. Similar maternal age relationships for 45,X SABs have been observed in Honolulu, Geneva (8), and Hiroshima (9).

Ferguson-Smith and Yates (10) reported from a collaborative European study of 52,965 amniocenteses on maternal age-specific rates for chromosome aberrations that the mean age of mothers with 45,X pregnancies is significantly reduced as compared to other numerical chromosome anomalies in mothers over 35. These authors comment that since the missing chromosome is paternally derived in 78% of cases, this would be expected to be due to maternal age-independent factors. Hassold et al. (11) have also determined the parental origin of X-chromosome monosomy using RFLPs in 10 spontaneously aborted conceptions and find the same general tendency. The mean age of the mothers of liveborn 45,X babies has also been reported by others to be similar to that of the general population—not elevated (12).

45,X/46,XX mosaicism is rarely seen in SABs. Some have suggested that the 45,X livebirths are all mosaics and have a different etiology from the pure 45,X karyotype found in SABs (5). In fact, there is a very recent suggestion that autosomal trisomies that survive are placental mosaics (13). This might also be true of 45,X fetuses.

Incidence of Turner syndrome in newborns has varied, with an average incidence of 1/2,500–1/10,000 female births. Hook and Warburton (5) summarized data from chromosome studies in New York and from four large-scale sex chromatin studies and found 9 cases in 76,474 females, or about 1/9000. Nielsen found 115 cases of Turner syndrome among 459,786 girls born in Denmark from 1955-1966, a prevalence of 3/10,000 (14).

My own studies in Denver revealed a somewhat higher incidence, which may be due to a more thorough assessment of the newborn population (using the amniotic membrane from every birth) and a more sensitive way of identifying sex chromosome mosaics. The advantage of using the amniotic membrane is that the sex chromatin body is large and easily seen and is present in 85-95% of cells in a 46,XX female. Hence, mosaics are more easily identified.

At any rate, by screening 19,705 consecutive female births by checking the amniotic membrane and confirming all discrepancies by chromosome analysis, we found an incidence of 45,X of 6 in 10,000 and an incidence of 45,X/46,XX mosaics of 8 in 10,000 (15). The fact that the 45,X mosaics had a greater incidence than the pure 45,X karyotype is different from most estimates of prevalence of mosaics because there was no bias of ascertainment, and screening for mosaicism was probably more thorough than in those studies where only 2-5 cells were checked.

However, I doubt that technique was the whole story. Alex Bell (16) screened 31,769 female newborns using our amniotic membrane method and found only one 45,X and five mosaics. Of particular interest, there were two different periods in which he screened 6,000 babies without finding any sex chromosomal anomaly (SCA) babies. This suggests that there may have been temporal or geographic variations in these incidences between Denver and Toronto. It may be recalled that in Denver we did find a significantly different seasonal incidence in birth of newborns with SCA. However, this was for *all* anomalies of the sex chromosomes (15). There is no evidence of a racial difference in occurrence of Turner syndrome.

Incidence of sex chromosome mosaicism (45,X/46,XX) in liveborns is really unknown, especially as it relates to the Turner phenotype, since the presence of Turner stigmata may vary greatly with the percentage of cells with a normal karyotype (17). Hook and Warburton say that at least 25% of all individuals with a 45,X cell line carry a chromosomally normal line (5), but that group had some bias of ascertainment. In our own experience, 45,X/46,XX mosaicism is fairly common among phenotypically normal women, especially those who have experienced recurrent abortions, and, as mentioned above, we found that about 60% of monosomic or partially monosomic newborns identified in a screening program were mosaics.

A variety of sex chromosome complements have been associated with the Turner phenotype. The Interregional Cytogenetics Registry System reported data on 651 such females as follows (18):

45,X	50%
45,X/46,XX; 45,X/47,XXX	13%
46,X,i(Xq); 45,X/46,X,i(Xq)	28%
45,X/46,XY	5.5%
45,X/mar	3%

Of interest is the feto-protective effect of the 46,X,i(Xq) karyotype, rarely seen in SABs, but not infrequent in liveborn individuals with Turner syndrome (3).

Little is known about the prevalence of Turner syndrome in the general adult population primarily because of methods of ascertainment, variability of expression, and differences at different ages. Turner syndrome is not in general a lethal condition after infancy, during which the hypoplastic left heart syndrome and inappropriately managed coarctation of the aorta may cause death.

One method of ascertainment has been primary amenorrhea in women over the age of 18. Two such studies, one by Philip et al. (19) and the other by Jacobs et al. (20), when combined found that 33 out of 133 amenorrheic women, or 25%, had SCA. Of these, 14% had 45,X, 6% had 45,X/46,XX, and 5% had 45,X/46,XY karyotypes. It should be stressed that these women were ascertained without regard to phenotype.

Anglani et al. (17) karyotyped females over 15 years of age with primary amenorrhea and divided them into those with no stigmata, short stature alone, and those with Turner syndrome phenotype (Table 1). It was surprising that only 80% of those with a Turner phenotype had an abnormal karyotype. Could some of the others have had Noonan syndrome?

A matter of some dispute is the incidence of Turner syndrome in populations of retarded individuals. Three different sex chromatin studies by Maclean et al. (21) de la Chapelle (22), and Harms (23), all in the 1960s, screened a total of 4,114 mentally retarded girls and found a prevalence of 1.2/1000 with Turner

Table 1 Primary Amenorrhea

1. Females >15 yr without short stature or Turner phenotype
   6/64 = 9.4% with abnormal karyotype (excluding 46,XY)
2. Females >15 yr with short stature
   20/36 = 55.5% with abnormal karyotype
   16/36 = 44% without Y chromosome
3. Females with Turner phenotype
   36/45 = 80%

Source: Ref 17.

syndrome. Yanagisawa and Shuto (24) surveyed a total of 24 sex chromatin studies of mentally retarded girls (12,849 in number) and found an incidence of 1.2/1000.

Nielsen (14) screened 2880 females in Danish institutions for mental retardation. The incidence was 1.8/1000 or about 6 times the expected frequency of Turner syndrome.

It may well be that mental retardation is slightly more common in females with Turner syndrome than in the general population. I would agree with Judith Hall that whereas mild to moderate mental retardation is common in Noonan syndrome, often a confusing entity in the differential diagnosis of Turner syndrome, it is uncommon in Turner syndrome (25). There is no question that there are other genetic and environmental factors which are rarely taken into account. I have seen several borderline mentally retarded girls with Turner syndrome who come from most disturbed families, all of whom have a below normal IQ. In addition, life is of course more stressful for these little girls, both because of their appearance and their perceptual problems.

Twinning has often been noted to be more common in the families of Turner syndrome probands. Carothers et al. (12) collected data on several studies which provided 20 twin births in 516 individuals with Turner syndrome or their siblings. The incidence of 3.9% is about three times the typical value for most Western populations. An apparent association between monozygotic twins rather than dizygotic twins and Turner syndrome within kindreds has been claimed several times, although I am unaware of conclusive data on the subject (26,27).

Finally, mention should be made of the 45,X/46,XY mosaic. The incidence of this karyotype in females with Turner phenotype is about 5%, and of course carries a need for special care because of the risk of gonadoblastomas. The use of Y chromosome probes has been helpful in this group, especially since on occasion the Y chromosomal material is present in a so-called marker chromosome which is not obviously of Y chromosomal origin.

In summary:

1. Incidence of TS in newborn females is between 1/3000 and 1/10,000. There may be temporal or geographic differences.
2. The incidence of 45,X/46,XX mosaics is probably underestimated.
3. The reason for the strong intrauterine selection against 45,X zygotes is unknown.
4. Mental retardation is not a prominent feature of the phenotype.

ACKNOWLEDGMENTS

Supported, in part, by U.S. Public Health Services Grant 5R01-HD10032 and The Genetic Foundation.

REFERENCES

1. Tjio JH, Levan A. The chromosome number of man. Hereditas 1956;42:1.
2. Hook EB. Prevalence of chromosome abnormalities during human gestation and implications for studies of environmental mutagens. Lancet 1981; 2:169–172.
3. Carr DH, Gideon M. Population cytogenetics of human abortuses. In Hook EB, Porter IH, eds. Population Cytogenetic Studies in Humans. New York: Academic Press, 1977:1–10.
4. Hamerton JL. Population cytogenetics: A Perspective. In Adinolfi M, Benson P, Giannelli F, Seller M, eds. Pediatric Research: A Genetic Approach. London: Spastics International Medical Publications, 1982:99–121.
5. Hook EB, Warburton D. The distribution of chromosomal genotypes associated with Turner's syndrome: Livebirth prevalence rates and evidence for diminished fetal mortality and severity in genotypes associated with structural X abnormalities or mosaicism. Hum Genet 1983;64:24–27.
6. Swain J, Stewart T, Leder P. Parental legacy determines methylation and expression of an autosomal transgene: A molecular mechanism for parental imprinting. Cell 1987;50:719–727.
7. Hassold T, Benham F, Kobryn C, Leppert M, Whittington F. Cytogenetic and molecular studies of sex chromosome monosomy. Am J Hum Genet 1987;41:A121.
8. Warburton D, Kline J, Stein Z, Susser M. Monosomy X: A chromosomal anomaly associated with young maternal age. Lancet 1980;1:167–179.
9. Kaju T, Ohama K. Inverse maternal age effect in monosomy X. Hum Genet 1979;51:147–151.
10. Ferguson-Smith MA, Yates JRW. Maternal age specific rates for chromosome aberrations and factors influencing them: Report of a collaborative European study on 52,965 amniocenteses. Prenatal Diagnosis 1984; Spring Vol. 4, special issue, 5–44.
11. Hassold T, Kumlin E, Takaesu N, Leppert M. Determination of the parental origin of sex chromosome monosomy using restriction fragment length polymorphisms. Am J Hum Genet 1985;37:965–972.
12. Carothers AD, Frackiewicz A, De Mey R, Collyer S, Polani PE, Osztovics M, Horvath K, Papp Z, May HM, Ferguson-Smith MA. A collaborative study of the aetiology of Turner syndrome. Ann Hum Genet 1980; 43: 355–368.
13. Kalousek DK, McGillivray B. Confirmed placental mosaicism and intrauterine survival of trisomies 13 and 18. Am J Hum Genet 1987;41:A278, supplement.
14. Nielsen J, Sillesen I. Turner's syndrome in 115 Danish girls born between 1955 and 1966. Acta Jutlandica LIV (Medicine Series), Aarhus, Denmark, 1981.
15. Goad WB, Robinson A, Puck TT. Incidence of aneuploidy in a human population. Am J Hum Genet 1976;28:62–68.

16. Bell AG, Corey PN. A sex chromatin and Y body survey of Toronto newborns. Can J Genet Cytol 1974; 16:239–250.
17. Anglani F, Baccichetti C, Artifoni L, Lenzini E, Tenconi R. Frequency of abnormal karyotypes in relation to the ascertainment method in females referred for suspected sex chromosome abnormality. Clin Genet 1984; 25:242–247.
18. Magenis RE, Breg WR, Clark KA, Hook EB, Palmer CG, Pasztor LM, Summitt, RL, Van Dyke D. Distribution of sex chromosome complements in 651 patients with Turner's syndrome. Am J Hum Genet 1980; 32:79A.
19. Philip J, Sele V, Trolle D. Primary amenorrhea: A study of 101 cases. Fert Steril 1965; 16:795–804.
20. Jacobs PA, Buckton KE, King MJ, Harnden DG, Court Brown WM, McBride JA, MacGregor TN, Maclean N. Cytogenetic studies in primary amenorrhea. Lancet 1961; 1:1183–1189.
21. Maclean N, Mitchell JM, Harnden DG, Williams J, Jacobs PA, Buckton KA, Baikie AG, Court Brown WM, McBride JA, Strong JA, Close HG, Jones DC. A survey of sex-chromosome abnormalities among 4514 mental defectives. Lancet 1962; 1:293–296.
22. de la Chapelle A. Sex chromosome abnormalities among the mentally defective in Finland. J Ment Defic Res 1963; 7:129–146.
23. Harms S. Anomalien der Geschlechtschromenzahl (XXX-und X0-zustrand) bei Hamburger Hilfsschulerinnen. Padiatr Padol 1967; 3:34–52.
24. Yanagisawa S, Shuto T. Sex chromatin survey among mentally retarded children in Japan. J Ment Defic Res 1970; 14:254–262.
25. Hall JG, Sybert VP, Williamson RA, Fisher NL, Reed SD. Turner's syndrome. West J Med 1982; 137:32–44.
26. Nance WE, Uchida J. Turner's syndrome, twinning and an unusual variant of glucose-6-phosphate-dehydrogenase. Am J Hum Genet 1964; 15:380.
27. Karp L, Bryant JI, Tagatz G, Giblett E, Fialkow PJ. The occurrence of gonadal dysgenesis in association with monozygotic twinning. J Med Genet 1975; 12:70–78.

DISCUSSION

DR. ROBERT BLIZZARD: Just repeat the figures on twinning, would you please? Give us a little speculation.

DR. ARTHUR ROBINSON: 3.9 percent of the individuals with Turner's had siblings who were twins. The majority of those, from what I can find out, were identical twins.

DR. ANDREA PRADER: You said that was three times more than expected?

DR. ROBINSON: That is right.

UNIDENTIFIED: Is there any correlation between XO karyotype in one family and other abnormalities of chromosomal disease? I just recall one family who has one Down's syndrome and one Turner.

DR. ROBINSON: Yes, I think everybody has had some experiences like that. I do not know that there is a specific correlation. As a matter of fact, another thing which is of interest, and that may have something to do with some of the data that were given this morning, is families where there has been more than one individual with 45X. I have recently seen a family with three individuals with 45X in different generations.

DR. MYRON GENEL: Aside from technique, is there anything that you can correlate between Toronto and Denver that would explain the difference in incidence?

Dr. ROBINSON: No.

DR. LARRY SHAPIRO: There is a little bit of data in the mouse system that would suggest there could conceivably be some genetic factors that might explain the difference, in that there is a strain of Balb-C, the Balb-CWT, which appears to have a high frequency of spontaneous postzygotic chromosome loss, presumably due to some abnormality of the Y chromosome in that strain. Maybe there are some Ys that are more predisposed to being lost in humans than others, and they may differ between Toronto and Denver.

Dr. Blizzard is at the University of Virginia at Charlottesville, Charlottesville, Virginia. Dr. Robinson is at the National Jewish Center and the University of Colorado Health Science Center, Denver, Colorado. Dr. Prader is at Kinderspital, Zurich, Switzerland. Dr. Genel is at Yale University, New Haven, Connecticut. Dr. Shapiro is at the University of California at Los Angeles School of Medicine, Los Angeles, California.

9

Prenatal Diagnosis and Fetal Loss

Mitchell S. Golbus

University of California at San Francisco, San Francisco, California

PRENATAL DIAGNOSIS

Recent advances in prenatal and neonatal care have improved perinatal mortality rates, and, consequently, birth defects represent a larger component of the residual mortality rate. Simultaneously, our ability to obtain information about the fetus has increased dramatically. This combination has produced great interest in the prenatal diagnosis of genetic defects. These techniques have made it possible, in many instances, to convert genetic counseling from an essentially passive endeavor to one in which the counselors and parents, in concert, can take the steps to alter the genetic risks to which the couple is exposed. As the name implies, the objective of prenatal diagnosis is to determine whether a fetus at risk for some genetic disease is or is not actually affected.

The test results are negative in more than 95% of cases, and in these cases some pregnancies that might have been terminated in the past because the fetus was at risk of being abnormal may now be completed. On the other hand, a positive diagnosis allows the expectant parents to choose their subsequent course of action: aborting the fetus, treatment of the fetus in the few cases where this is possible, continuing the pregnancy and treating the neonate, or continuing the pregnancy and having the neonate adopted or institutionalized. This decision ultimately is the right and responsibility of the prospective parents and will be influenced by their social and ethical concepts. Although the ultimate goal of prenatal diagnosis is the treatment and care of the genetically ill fetus, this goal is still distant. In the interim, difficult decisions will have to be made by couples who find that they have conceived a genetically abnormal fetus.

Prenatal diagnosis has usually relied upon the cytogenetic or biochemical analysis of cultured amniotic fluid cells. Amniocentesis was introduced initially in the 1930s, and by 1950 it was being utilized for the management of erythroblastosis fetalis (1). The technique gained widespread acceptance for studying Rh isoimmunization, because it caused minimal maternal or fetal morbidity. Fuchs and Riis (2) demonstrated the prenatal diagnosis of fetal sex by examination of X-chromatin bodies in amniotic fluid cells. The ability to grow amniotic fluid cells in tissue culture and acquire sufficient viable cells for karyotype analysis and biochemical studies was demonstrated in 1966 (3). Since that time amniocentesis at 16 menstrual weeks has become the traditional approach to prenatal diagnosis of genetic defects. Because of the lateness of availability of the diagnosis, efforts have been directed toward developing an earlier method of prenatal diagnosis.

Chorionic villus sampling (CVS) involves obtaining a small amount of the developing trophoblast as early as 9 menstrual weeks. This tissue is of fetal origin and can be used for a wide range of prenatal diagnostic studies. The first attempt to obtain chorionic villus cells was reported in 1968 using transcervical hysteroscopy (4). However, there was an extremely low yield of villus material and difficulty in culturing what little tissue was obtained. The first series of CVS in ongoing pregnancies was performed in China (5). One hundred patients underwent transcervical CVS without ultrasound guidance for the prenatal diagnosis of fetal sex. Ninety-four patients were diagnosed correctly. Direct tissue preparations were used for sex chromatin analysis, and thus this study did not contribute to solving the problem of culturing the villus material. In 1981 a technique was devised to culture chorionic villi by trypsinization to expose the villus inner mesenchymal core (6). These studies laid the groundwork for the large collaborative clinical studies of CVS in ongoing pregnancies which are currently in progress.

Amniocentesis or chorionic villus sampling must be preceded by the careful recording of a family pedigree and appropriate genetic counseling. The counselor should be able to verify the diagnosis of previously affected relatives, determine the applicable genetic facts, and be able to recognize and deal with the psychosocial implications of the material with which he or she is dealing. The genetic counseling should include discussion of the risks of having a genetically defective fetus, the dangers of amniocentesis and chorionic villus sampling, and any reservations about the results that may be obtained.

The UCSF Prenatal Diagnosis Program has performed 15,000 amniocenteses and 3000 chorionic villus samplings. Table 1 indicates a 2.3/1000 incidence of 45,X karyotypes and a 2.7/1000 incidence of 45,X mosaics among chorionic villus samplings performed at 9–12 menstrual weeks. There was a 0.8/1000 inci-

Table 1 UCSF Prenatal Diagnosis Program Experience

Chorionic Villus Sampling (n = 3,000)	no. of cases
45,X	7
45,X Mosaics	8
Amniocentesis (n = 15,000)	
45,X	12
45,X Mosaics	20

dence of 45,X karyotypes and a 1.3/1000 incidence of 45,X mosaics among amniocenteses done at 16-18 menstrual weeks. This suggests that approximately 67% of 45,X and 50% of 45,X mosaic embryos will be spontaneously aborted between 9-12 and 16-18 menstrual weeks.

FETAL LOSS

Chromosome heteroploidy is responsible for a substantial segment of birth defects and reproductive inefficiency. Sterility, reduced fertility, embryonic or fetal death, stillbirths, and/or congenital malformation may result from an aberration in chromosome number. One of the most common of clinically significant aneuploidies is the 45,X chromosome complement.

To collect data on early human gestations, a number of cytogenetic surveys have been conducted on induced abortuses (7-9). Table 2 shows that 2.6% of first trimester-induced abortions were chromosomally abnormal. That this represents a low estimate is seen in that the early studies devoted themselves to complete specimens containing both membranes and an embryo and found a 1.1% incidence of chromosome abnormality, while more recent studies which

Table 2 Chromosome Abnormalities in Induced Abortions

Author	Incidence of abnormality	Mean developmental age (days)	Mean maternal age (yr)
Sasaki	16/1297	39	26.6
Tonomura	11/609	36	27.1
Yasuda	5/188	37	29.0
Ford	0/307	51	27.7
Kajii	23/728	49	28.4
Hahnemann	6/172	73	26.5
Yamamoto	80/1250	45	28.0
Klinger	9/1233	–	24.7
Total	150/5784 (2.6%)		

Table 3 Chromosome Abnormalities in Induced Abortions by Developmental Age

Developmental age (weeks)	Number of karyotypes	Chromosome abnormalities
3-4	108	10 (9.3%)
5-10	1558	90 (5.8%)
> 10	259	2 (0.8%)

Source: Refs. 8 and 9.

have included incomplete anembryonic specimens found a 5.0% incidence of chromosome anomaly. The rate of karyotype abnormality is also a function of the developmental age of the embryo (Table 3), and these data suggest an abnormality rate of approximately 10% in the early postimplantation human embryo.

A second source of information regarding human fetal aneuploidy has been karyotypes of spontaneously aborted first-trimester fetuses. A number of such surveys have been published and, as seen in Table 4, it is generally agreed that about 50% of unselected clinically recognized spontaneous abortions are chromosomally aberrant (10). Of these, the most common single anomaly is 45,X, which occurs in approximately 20% of the chromosomally abnormal fetuses. A study of the incidence and distribution of cytogenetic abnormalities as a function of race found no significant differences among the different racial groups (10).

The fact that only 0.59% of newborns are chromosomally abnormal indicates that the spontaneous abortion mechanism selectively removes 92% of the aneuploid conceptions. Assuming a 10% incidence of 45,X among spontaneous

Table 4 Results of Five Cytogenetic Surveys of Spontaneous Abortions

Total abortuses karyotyped	3080			
Normal karyotypes	1541	(50%)		
Abnormal karyotypes	1539	(50%)		
Trisomic			810	(26%)
45,X			287	(9%)
Triploid			260	(8%)
Tetraploid			92	(3%)
Structural Abnormalities			61	(2%)
Mosaics			25	(1%)
Other			4	—

Source: Adapted from Ref. 10.

Table 5 Frequency of 45,X Gestations Among Spontaneous Abortions

Weeks of gestation	Total abortions	45,X abortions	Percent
0–7	49	0	0.0
8–11	252	16	6.3
12–15	299	20	6.7
16–19	124	1	0.8
20+	152	1	0.7

Source: Adapted from Ref. 12.

abortuses (10), a 15% incidence of spontaneous abortions among recognized pregnancies, and a 1:5000 incidence of 45,X among liveborns (11), one can compute that more than 98% of 45,X conceptions are spontaneously aborted. The decrease in the prevalence of 45,X pregnancies as gestation progresses is demonstrated both in Table 5 and in the UCSF Prenatal Diagnosis Program data (see above). Clearly, spontaneous abortion serves as a mechanism preventing the birth of a much larger number of 45,X neonates.

REFERENCES

1. Bevis DCA. Composition of liquor aminii in hemolytic disease of the newborn. Lancet 1950; 2:443.
2. Fuchs F, Riis P. Antenatal sex determination. Nature 1956; 177:330.
3. Steele MW, Breg WT. Chromosome analysis of human amniotic fluid cells. Lancet 1966; 1:383-5.
4. Hahnemann N, Mohr J. Genetic diagnosis in the embryo by means of biopsy from extraembryonic membranes. Bull Eur Soc Hum Gen 1968; 2:23-9.
5. Department of Obstetrics and Gynecology, Tietung Hospital, Anshan Iron and Steel Company. Fetal sex prediction by sex chromatin of chorionic villi cells during early pregnancy. Chin Med J 1975; 1:117-26.
6. Niazi M, Coleman DV, Loeffler FE. Trophoblast sampling in early pregnancy. Culture of rapidly dividing cells from immature placental villi. Br J Obstet Gynaecol 1981; 88:1081-5.
7. Kajii T. Chromosome anomalies in induced abortions. In: Boue A, Thibault C, eds. Chromosomal Errors in Relation to Reproductive Failure. Paris: INSERM, 1973:57-66.
8. Kajii T, Ohama K, Mikamo K. Anatomic and chromosomal anomalies in 944 induced abortuses. Hum Genet 1978; 43:247-58.
9. Yamamoto M, Watanabe G. Epidemiology of gross chromosomal anomalies at the early embryonic stage of pregnancy. Contr Epidemiol Biostat 1979; 1:101.

10. Hassold TJ, Matsuyama A, Newlands IM, et al. A cytogenetic study of spontaneous abortion in Hawaii. Ann Hum Genet 1978;41:443–54.
11. Stein Z, Susser M, Warburton D, et al. Spontaneous abortion as a screening device. Am J Epidemiol 1975; 102:275–90.
12. Warburton D, Stein Z, Kline J, Susser M. Chromosome abnormalities in spontaneous abortion: data from the New York City study. In: Porter IH, Hook EB, eds. Human Embryonic and Fetal Death. New York: Academic Press, 1980:261–87.

DISCUSSION

DR. MELVIN M. GRUMBACH: I wonder if you would say something else about prenatal diagnosis, including alpha fetoprotein studies.

DR. MITCHELL S. GOLBUS: Just a general statement; many of you are aware that back in the early '70s it became obvious that the amniotic fluid alpha fetoprotein was elevated when the fetus had a lesion that exposed capillaries basically to the amniotic fluid. This was originally thought to be a way of looking for neural tube defects, and that was what the British were after. But it quickly turned out that other things, like gastroschisis, omphalocele, and cystic hygromata gave you high alpha fetoproteins in the amniotic fluid. Some of the highest alpha fetoproteins, by the way, came from people who were doing an amniocentesis on a fetus with cystic hygroma and hit the cystic hygroma and therefore drew out cystic hygroma fluid, and it had sky-high alpha fetoprotein levels. What has come out of that more recently is maternal serum alpha fetoprotein screening programs, again to try to find in the general population women at higher risk of having a neural tube defect fetus, but again, it is turning out that women who are carrying a fetus with a cystic hygroma, omphalocele, or gastroschisis may well have a high maternal serum AFP, probably derived from their high amniotic fluid AFP. The kicker to that program, which we did not anticipate ahead of time but has now fallen out, is that fetuses with trisomy appear to have a lower maternal serum alpha fetoprotein, and it probably is going to be as effective a mechanism for finding trisomy as using the high maternal age-screening mechanism. It is not at all clear that women who are carrying a fetus with 45X are at more risk of having a low serum AFP, and I think there is just

Drs. Grumbach and Golbus are at the University of California at San Francisco, San Francisco, California. Dr. Shapiro is at the University of California at Los Angeles School of Medicine, Los Angeles, California. Dr. Saenger is at Montefiore Medical Center/Albert Einstein College of Medicine, Bronx, New York. Dr. Robinson is at the National Jewish Center and the University of Colorado Health Science Center, Denver, Colorado.

not enough data to answer that question, but it is one of the things that may come out of programs such as the California state program.

DR. LARRY J. SHAPIRO: Dr. Golbus, you have lumped together in many ways mosaicism information derived from direct karyotyping of villi with those of cultures. My suspicion is that we are looking at very different cells when we do that. I mean, we are looking at the cytotrophoblast when we do the direct preparations, which is trophoblastic in its lineage, whereas those cells which grow in culture 2 to 3 weeks later are probably embryonic in their origin and derive from the fetal invasion of the trophoblast. Is there a real difference?

DR. GOLBUS: That would be nice, but it is not. This is all cultured material.

DR. SHAPIRO: This is all cultured material?

DR. GOLBUS: Yes, so that it is there and it is mosaic in the cultured material. The direct prep has led to other errors. In fact, there are now a fair number of trisomies that have been missed on direct preparation, and I think virtually all the programs are leaving direct preparations for the cultured material at this point.

DR. PAUL SAENGER: The AFP levels seem to be also lower in obesity, in over-weight pregnant ladies, so that should be also added on so it does not confuse the issue. Isn't that so?

DR. GOLBUS: Yes, it has to do with plasma volume. You have to correct AFP levels for weight, for race, and for insulin-dependent diabetes. All of those things influence the level.

DR. ARTHUR ROBINSON: You mentioned the fact that the maternal serum AFP is lowered in the case of trisomies, autosomal trisomy. I have had calls from around the country of about eight cases of individuals who had an amniocentesis because of a high maternal serum alpha fetoprotein, and there was sex chromo-somal trisomy. I do not know of any case which was 45X, though. I am not sure—is that just an accident, or is that something which you have heard of, too?

DR. GOLBUS: No, the only ones that I would expect to be high and found would be those with cystic hygromata. I do not know of any other association.

DR. ROBINSON: The ones I know of are triple-Xs or XXYs, not 45X.

DR. GOLBUS: I do not know of any such association.

10

Oocyte Donation in Ovarian Failure

Zev Rosenwaks* and Daniel Navot

The Jones Institute for Reproductive Medicine
Eastern Virginia Medical School
Norfolk, Virginia

INTRODUCTION

The year 1978 marked the beginning of a new era in reproductive physiology and infertility therapy (1). In vitro fertilization (IVF) and related technologies have allowed the probing of the ovarian follicle, offering access to the microenvironment of the oocyte, the subtleties of gamete interaction, and the intricacies of syngamy and early embryonic development. Egg and embryo donation is an obvious outgrowth of IVF. Essentially the technique involves the transfer of embryo(s) or oocyte(s) from a fertile donor into the uterus of a phenotypically matched infertile recipient (2-4). Successful transfer of donor embryos (4-6) and in vitro fertilized donor oocytes (2-3) has extended our ability to treat female infertility due to ovarian agenesis, oocyte depletion, inaccessibility of oocytes, and genetic abnormalities which preclude the use of disease-carrying gametes (2,3,7).

Although oocyte donation is medically analogous to sperm donation, the relative inaccessibility of female gametes and the relative difficulty of synchronizing the ovulatory process in the donor with endometrial maturation in the recipient make the procedures quite different technically. Because the temporal window of endometrial receptivity and the window of transfer in the human is unknown,

---

Current affiliation: Cornell University Medical Center–The New York Hospital, New York, New York

there is a tremendous clinical and scientific challenge—and reward—inherent in the practice of oocyte donation.

HISTORICAL PERSPECTIVES

Although the use of embryo transfer (ET) technology to alleviate infertility is relatively recent, this technology has been under investigation for a century. The first successful ET was performed in rabbits nearly a century ago (8). This transfer was followed by experimentation in many species, with the greatest number of studies performed in the mouse, rabbit, sheep, and cow. Indeed, the first successful bovine ET was reported in 1951 (9). Since then, many advances and refinements have led to a high success rate and the routine use of this technique in the cattle industry (10). Briefly, the procedure involves the following steps: superovulation of the donor with gonadotropins, insemination (allowing fertilization to occur in vivo), embryo recovery, isolation of the embryo(s), and transfer of the embryo(s) to a recipient uterus. Thus, the donor is the genetic mother, while the host or recipient is the surrogate who carries and gives birth to the young.

It is evident that to optimize success in the bovine model, the recipient must be at the same stage of the estrous cycle as the donor. Asynchrony between the donor and recipient estrous cycle of 2 days or more in the luteal phase results in poor pregnancy rates (11). In mice, synchrony between donor and recipient must be within 6 hours for implantation to take place (12). In sheep, when synchronization of donor and recipient is exact, 75% of all recipients become pregnant; a relatively high pregnancy rate is also obtained when there is asynchrony of up to 2 days. When there is a difference of 3 or more days, however, only 8% of ewes become pregnant (13). In cattle, transfer efficiency approaches 70% (14). Hodgen reported a 36% pregnancy rate (4 of 11) in oophorectomized recipient monkeys replaced with subcutaneous estradiol (E_2) and progesterone (P) capsules (15) with a tolerance of 3 days of asynchrony between embryo and endometrium.

PATIENT SELECTION AND INDICATIONS

Women in their reproductive life span who lack ovaries or have ovaries which are not functional make up an important group of sterile patients who may benefit from ovum donation (Table 1). By far the most common complaint that brings infertile couples to request ovum donation is the idiopathic form of premature ovarian failure (POF) or "premature menopause." The latter is defined as permanent ovarian failure, characterized by elevated gonadotropins and occurring after menarche but before the age of 35 or 40 years (16,17). POF is rela-

Table 1   Etiological Diagnoses and Indications for Ovum Donation

---

  I. Ovarian agenesis or dysgenesis
     a. Pure gonadal dysgenesis (46XX)
     b. Turner syndrome (45,X)
     c. Turner-like mosaics (variable karyotype)
     d. Swayer syndrome (46XY)
 II. Premature ovarian failure
     a. Idiopathic (premature menopause)
     b. Autoimmune ovarian failure
     c. Iatrogenic (surgical ablation, x-ray, or chemotherapy) or environmental
        (infections, drugs)
     d. Resistant ovary syndrome
     e. Genetic predisposition
III. Genetically transmitted diseases
     a. Maternal autosomal dominant
     b. Autosomal recessive—both partners
     c. X linked recessive
 IV. Surgically inaccessible ovaries
  V. Oocyte abnormalities
 VI. The perimenopausal period

---

tively rare; however, approximately 4% of women reach menopause before the age of 30 years (17). Undoubtedly a sizable proportion of these may not have completed their families. A very important subgroup of patients—who need meticulous pretreatment evaluation—are those with Turner syndrome and various other major chromosomal aberrations.

There is a strong correlation between autoimmune phenomena and POF; POF has been linked to Addison's disease (18,19). Hashimoto's thyroiditis, myasthenia gravis, and systemic lupus erythematosus (17). Further support of an autoimmune phenomenon is given by numerous reports on the presence of antibodies to specific ovarian components (20,21). There are numerous other possible indications for ovum donation, most of which are self-explanatory (Table 1).

The list of etiological diagnoses in Table 1 discriminates two subgroups in regard to treatment strategy. Groups III through V are normally cycling women, in whom an attempt at ovum donation takes place during a natural cycle. In contrast, groups I and II need exogenous hormonal replacement, since they are acyclic and lack any endogenous ovarian activity. Group VI may still have cyclicity which may be inadequate, and hormone replacement or augmentation may be needed.

EVALUATION OF THE INFERTILE COUPLE PRIOR TO OVUM DONATION

Prerequisites for ovum donation include a normal uterus in the female, an adequate spermogram in her partner, and the absence of any contraindication for pregnancy.

Table 2 outlines the general guidelines for pretreatment evaluation. As a rule, programs which practice ovum donation are referral centers, and the patients referred have already been through at least a preliminary diagnostic workup. Still, the need may arise to complete such a workup. In primary ovarian failure patients, the karyotype should be scrutinized for the existence of a Y chromosome or fragment which, if found, requires gonadectomy. In the face of Turner syndrome or a Turner-like mosaic, a thorough cardiopulmonary workup is warranted. The detection of associated congenital abnormalities should raise doubts about the advisability of pregnancy. The possible adverse effects on the already compromised cardiovascular system should be carefully assessed. In secondary ovarian failure of any etiology, the irreversibility of the phenomenon should be reassessed. Finally, for optimal patient care and better clinical outcome, preparatory cycles should be evaluated for adequacy of the natural or exogenously stimulated endometrial cycle. During these preparatory cycles (3,7) serial hormone studies and dated endometrial biopsies should be carried out. In the natural cycle, a day 26 biopsy is needed to rule out an inadequate luteal phase.

Table 2 Workup of Couples Who Are Candidates for Ovum Donation

Female with ovarian failure	Male partner
Baseline hormonal study	Spermatogram
Karyotype[a]	
Hysterosalpingography	
Anti ovarian antibodies[a]	
Cardiopulmonary workup[a]	
Blood chemistry and hemotalogic profile	
Rubella AB	
VDRL, hepatitis screen, HTLV-III	Tay-Sachs[a]
HLA-AB typing	HLA-AB typing
Preparatory cycle(s)	
	Psychiatric and Social Evaluation
	Informed Consent

[a]If indicated

During an exogenously supplemented cycle, a periimplantation (day 20 to 22) and a late luteal (day 26) biopsy should ascertain normalcy of the artificially induced cycle.

ARTIFICIALLY INDUCED ENDOMETRIAL CYCLES IN OVARIAN FAILURE RECIPIENTS

Although various replacement protocols have been reported, they all endeavor to mimic the steroidal milieu of the normal menstrual cycle (2,3,7). Essentially, estrogen (E) and E + P are administered sequentially.

Lutjen et al., who reported the first pregnancy in a POF patient, used oral estradiol valerate (E_2V) (Progynova, Schering) and vaginal P suppositories for steroid replacement (2). Following ET, they utilized intramuscular P injections and oral E_2V for the maintenance of pregnancy. A slight modification of Lutjen's protocol resulted in satisfactory serum levels of both steroids and an adequate endometrial development, as judged by luteal biopsy. Figure 1 details the protocol which we used initially (3). Briefly, E_2V (1 mg/day) was administered orally on days 1 through 5. The dosage was increased to 2 mg/day on days 6 through 9 and to 6 mg/day on days 10 through 13. The dosage was reduced to 2 mg/day on days 14 through 17, increased to 4 mg/day on days 18 through 26, then reduced to 1 mg/day on days 27 and 28. It should be noted that the reduction on days 14 through 17 was used to mimic the drop in E_2 which one observes in the natural cycle after the LH surge. P was administered in a single intramuscular dose of 25 mg/day on days 15 and 16, increased to 50 mg/day on days 17 through 26, then reduced to 25 mg/day on days 27 and 28.

Intramuscular P appears to be more consistently absorbed, offering a more predictable serum level and an invariable action at the level of the target organ, the endometrium. Indeed, serum E_2 and P levels closely simulated those of a normal 28-day cycle. The E_2 level rose gradually from a mean of 120 pg/ml in the early follicular phase to 900 pg/ml during the preovulatory phase. After a decrease in E_2 in the early luteal phase, a secondary rise corresponding to the mid-luteal phase was observed (Fig. 1). Serum P likewise reached a peak at a mean level of 27 ng/ml. Endometrial thickness gradually increased from about 6 mm on day 6 to 12 mm on day 18 and remained constant thereafter (Fig. 1).

A similar protocol using micronized E_2 (Estrace, Mead Johnson) was used in the donor egg program in Norfolk (Fig. 2) (7). An adequate luteal phase was induced by P vaginal suppositories (75 to 150 mg/day) or an intramuscular regimen. Additional acceptable routes of E_2 administration include vaginal rings (7) and transdermal patches (Estraderm, CIBA Pharmaceutical Co., Summit, NJ).

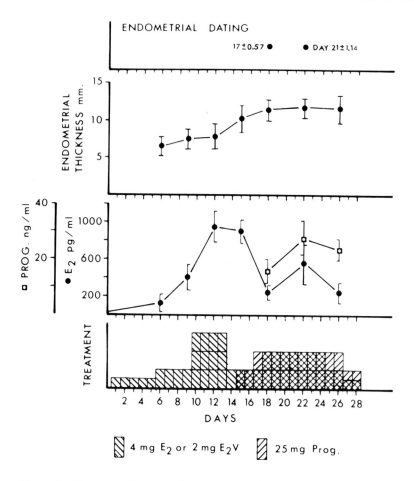

Figure 1 Exogenous hormonal treatment and serum E and P levels throughout the preparatory cycle in eight patients. The endometrial response was evaluated both ultrasonographically and morphologically. Values are means ± SD. E_2 denotes estradiol; $E_2 V$ denotes estradiol valerate. (From Ref. 3.)

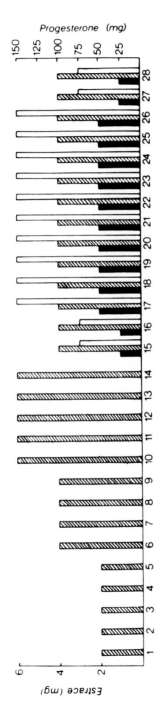

Figure 2 Sequential E (estrace) and P (intramuscularly or as vaginal suppositories) as utilized for steroid replacement. (From Ref. 7.)

ENDOMETRIAL MORPHOLOGY

Endometrial biopsies are performed during two replacement cycles. A preimplantation phase biopsy (day 20 to 22) is followed by a late (day 26 to 27) biopsy in a second E + P replacement cycle.

We have observed that biopsies performed on days 20 to 22 display day 17 to 18 glandular architecture, along with a characteristic day 21 to 23 stroma. A typical early biopsy performed on day 21 is depicted in Figure 3. The subnuclear vacuolization and linear arrangement of nuclei characteristic of day 18 architecture are juxtaposed with edematous stroma suggestive of day 21 to 22 endometria. This asynchrony occurs despite seemingly adequate P absorption. In contrast, biopsies performed on day 26 revealed the characteristic pseudodecidual changes in the stroma of day 25 to 26 endometria. Thus, early endometrial gland development seems to lag behind the stroma, although the endometrium appears to catch up in the late luteal phase.

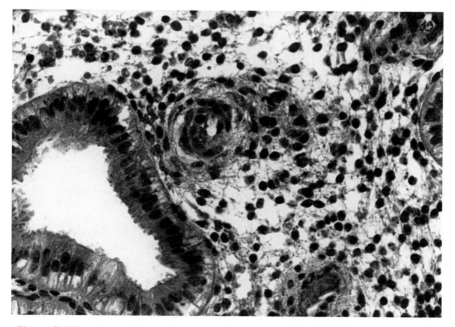

Figure 3 Histology of day 21 endometrial biopsy after E + P replacement of an ovarian failure patient. Note the subnuclear vacuolization and linear arrangement of nuclei characteristic of day 18 glands juxtaposed with edematous stroma and prominent arteriols characteristic of days 22 and 23 endometrium.

OOCYTE DONORS

Patients who undergo IVF and have excess oocytes are potential candidates for ovum donation. Prior to the availability of cryopreservation, patients were advised not to attempt fertilization of more than 5 oocytes, to minimize the occurrence of multiple gestations. The term "excess oocytes," however, became obsolete with successful cryopreservation of human embryos. Patients may now choose to inseminate all of their oocytes, transfer a prechosen number, and freeze any remaining concepti. Consequently, the donor program depends on the availability of specific donors. In some instances a sister has provided oocytes. At other times a patient requesting tubal sterilization agrees to undergo gonadotropin stimulation before her surgical procedure.

Payment to donors should be discouraged, as recommended by the Ethics Committee of the American Fertility Society (22).

A prospective donor and recipient are phenotypically matched. The donor should undergo a complete psychological and medical evaluation, and should be screened for hereditary and sexually transmitted diseases, as detailed in Table 3.

To secure multiple fertilizable oocytes, ovarian stimulation must be carried out. Any stimulation of proven efficacy may be used (2,3,7).

TEMPORAL WINDOW OF ENDOMETRIAL RECEPTIVITY IN THE HUMAN

In the natural cycle, ovum transport is programmed in a way that allows fertilization, embryo transport, and development to be synchronous with endometrial receptiveness. During IVF the embryo available for transfer is usually at the stage of 4 to 8 blastomeres. For this early developmental stage the optimal window of transfer or optimal endometrial receptivity has not been defined. At the inception of our donor egg program (3,7), a clinical experiment was devised which would define this temporal window. In this experimental model, complete

Table 3 Guidelines for Selection and Workup of Prospective Ovum Donors

Clinical appraisal	Laboratory studies
Age (less than 35 years)	CBC and chemistry panel
Phenotype	HTLV III
Complete history and physical	Hepatitis screen
Family history of congenital or hereditary diseases	Tay Sachs[a]
Detailed informed consent	Sickle cell screen[a]
Psychiatric interview	HLA-AB[b]

[a] As indicated
[b] Optional

dissociation between the events leading to embryogenesis (donor) and endometrial development (recipient) allowed replacement of embryos of a definite
blastomeric stage into endometria at variable maturational stages. Endometrial
receptivity was tested by replacing 2- to 16-cell embryos between days 16 and
24 of hormonally and histologically defined cycles (3,7). In our preliminary experience (Table 4) (3), 2 of 8 recipients transferred on days 16 to 21 conceived.
Two conceptions occurred on days 18 and 19; others failed to occur on days 16,
17, 18 (2), 19, and 21. Additional experience (7) has confirmed endometrial receptivity on days 18 to 19 and has extended the window of transfer to day 17.
Of 21 transfers performed with multiple concepti derived from mature oocytes,
7 patients became pregnant. All 7 (or 7 of 14) were transferred on day 17 to 19
of an idealized cycle, while none of the remaining 7 patients transferred on day
20 or later did so.

The Monash group (2,23) typically performed ET on day 17 ± 1 of the replaced cycle. Most of their transfers were of embryos derived from IVF patients
who were willing to donate excess oocytes. Thus, they transferred single
embryos in most donation cycles. Since it has been shown that the IVF success
rate is increased by transfer of increasing numbers of embryos (24), it is expected that transfer of multiple concepti to recipients would result in an improved success rate. Perhaps more importantly, excess oocytes obtained from
IVF patients tend to be the least desirable morphologically, because the oocytes

Table 4 Pregnancies Achieved by Ovum Donation According to Diagnosis and
Timing of Transfer

Primary diagnosis	Day of embryo transfer	Number of embryos replaced	Stage of embryonic cleavage[b]
Surgically castrated[b]	19	4	(4)2 (6)2
Gonadal dysgenesis[b] (46XX)	18	4	(4)3 (6)1
Premature menopause	18	2	(6)1 (8)1
Premature menopause	21	3	(4)2 (3)1
Premature menopause	19	2	(5)1 (6)1
Premature menopause	17	2	(5)1 (6)1
Balanced translocation	18	2	(2)1 (2PN)1
Turner syndrome	16	3	(4)3

[a]Cell stage in parentheses, followed by number of embryos attaining that stage of embryonic cleavage PN, pronucleus
[b]Conceived after ET

with the best morphology are saved for the IVF patient. Therefore, clinics using excess oocytes may have a lower pregnancy rate than clinics using designated fertile donors. For the most part, the Norfolk program has used excess oocytes, although sisters and women undergoing sterilization have also been donors.

A recent report by Van Stierteghem et al. (25) on the transfer of a frozen/ thawed embryo has further extended the period of successful ET to day 16. Formigli (26) has successfully transferred a blastula into a day-22 endometrium. However, his report lacked precise delineation of the occurrence of the LH surge and ovulation, thus making his conclusions somewhat speculative.

If one considers that a 2- to 12-cell embryo requires approximately 3 or 4 days to reach the blastocyst stage, a stage at which implantation takes place, then ET on day 19—the limit of the transfer window—would lead to implantation on day 22 or 23. It can therefore be speculated that after day 23, the endometrium is incompatible with embryo implantation. It appears that ET as early as day 16 allows embryonic development to continue within the uterine cavity, enabling implantation to occur at a later stage when endometrial maturation catches up with embryonic development.

The temporal window for human ET extends between days 16 and 19 of a hormonally and morphologically defined 28-day cycle. Whether there is an optimal day of transfer within that time frame, or whether embryonic or endometrial tolerance for asynchrony is even greater, must await the availability of additional data.

SYNCHRONIZATION BETWEEN DONOR AND RECIPIENT

The relatively restricted period available for implantation demands precise synchronization between donor and recipient. The strategy for synchronization is completely different for natural cycles and stimulated cycles.

Stimulation for multiple follicular recruitment and multiple ovulation is an obligatory step in the prospective ovum donor. When the donor is aligned with a recipient who has natural cycles, the problem of synchronization is further complicated by the fact that in the stimulated cycle the follicular phase is shortened by as much as 4 to 5 days. In a typical gonadotropin-stimulated cycle, hCG—as a surrogate LH surge—is given on day 9 of the cycle (27). Figure 4 illustrates the point precisely. The recipient's menstrual cycle started 6 days prior to the donor's cycle. However, because of a shortened follicular phase in the donor, at the time of the natural and surrogate LH surges, there was a lag of only 1 day in the recipient. ET on day 19 of the recipient resulted in a pregnancy that carried to term.

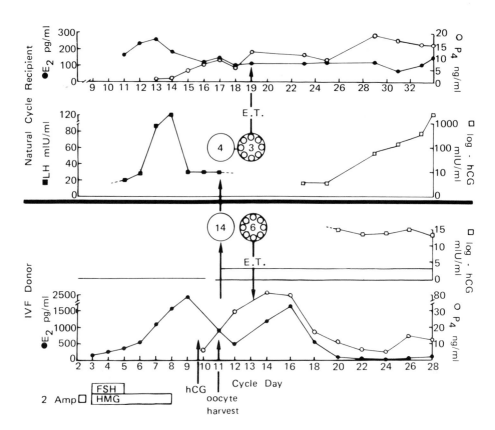

Figure 4 Oocyte donation of excess oocytes to a natural cycle recipient. The day of LH surge is arbitrarily defined as day 14. Four excess oocytes were inseminated with the sperm of the recipient's husband. Embryo transfer of 3 concepti was accomplished on day 19. An 8-cell conceptus was the most advanced embryo transferred. (From Ref. 7.)

PREGNANCY AND ITS MAINTENANCE IN OVARIAN FAILURE

As of May 1987, 18 centers around the world reported on 69 pregnancies resulting from ovum donation; 56 pregnancies were achieved in patients with POF and 13 in natural cycles (28).

Detailed experience describing the requirements for pregnancy maintenance has been reported by several investigators (2,3,7). A positive beta-hCG titer can be expected approximately on day 28: 10 days after ET. If the pregnancy test is negative, one tapers the E + P dosage to allow endometrial shedding and menstruation to occur. If the test is positive, most investigators immediately and substantially increase the E dosage. Lutjen (2) maintained his patients on 2 mg of E_2V in the luteal phase of the transfer cycle, increasing the dosage to 8 or 9 mg/day as soon as the beta-hCG titer became positive. At the same time he placed the patient on intramuscular P (50-100 mg/day). He suggested that this regimen maintained the plasma steroid levels at concentrations which were within the normal ranges for pregnancy. His goal was to maintain E_2 concentrations at 100-500 pmol/L and P within the 100-200 nM/L range. Lutjen discontinued E treatment at 12 weeks of pregnancy, whereas P injections were maintained through week 16.

Navot et al. (3) rapidly increased exogenous E + P when pregnancy was diagnosed (Figure 5). From weeks 7 and 8, when E + P were kept at a fixed dosage, relatively stable blood levels were obtained. It was assumed that notable endogenous production of steroids would be reflected by a net increase in the artificially achieved steady state. During week 11 the anticipated surge in E_2 was observed, and stepwise withdrawal of exogenous E was begun. In the first 2 patients there was a rise in P during week 12, and a stepwise withdrawal of exogenous P was begun. By week 16, both pregnancies were maintained solely by placental E_2. By week 18, one patient no longer required exogenous P.

These preliminary observations dated placental takeover to week 12 of gestation (3). In contrast, our more recent data (unpublished) suggest that significant placental steroidogenesis may begin earlier. It appears that in the human, E + P dosage required for implantation and early pregnancy maintenance may be less than has been previously used. Nevertheless, gravid patients who lack ovarian function should be regarded as in vivo models for the study of placental steroidogenesis isolated from ovarian hormonal function. These models should be used to determine specifically the time of luteo-placental shift and the exact E + P requirements for the initiation and maintenance of pregnancy in POF patients.

E + P replacement in ovarian failure patients allows assessment of the relative roles of these steroids in endometrial proliferation and differentiation. The transfer of concepti of a defined stage into a specific endometrium has made possible the assessment of the human window of implantation. Precise manipulation of endometrial proliferation and differentiation, by varying the E + P regimen in POF patients, will allow the separation of endometrial from ovarian factors. The ability to manipulate E + P dosage during pregnancy in POF patients will precisely define the role of these steroids in the establishment and maintenance of pregnancy.

A donor oocyte program, while it is an exciting and gratifying treatment modality for infertility, has provided a unique human model for the study of conceptus/endometrial/steroidal interaction. It may also elucidate previously unapproachable questions of human reproduction and infertility.

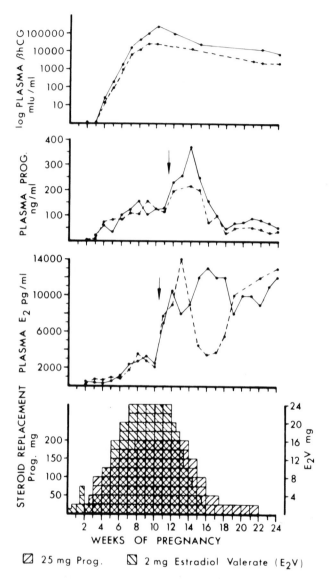

Figure 5 Exogenous hormonal treatment and plasma E$_2$, P, and hCG levels during two pregnancies. The anticipated rise in E$_2$ was observed during week 11 (arrow), and endogenous production of P was observed in week 12 (arrow). P was gradually withdrawn by week 18 in one patient (solid line) and by week 22 in the other patient (broken line). (From Ref. 3.)

REFERENCES

1. Steptoe PC, Edwards RG. Birth after the reimplantation of a human embryo. Lancet 1978; 2:336.
2. Lutjen P, Trounson A, Leeton J, Findlay J, Wood C, Renou P. The establishment and maintenance of pregnancy using in vitro fertilization and embryo donation in a patient with primary ovarian failure. Nature 1984; 307:174.
3. Navot D, Laufer N, Kopolovic J, Rabinowitz R, Birkenfeld A, Lewin A, Granat M, Margalioth E, Shenker JG. Artificially induced endometrial cycles and establishment of pregnancies in the absence of ovaries. N Engl J Med 1986; 314:806.
4. Buster JE, Bustillo M, Thorneycroft IH, Simon JA, Boyers SP, Marshall JR, Louw JA, Seed RW, Seed RG. Nonsurgical transfer of in vivo fertilized donated ova to five infertile women: report of two pregnancies. Lancet 1983; 2:223.
5. Bustillo M, Buster JE, Cohen SW, Thorneycroft IH, Simon JA, Boyers SP, Marshall JR, Seed RW, Louw JA, Seed RG. Nonsurgical ovum transfer as a treatment in infertile women: preliminary experience. JAMA 1984; 25:1171.
6. Bustillo M, Buster JE, Cohen SW, Hamilton F, Thorneycroft IH, Simon JA, Rodi IA, Boyers SP, Marshall JR, Louw JA. Delivery of a healthy infant following nonsurgical ovum transfer. JAMA 1984; 251:889.
7. Rosenwaks Z. Donor eggs: their application in modern reproductive technologies. Fertil Steril 1987; 47:895.
8. Heape W. Preliminary note on the transplantation and growth of mammalian ova within a uterine foster mother. Proc R Soc London 1890; 48:457.
9. Wilett EL, Black WG, Casida LE, Stone WH, Buckner PJ. Successful transplantation of a fertilized bovine ovum. Science 1951; 113:247.
10. Seidel GEJ Jr. Superovulation and embryo transfer in cattle. Science 1981; 211:351.
11. Newcomb R, Rowson LE. Conception rate after uterine transfer of cow eggs in relation to synchronization of oestrus and age of eggs. J Reprod Fertil 1975; 43:539.
12. Beatty RA. Transplantation of mouse eggs. Nature 1951; 168:2995.
13. Rowson LEA, Moor RM. Embryo transfer in the sheep: the significance of synchronizing oestrus in the donor and recipient animal. J Reprod Fertil 1966; 11:201.
14. Rowson LEA, Lawson RAS, Moor RM, Baker AA. Egg transfer in the cow: synchronization requirements. J Reprod Fertil 1972; 28:427.
15. Hodgen GD: Surrogate embryo transfer combined with estrogen-progesterone therapy in monkeys, implantation, gestation and delivery without ovaries. JAMA 1983; 250:2167.
16. Friedman C, Barrows H, Kim MH. Hypergonadotropic hypogonadism. Am J Obstet Gynecol 1983; 145:360.

17. Tulandi T, Kinch RAH. Premature ovarian failure. Obstet Gynecol Surv 1981;36:521.
18. Turkington RW, Lebovitz HE. Extra-adrenal endocrine deficiencies in Addison's disease. Am J Med 1967;43:499.
19. Irvine WJ, Chan MMW. Immunological aspects of premature ovarian failure associated with idiopathic Addison's disease. Lancet 1968;1:883.
20. De Moraes-Ruehsen M, Blizzard RM, Garcia-Bunuel R, Jones GS. Autoimmunity and ovarian failure. Am J Obstet Gynecol 1972;112:693.
21. Caldwell BV, Luborsky-Moore JL, Kase N. A functional LH agonist and LH receptor antagonist in serum from a patient with premature ovarian failure syndrome. Endocrine Society Meeting, Miami, FL, June 15, 1978. Abstract.
22. Jones HW Jr, ed. Ethical Considerations of the New Reproductive Technologies. Fertil Steril 1986;46:supp 1.
23. Lutjen PJ, Findlay JR, Trounson AO, Leeton JF, Chan LK. Effects on plasma gonadotropins of cyclic steroid replacement in women with premature ovarian failure. JCEM 1986;62:419.
24. Jones HW Jr, Acosta AA, Andrews MC, Garcia JE, Jones GS, Mayer J, McDowell JS, Rosenwaks Z, Sandow BA, Veeck LL, Wilkes CA. Three years of in vitro fertilization at Norfolk. Fertil Steril 1984;42:826.
25. Van Stierteghem AC, Van den Abbeel E, Braeckmans P, Camus M, Khan I, Smitz J, Staessen C, Van Waesberghe L, Wisanto A, Devroey P. Pregnancy with a frozen-thawed embryo in a woman with primary ovarian failure. N Engl J Med 1987;317:113.
26. Formigli L, Formigli G, Roccio C. Donation of fertilized uterine ova to infertile women. Fertil Steril 1987;47:162.
27. Rosenwaks Z, Muasher SJ. Recruitment of fertilizable eggs. In Jones HW Jr, Jones GS, Hodgen GD, Rosenwaks Z, eds. In Vitro Fertilization—Norfolk. Baltimore: Williams and Wilkins, 1986, p 30.
28. Schenker JG. Ovum donation: state of the art. NY Acad Sci (in press).

DISCUSSION

DR. LINDA GIUDICE: I would like to briefly discuss some of the screening of oocyte donors, and before I do that I know Dr. Rosenwaks did mention the two alternative methods for ovum donation.

Advances in fertility technology have been such that women with premature or primary ovarian failure can now achieve pregnancy, and there are essentially three methods. One is in vitro fertilization using donor oocytes which Dr. Rosenwaks has so eloquently presented. The two in vivo fertilization methods include GIFT or gamete intrafallopian tube transfer. This involves obtaining the oocyte from the donor and putting it into the fallopian tube of the recipient along with the sperm from the recipient's partner, so that fertilization can occur in the fallopian tube, where it normally does, presumably in the ampullary region. The rationale for this is that the transit of zygote would be in a more natural environment from its place of fertilization to the uterus, where it is going to implant.

The problem with GIFT for ovum donation obviously is that the recipient undergoes a surgical procedure, either laparoscopy or minilaparotomy.

The second type of in vivo fertilization is the so-called nonsurgical ovum donation and embryo transfer which was pioneered by Buster and his colleagues in Southern California.

This involves artificially inseminating a donor with the sperm of the recipient's husband and then, just before the embryo implants, to lavage the embryo out of the donor and place it into the recipient, who has undergone hormonal replacement as Dr. Rosenwaks has described.

One of the major problems with this is that there is about a 10% rate of retention of the embryo in the donor, and this is unacceptable.

I would like to emphasize that there is a triad in the ovum donation program, and that involves not only the donor and the recipient, but also the fetus. We must all keep in mind what we learned in medical school, and that is primum no noceri, or first do no harm, because all of these procedures do have some inherent risks.

In the screening of oocyte donors, it is very important that we take a thorough medical history, a family genetic history, social and ethnic history, and sexual history. The American Fertility Society has some guidelines for sperm

Drs. Giudice and Rosenfeld are at the Stanford University School of Medicine, Stanford, California. Dr. Rosenwaks is at Cornell University Medical Center–The New York Hospital, New York, New York. Dr. Prager is at Kinderspital, Zurich, Switzerland. Drs. Grumbach and Golbus are at the University of California at San Francisco, San Francisco, California. Dr. Erhardt is at Columbia University College of Physicians and Surgeons and New York State Psychiatric Institute, New York, New York. Dr. Simpson is at the University of Tennessee at Memphis, Memphis, Tennessee. Dr. Hall is at the University of British Columbia, Vancouver, Canada.

donor screening. However, the oocyte donor program is so new that the Fertility Society has not come out with guidelines for this particular group.

However, we can extrapolate from the sperm donors, and that is what I have done here. Most programs require that the donor be less than 30 years old, for obvious reasons. Her health, in general, should be good and she should not have any major medical problems or any psychiatric problems. It is preferable that she has had proven fertility and that her gynecologic history is benign. It is also important that she doesn't have any estrogen-dependent neoplasms because of the high levels of estrogen that are generally found in ovulation induction protocols.

The family and genetic history are obviously very important and the social and ethnic history is also important for reasons of any risks of transmission of any hereditary disorders.

Very recently, in the *Journal of Fertility and Sterility*, it has been shown that women who are chronic carriers of hepatitis B have very high levels of hepatitis B surface antigen in their follicular fluid surrounding the egg and, therefore, it is important that donors who give oocytes also are not carriers of hepatitis or any of the other transmitted diseases, such as, obviously, HIV or CMV.

It is also important that the oocyte donor be karyotyped and that the ABO-Rh is compatible with the recipient's husband.

This is the obvious goal of all of the donor oocyte programs, that is, normal healthy babies. We must also focus, however, on having a normal healthy pregnancy in the recipient. This is particularly germane to women with Turner's syndrome, because of associated abnormalities that they may have.

It is somewhat of a problem to present a slide like this with a group like this. I am sure you are all aware of the various problems in Turner's syndrome, but I have put an asterisk next to those that can predispose to a high-risk pregnancy, particularly coarctation of the aorta. There is an increased risk of aortic dissection, bacterial endocarditis, intracranial aneurysms, and in women who do become pregnant with long-standing coarctation, there is a maternal mortality of 5 to 8% and a fetal loss which is quite high, at 11%.

So this really brings us back to: We must be very careful that we do no harm.

Women who have Turner's syndrome or any agonadal woman who has a recipient egg, but particularly Turner's patients, should be followed by the appropriate maternal-fetal specialist during her pregnancy.

I would also like to make a pitch for the adult follow-up of women with Turner's syndrome who are not pregnant. Very often they are very carefully followed by pediatricians throughout their childhood and teen years and then seem to get lost in the medical system in their early 20s.

At Stanford the reproductive endocrinologists have been essentially vying for the pediatric population of Turner's syndrome, and I would encourage you to refer Turner's patients to reproductive endocrinologists for their routine gynecologic care.

DR. RON G. ROSENFELD: One of the questions which we are being asked now is, is there any feasibility, if the diagnosis of Turner's is made in very early childhood, of actually removing potentially functional oocytes from the young child and freezing them for later fertilization? Is that at all a possibility in the future?

DR. ZEV ROSENWAKS: The answer is yes and no. The question was asked actually during our break. You know there have been babies born as a result of frozen thawed oocytes fertilized in vitro. There are at least two babies from Australia that have been born and have been healthy, although the efficiency of this procedure at the moment, or this technique, is very low. At this point, the risk versus benefit is such that we cannot offer it to the patient at the moment. I can foresee a time, and not in the too distant future, as we develop the cryopreservation technology, and it is improving, well, I would say yearly, that the cryopreservation oocytes will be so efficient that this could be offered, especially now since the majority of the aspiration techniques, the oocyte harvest, oocyte pickup is by transvaginal retrieval with local anesthesia. So that the risk to the patient is relatively low compared to a general anesthetic and a laparoscopy. So yes, the answer is yes, in the future, perhaps not right now.

DR. ANDREA PRADER: Dr. Rosenfeld, at what age did you think that could be done; was your question in the newborn?

DR. ROSENFELD: Potentially in infancy or early childhood? It may be hard to do a local anesthesia.

DR. ROSENWAKS: Let me tell you what we are working on at the General Institute. Gary Hodgin is looking into the ovarian follicle in vitro and its development, and it is hoped that many years from now, hopefully sooner than later, that we will be able to take a piece of ovary, cryopreserve it and at some later time with in vitro manipulation, get follicular development in an in vivo model, in an in vitro, perfusion model and then provide it for the particular patient. So you can theoretically do it at any age. At the moment, I think, and speaking about cryopreserved oocytes, this should only be reserved to those few gonadal dysgenesislike patients who have remaining oocytes. Perhaps as a teenager, one can perform a stimulation. Although I think there is a note of caution there also, since generally these patients have very few follicles, and even if you stimulate them, you will get one or two at most, and the efficiency is so low that at the moment I certainly do not think you can do it. This is theory; this is not practical.

DR. MELVIN M. GRUMBACH: It sure is, and I am afraid the impression has been left that it is common to find a lot of oocytes in these streaks, and in my experience it is not. There are very few, and they are not very healthy-looking. I think those in which they may have some, with few exceptions, are probably mosaics, and I think in the mosaic you have a crack at it.

DR. ROSENWAKS: Right. For the most part it is a theoretical discussion.

DR. ANKE A. ERHARDT: I am glad you added a word of caution, because there is really a misunderstanding now among patients who often at least think that they hear the endocrinologist say that the new reproductive technologies are readily available to anybody. I think that is a set-up for disappointment, because obviously we are far away from thinking of that as a routine procedure, and since so many adult patients with Turner syndrome are very eager to have children, let us be sure not to raise hopes which cannot be fulfilled in the next 10 or 15 years.

DR. ROSENWAKS: I believe your statement is true in regard to the availability of donors, because that has really been the stumbling block of the program rather than the ability and the feasibility of doing it. I think that the IVF technology has reached a point where this can be provided fairly routinely for the patient with ovarian failure. At Norfolk now, we have close to 100 women in the donor egg program. The difficulty is not preparing them. The difficulty is obtaining a suitable phenotypically matched donor who has been screened psychologically and medically for HIV, hepatitis, and all the other things that were just mentioned. But I really do see the day, especially with cryopreservation now, where we can provide, have an embryo waiting for a patient and believe that within the next 5 years this will be as common as in vitro fertilization. And I believe in vitro fertilization is common right now.

DR. PRADER: Yes, Dr. Simpson.

DR. JOE L. SIMPSON: Just to put it in context, it is probably worth pointing out, that if anything, the success rate of patients who are agonadal in donor embryo transfer is superior to that of regular patients who utilize in vitro fertilization as a last resort. So I think the technology is here, and as you said, the rate-limiting step is the availability of the donors. If anything, it works better than IVF, which is routine.

DR. PRADER: If you transfer multiple embryos, do you get multiple pregnancies?

DR. ROSENWAKS: Yes. I probably did not mention why we do not inseminate more than four eggs now, because 25% of all our ongoing pregnancies in Norfolk are multiple. And we have placed four embryos in and have gotten quadruplets. Up to about 3 months ago, the limit was five, and we were always worried that we will get quints one of these days. In the donor egg program, at least in our program, generally the average number of embryos we put in for the whole program is less than two. We have had 14 single embryo transfers. I did not show you that slide, but only 1 has become pregnant, whereas in multiple embryo transfers, which the average is 2.5 for the multiple transfers, the pregnancy rate is almost 50%. I should mention, because the GIFT procedure has been touted as a potential easy way of treating the ovarian failure patient because the pregnancy rate is better than 50% with GIFT, that GIFT requires a surgical procedure, where you take the egg and the sperm and place it into the fallopian tube on the day that you start progesterone treatment. However, instead of multiple concepti transfer, you really get the same success rate with IVF, and you will get multiple pregnancies as you put more than two embryos in, no doubt. The majority of the time, although we stimulate patients, we generally have only one or two embryos that are viable at time of transfer. Therefore there is not a great risk of having triplets and quadruplets. There is a good risk, at least some risk, of having twins.

DR. JUDITH G. HALL: I wanted to ask how it really is working in Turner's syndrome. In other words, you showed a number of ovarian failures, but I would have thought that Turner's women might be slightly different, having not had estrogen during childhood, maybe having smaller uteruses. Of the women with Turner who have tried this worldwide, how successful is it? How many cases have actually gone through pregnancy?

DR. ROSENWAKS: It is interesting. I tried to find out those figures for this symposium. Dr. Shankar from Israel updated the world experience on oocyte donation as of last March and there are approximately 60 pregnancies in ovarian failure patients, perhaps. To my knowledge in the programs that I know of that have had gonadal dysgenesis, 45 X patients, their ongoing pregnancy rate in Turner's was 25%. I should tell you that it is interesting, we have lots and lots of data on the endometrial response to first, second, and third cycle of priming, and it is interesting that it is not different with or without previous exposure, to our amazement. So that the first exposure to adequate estrogen milieu gives you a proper response, at least according to comparison with women who have secondary ovarian failure, and this surprised us to some degree.

DR. MITCHELL S. GOLBUS: I will just comment on the multiple gestations after putting back in multiple embryos. There have now been a fair number of pregnancies with three and more embryos from IVF that have been reduced back to twins for obstetrical reasons and have successfully gone on.

11

Spontaneous Puberty and Fertility in Turner Syndrome

Robert L. Rosenfield

The University of Chicago Pritzker School of Medicine
Chicago, Illinois

Gonadal dysgenesis is so characteristic of Turner syndrome that the term "gonadal dysgenesis" is often used as a synonym for Turner's.

Nevertheless, it is well recognized that some patients with Turner syndrome demonstrate evidence of ovarian function at puberty. Lippe (1) concludes from her review of the literature that

> in as many as 5 to 10% of patients ... the estrogen secretion is sufficient to initiate breast development ... and in a small percentage of (these), it is sufficient to initiate menses. . . A very few ... will maintain normal ovarian function, so that ovulatory menses will occur and pregnancy may result. While maintenance of ovarian function is more often reported in patients with mosaic karyotype, it may occur in the 45,X individual as well.

Grumbach and Conte (2) note that conceptions have been documented in 11 women with Turner syndrome in whom extensive karyotypic analysis has revealed only a 45,X cell line in more than one tissue.

A case is presented, some features of which have been reported (3), to illustrate the typical features of these atypical Turner syndrome patients who spontaneously enter puberty and are potentially fertile. The implications of such cases for concepts of ovarian development, endocrinologic diagnosis, and growth are then discussed.

CASE REPORT

KB, UCMC #93-45-28, underwent an endocrinologic evaluation by an internist at 9.5 years of age for short stature. She was 118.75 cm tall and weighed 32.4 kg. Buccal smear was 25% chromatin positive. Thyroid tests showed positive antimicrosomal antibodies and a slightly low free thyroxine index (PB1 5.8 μg/dl and resin T3 uptake 23%). When a trial of thyroid hormone replacement therapy did not improve her growth rate, she was referred to pediatric endocrinology. Upon initial evaluation at 10.67 years of age, her height was 121.9 cm and weight 36.8 kg. She had multiple pigmented nevi, a highly arched palate, cubitus valgus, hypoplastic areolas, and a short right 5th metacarpal. At 11.33 years of age, her height was 126.0 cm, she had no secondary sexual characteristics, bone age was 11.0 years, LH was 126, and FSH 280 ng LER-907/ml. Because of her Turner phenotype, karyotype was advised. Eighty-two peripheral lymphocytes were examined, 25 by G-banding, and all showed an isochromosome of the long arm of the X chromosome (karyotype 46,XXqi). A diagnosis of Turner syndrome was therefore made in this prepubertal child. The patient was accordingly advised that she had a height potential of only 139 cm, which treatment could not change, and, incorrectly as events were to subsequently prove, that she would require sex hormone replacement treatment to go into puberty.

At 13.25 years of age, she defied a part of the prediction: she had spontaneously entered puberty. Concomitantly, she underwent a pubertal growth spurt (Fig. 1). Breast diameters were 3.5-4.0 cm and sexual pubic hair had appeared.

At 13.9 years, menarche occurred and menses subsequently recurred monthly. At 15.3 years of age, she was sexually mature (Fig. 2). Menses continued to occur at monthly intervals. However, these cycles were apparently anovulatory over the next 2 years. This was indicated on five occasions by basal body temperature records, lack of vaginal cornification, and by a low plasma progesterone level on day 19 of a menstrual cycle. This did not presage menopause, however.

At 16.5 years of age, laparascopy (Fig. 3) revealed her to have ovaries bilaterally: these were small, measuring about $1 \times 1 \times 1.5$ cm. Follicular activity and a corpus luteum were visible. Biopsy of the latter was consistent with a late corpus luteum, but no other follicles were found in the biopsy field. Simultaneous plasma progesterone was 192 ng/dl and endometrial currettings showed late secretory endometrium. These findings were consistent with recent ovulation from an ovary with a marked paucity of follicles.

At 17.75 years of age she was 137.9 cm tall, menstrual cycles were normal and ovulatory as indicated by finding a progesterone level of 700 ng/dl and 17% vaginal cornification.

A gonadotropin releasing hormone (GnRH) test was then performed when plasma estradiol was 79 pg/ml and serum LH averaged 72 ± 11 and FSH 73 ± 26 ng/ml. In response to 100 μg LHRH, LH rose by 198 and FSH by 327 ng/ml, responses which were about 2-fold greater than those of normal follicular phase

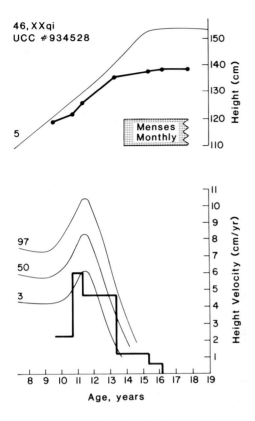

Figure 1 Growth chart during spontaneous puberty of patient KB with ovulatory Turner syndrome due to isochromosome of the long arm of an X chromosome. Normal percentiles from Tanner and Davies (4); 5th percentile for height is that for delayed girls.

controls. This exaggerated gonadotropin response to LHRH is typical of partial ovarian failure.

At 17.9 years of age, clomiphene citrate 50 mg bid was administered commencing on day 5 of the menstrual cycle: after 5 days plasma immunoreactive estrogen was >500 pg/ml, LH 10–30, and FSH 980–1250 ng/ml. This exaggerated FSH response with a normal estrogen rise is typical of diminished ovarian reserve (5).

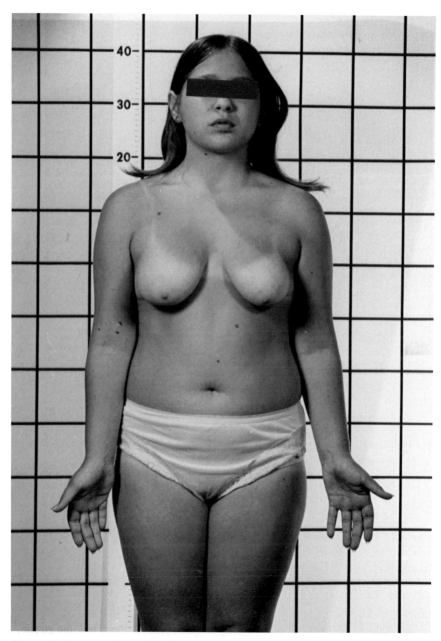

Figure 2 Patient KB with Turner syndrome after undergoing spontaneous puberty and menarche. Note short stature, cubitus valgus, hypoplastic areolae, multiple nevi.

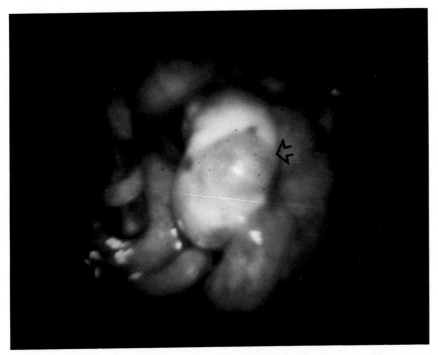

Figure 3 The small right ovary, as viewed through a laparoscope, of patient KB with ovulatory Turner syndrome. Note the prominent late corpus luteum (arrow). Photograph courtesy of Dr. Moon H. Kim.

OVARIAN DEVELOPMENT IN TURNER SYNDROME

Normally, after repeated mitoses, sex-chromatin-negative oogonia differentiate into oocytes which enter meiotic prophase commencing during the third month of fetal life (6). Reactivation of the inactive X chromosome then occurs so that two functional X chromosomes are present in each oocyte (7). Contact of the oocyte with follicular cells then seems necessary to forestall further maturation, whether it be directed toward degeneration or toward completion of meiosis (6). Degeneration becomes the predominant fate of germ cells by the fifth month of gestation (Fig. 4) (8). At birth about half of the germ cells are normally atretic. The number of germ cells normally declines steadily throughout life, and menopause ensues when their total number falls below about 10^4 (9,10). Atresia is the destiny of the vast majority of germ cells: millions become atretic, while only a few hundred develop to the point of ovulation. One to two antral (Graafian) follicles typically appear in late gestation, and a few are often found

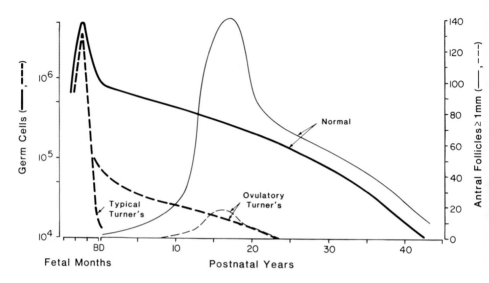

Figure 4 Model of development and atresia in normal and Turner syndrome ovaries. Normal curve smoothed from data of Baker (8) and Block (9,10). Curve for "typical" Turner syndrome estimated from data presented by Carr and associates (16,17). Curve for "ovulatory" Turner syndrome estimated from Carr et al. finding approximately 1/50 of a normal complement of germ cells in recognizable ovaries from a 45,X neonate (17) and the assumption of a menopausal complement of germ cells in such patients at about 25 years of age.

in mid-childhood (9-11). Then under the influence of pubertal gonadotropins, more primary follicles are induced to grow (12). It is the growing antral follicles of 1 mm diameter or more that produce estradiol (13). There appears to be a tremendous surge in the number of such follicles at puberty as a consequence of mature levels of gonadotropins, perhaps of maximal bioactivity (15), acting on a greater population of germ cells than is present at any other time during reproductive life.

In spite of the previous concept that "the gonad does not develop" in Turner syndrome (15), Carr and associates recognized that the ovaries are normal in early fetal life. Singh and Carr found no significant difference between the gonads of 45,X and 46,XX fetuses up to the third intrauterine month (16). Carr et al. then noted that at approximately the time granulosa cells begin to organize into follicles around germ cells and degeneration normally occurs (8), the gonocyte population of 45,X ovaries begins to fall (17). They concluded that the ovarian picture at term was highly variable in the seven cases on whom data were available. Of the 45,X newborns they reviewed, about half had streak gonads devoid of germ cells. The remainder had recognizable ovaries which contained primordial follicles, and about half of these cases had nearly normal ovaries, in which early preantral follicles were sometimes described (18). Carr and associates promulgated the concept which stands to this day, supported by Ohno and Smith (6), that the 45,X germ cells may not be able to organize primordial follicles, with degeneration of germ cells being the consequence. This high degree of follicular atresia with the accompanying increase in connective tissue at a very early age leads to the streak gonad of typical Turner syndrome.

However, in some cases germ cells appear to be lost more gradually. When this happens, ovarian development is sufficient to bring about feminization at puberty. This was first recognized by Weiss, who reported a 14½-year-old Turner syndrome patient who entered puberty at 10 years of age, experienced menarche at 11 years, and had regular menses thereafter (19). She had a 45,X karyotype in lymphocytes and skin fibroblasts. At laparoscopy, one ovary was normal in size, the other small. Both contained primitive follicles, and one contained a regressing corpus luteum.

Philip and Sele reported a similar ovarian picture in a fertile patient with 45,X Turner syndrome (20). At laparoscopy, one ovary was very small, and the biopsy contained two primary follicles and an atretic follicle, whereas the other gonad was a streak. King et al., however, reported unequivocally normal ovaries in a 45,X Turner syndrome patient of proven fertility and a normal menstrual history (21). Laparotomy revealed ovaries which were grossly normal and contained a normal complement of follicles. Mosaicism was not found in a search through four tissues.

One must conclude that there is a spectrum of ovarian development in Turner syndrome (Fig. 4). The problem is not one of lack of development of germ cells, but rather one of maintenance of the germ cell population. In most cases, the process of atresia is so tremendously accelerated that the gonads become devoid of germ cells within months to years: these become dysgenetic, devolving into streaks during this time. In about 5 to 10% of cases, it appears that the number of germ cells persisting into the second decade of life is above the critical level (about 10^4) at which sufficient antral follicles capable of secreting estrogen will emerge under gonadotropic stimulation. In the vast majority of these cases, the margin is so narrow that atresia overtakes follicular development so that ovarian failure commences at about the time puberty begins. However, in atypical cases, the number of germ cells is sufficient to result in more normal ovarian development. In most such cases, the gonads are clearly small ovaries (Fig. 3) with a clear paucity of primordial and primary follicles, and biopsy reveals a smattering of corpora albicans or a corpus luteum as evidence of past ovulatory activity (Fig. 5). In exceptional patients, the ovaries have been reported to be normal.

The basis for the rare preservation of ovarian function in Turner syndrome is unclear. It is commonly supposed that ovulatory 45,X patients may be unrecog-

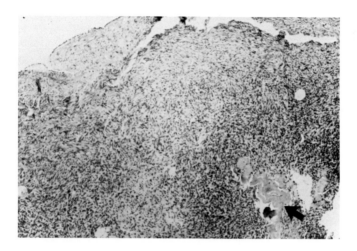

Figure 5 Biopsy specimen from the small ovary of a patient with secondary amenorrhea due to an isochromosome of the short arm of an X chromosome. The specimen contained only two primordial follicles and a corpus albicans (arrow). Photograph courtesy of Dr. Moon H. Kim.

nized mosaics. A variation on this theory has been that a germinal 46,XX mosaic cell line has disappeared over time (22). Another explanation has been that some single X germ cells may undergo mitotic nondisjunction with the formation of XX oogonia (2). The evidence, subject to ascertainment bias, that about one half of newborns with Turner syndrome have recognizable ovaries (17) and that fertile Turner's have a relatively high incidence of 45,X offspring (21) belies the possibility that germ cell survival and ovarian development have an absolute requirement for two X chromosomes. Rather, an alternate explanation seems necessary. A model is proposed in which accelerated atresia as a consequence of an absent X is mediated by interaction with an autosomal message. This model proposes that an autosome produces an "atresia factor," the production or action of which is normally blocked in the presence of two X chromosomes, but permitted in 45,X gonads. However, the occasional individual with an autosomal mutation would be unable to make or respond to such a factor even in the absence of the signal from a double-X.

THE ENDOCRINOLOGIC CHARACTERISTICS OF OVULATORY TURNER SYNDROME

The typical course of fertile Turner syndrome is to undergo normal pubertal maturation and menarche and then to go on to premature menopause. The period of normal menstrual cycles is variable; it ranges from nil to decades. The diagnosis of primary ovarian failure as the basis for the eventual secondary amenorrhea is not difficult in postmenopausal patients with the typical Turner phenotype if one knows of this syndrome. Hypergonadotropinism is the hallmark of the diagnosis of these cases (23), as it is of other cases without ovarian follicles (24). This should then direct the diagnostician to perform a karyotype in patients with unexplained premature menopause whether or not Turner stigmata are present (25).

However, random gonadotropin levels are usually normal in premenopausal women with 45,X Turner syndrome (19-21,26,27). Consequently, before menopause the diagnosis of primary ovarian insufficiency is more difficult in patients with oligomenorrhea and minimal physical stigmata. Recognition of the diagnosis is hindered because major textbooks (15,28) do not consider Turner syndrome, or other forms of primary ovarian failure for that matter, in the differential diagnosis of oligo/amenorrhea when gonadotropin levels are normal.

The gonadotropin dynamics in ovulatory Turner's seem like those in any premenopausal woman. Sherman and Korenman demonstrated that as menopause approaches, the menstrual cycles are characterized by a slight elevation of serum FSH and a blunting of plasma estradiol (29). These hormones fluctuate substantially, yet the baseline FSH and estradiol levels usually lie within the broad range of normal. An elevated responsiveness of FSH to GnRH stimulation (3,30) or clomiphene administration (5) is more characteristically found in early/partial ovarian failure than is an elevated baseline FSH.

Serum gonadotropins are sometimes normal several years after the amenorrhea of premature menopause has set in, even the presence of profound hypoestrogenism (3). We have observed this situation in a patient with 46,XXpi Turner syndrome variant. In spite of plasma estradiol below 9 pg/ml, this patient had normal baseline serum LH and FSH, but an excessive FSH responsiveness to GnRH. Her ovaries were small (1 X 1 X 2 cm), and a laparoscopic biopsy specimen (approximately 2 X 3 X 5 mm in diameters) contained only two primordial follicles and a corpus albicans (Fig. 5). To explain the absence of gonadotropin elevation in cases with rare follicles who are hypoestrogenic, we have postulated that sufficient inhibin is still being produced by the ovaries to prevent a rise in FSH. Inhibin is now established to be secreted by granulosa cells (31). In analogy to the male, in whom basal FSH levels rise to clearly abnormal levels only in the virtual absence of spermatogonia (32), it seems likely that clearly and persistently elevated FSH levels are only found in Turner syndrome and other types of partial ovarial failure in the virtual absence ($<10^2$-10^3?) of follicles.

The clinical features of the patients with ovaries have not always been straightforward. Two became pregnant after long periods of amenorrhea for which they were treated by intermittent cycling with estrogen (20,33). One of these was resistant to gonadotropin stimulation during this time (20). Another had dysfunctional uterine bleeding (27). These phenomena, however, are not unusual in menopausal women or women with premature ovarian failure from other causes (34).

GROWTH IN OVULATORY TURNER SYNDROME

It is commonly accepted that short stature is an intrinsic abnormality in Turner syndrome, rather than a result of sex hormone deficiency, because these patients grow up to be short as adults in spite of sex hormone replacement therapy. However, it could be argued that current therapeutic regimens are not optimal. Consequently, it seems important to know how well patients with ovulatory Turner syndrome fare when the pubertal growth results from endogenous sex hormone secretion.

The pubertal growth record of our patient, who lacked the statural determinants mapped to the short arm of the X (see Chapter 6), shows that growth velocity dropped to a subnormal level in the late prepubertal years and rose to approximately the third percentile during puberty (Fig. 2). She reached a subnormal final height, only 1 cm below that which had been predicted in the prepubertal years from the Bayley-Pinneau tables (35).

Table 1 Adult Height of 45,X Patients with Ovulatory Turner Syndrome

Height	Fetal outcome	Author	Reference
129.0	no pregnancy	Weiss	19
142.0	normal X 1, abortion X 1	Philip	20
138.0	normal X 1	King	21
136.0	normal X 1	Bahner	21
140.0	abortions X 2	Kohn	23
156.2[a]	normal X 1, abortion X 1	Groll	27
149.9[a]	no pregnancy	Groll	27
137.0[a]	normal X 1	Grace	33
137.5	abortion X 1	Shokier	36
140.0	normal X 1	Shokier	36

140.6 ± 7.6 (mean ± SD)

[a]Only peripheral lymphocytes were karyotyped; buccal smears were chromatin negative.

Table 2 Growth Outcome of 45,X Patients Treated with Physiologic Doses of Depot Estradiol (E_2)

ID	Pretreatment CA	Height	Pred. height	Yr. E_2 therapy	Final height	Other therapy
SS	14.5	144.3	150.4	3.2	151.9	
LM	16.1	125.2	135.3	3.5	129.8	
DH	16.2	142.2	146.6	2.5	149.9	
GK	16.6	149.9	158.2	2.1	157.0	T
SN	17.1	141.7	146.1	1.7	146.1	
JB	18.0	137.1	140.5	2.8	140.5	T
KS	12.8	122.7	132.6	4.2	135.4	A
LS	13.7	122.2	137.4	3.8	132.1	T
NR	14.2	135.1	144.8	4.5	148.2	T
RM	14.7	142.5	148.1	3.5	150.1	T
MA	14.7	136.4	145.5	3.7	144.5	T
SM	14.8	132.3	141.7	4.8	144.3	T
	15.3 ± 1.5	136.0 ± 8.9	143.9 ± 7.0	3.4 ± 0.9	144.2 ± 8.3	

ID = patient identification; CA = chronologic age (yr), height (cm), and predicted height by Bayley-Pinneau method before steroid therapy; other therapy = one to two 6-month courses of steroid given intercurrently (T = depot testosterone in average monthly dose 28 mg/m² (39); A = oxandrolone 0.1 mg/kg/day).
Source: Ref 37.

Although no pubertal growth data are available, the final heights reported in 45,X ovulatory Turner syndrome have been tabulated (Table 1). They are compared to final heights of the 45,X patients with typical Turner syndrome whom we have treated using a physiologic sex hormone replacement regimen (Table 2) (37,38). It can be seen that spontaneous puberty did not appear to normalize their height or to improve it above that which can be achieved therapeutically.

SUMMARY AND CONCLUSIONS

The ovaries are normal in early fetal life in Turner syndrome. Atresia, which normally commences in mid-fetal life to become the predominant fate of follicles, commences at an accelerated rate in Turner syndrome when primordial follicles do not efficiently organize about the oöcytes. Nevertheless, at birth some patients with Turner syndrome have recognizable ovaries. In the vast majority of cases the high rate of follicular atresia devolves into the dysgenetic streak gonad typical of Turner syndrome early during the first decade of life.

However, in some cases follicular loss is more gradual, and varying numbers of ovarian follicles persist longer.

The number of follicles is sometimes sufficiently great that antral follicles capable of secreting estrogen emerge at puberty. This results in initiation of feminization in perhaps 5 to 10% of cases of Turner syndrome. Usually the number of antral follicles is at a menopausal level at this time and puberty does not progress to menarche.

In rare cases, enough ovarian development persists that the Turner syndrome patient undergoes normal pubertal maturation (with a modest growth spurt) and menarche, and then goes on to premature menopause. The duration of normal menstrual cycles in the interim is highly variable and ranges from nil to decades. If it is long enough, fertility is possible. Fertile patients apparently have a relatively high incidence of fetal wastage and chromosomal nondisjunctional abnormalities, including both Turner syndrome and Down syndrome (21).

Ovulatory Turner syndrome patients are usually found to have small ovaries with a paucity of follicles. Endocrinologic findings are characteristically similar to those of the premenopause: baseline gonadotropin levels are normal, even in the face of varying degrees of hypoestrogenism, and the FSH responses to GnRH and clomiphene stimulation tests are exaggerated.

The evidence, though scanty, suggests that ovarian development in Turner syndrome can (rarely) develop in the absence of two X chromosomes. To explain the development of ovaries in apparently 45,X individuals, a model is postulated in which the double-X constitution is normally necessary to inhibit the production or function of an autosomally controlled atresia factor.

Because there is currently not a means of determining prepubertally which patients with even 45,X Turner syndrome have gonadal dysgenesis, except possibly for elevated FSH levels in infancy (2), counseling of these patients should not convey anticipation of inevitable gonadal failure and infertility. In fact, it may ultimately prove possible to collect eggs from some of these patients in the prepubertal years and store them for eventual in vitro fertilization.

ACKNOWLEDGMENTS

The author's studies were supported in part by USPHS grants MO1 RR-00055 and HD-06308. The manuscript was typed by Jean Moore.

REFERENCES

1. Lippe B. Primary ovarian failure. In Kaplan SA, ed. Clinical Pediatric and Adolescent Endocrinology. Philadelphia: WB Saunders, 1982, 269-299.
2. Grumbach MM, Conte FA. Disorders of sexual differentiation. In Wilson JD, Foster DW, eds. Williams' Textbook of Endocrinology, 7th ed. Philadelphia: WB Saunders, 1985:312-404.

3. Razdan AK, Rosenfield RL, Kim MH. Endocrinologic characteristics of partial ovarian failure. J Clin Endocrinol Metab 1976; 43:449-452.
4. Tanner JM, Davies PSW. Clinical longitudinal standards for height and height velocity for North American children. J Pediatr 1985; 107:317-329.
5. Navot D, Rosenwaks Z, Margalioth EJ. Prognostic assessment of female fecundity. Lancet 1987; 2:645-647.
6. Ohno S, Smith JB. Role of fetal follicular cells in meiosis of mammalian oocytes. Cytogenetics 1964; 3:324-333.
7. Gartler SM, Andina R, Gant N. Ontogeny of X-chromosome inactivation in the female germ line. Exp Cell Res 1975; 91:454-458.
8. Baker TG. A quantitative and cytological study of germ cells in human ovaries. Proc Roy Soc B 1963; 158:417-433.
9. Block E. Quantitative morphological investigations of the follicular system in women. Acta Anatom 1952; 14:108-123.
10. Block E. A quantitative morphological investigation of the follicular system in newborn female infants. Acta Anatom 1953; 17:201-206.
11. Peters H, Byskov AG, Grunsted J. Follicular growth in fetal and prepubertal ovaries of humans and other primates. Clin Endocrinol Metab 1978; 7:469-483.
12. Ross GT. Gonadotropins and preantral follicular maturation in women. Fertil Steril 1974; 25:522-543.
13. McNatty KP, Smith DM, Makris A, Osathanondh R, Ryan KJ. The microenvironment of the human antral follicle: interrelationships among the steroid levels in antral fluid, the population of granulosa cells and the status of the oocyte in vivo and in vitro. J Clin Endocrinol Metab 1979; 49:851-860.
14. Lucky AW, Rich BH, Rosenfield RL, Fang VS, Roche-Bender N. LH bioactivity increases more than immunoreactivity during puberty. J Pediatr 1980; 97:205-213.
15. Jaffe RB. Disorders of sexual development. In Yen SSC, Jaffe RB, eds. Reproductive Endocrinology, 2nd ed. Philadelphia: W.B. Saunders, 1986: 283-312.
16. Singh RP, Carr DH. The anatomy and histology of XO human embryos and fetuses. Anat Rec 1966; 155:369-384.
17. Carr DH, Haggar RA, Hart AG. Germ cells in the ovaries of XO female infants. Am J Clin Path 1968; 49:521-526.
18. Conen PE, Glass IH. 45/XO Turner's syndrome in the newborn: report of two cases. J Clin Endocrin Metab 1963; 23:1-10.
19. Weiss L. Additional evidence of gradual loss of germ cells in the pathogenesis of streak ovaries in Turner's syndrome. J Med Genet 1971; 8:540-544.
20. Philip J, Sele V. 45,XO Turner's syndrome without evidence of mosaicism in a patient with two pregnancies. Acta Obstet Gynecol Scand 1976; 55: 283-286.
21. King CR, Magenis E, Bennett S. Pregnancy and the Turner syndrome. Obstet Gynec 1978; 52:617-624.

22. Taysi K, Kohn G, Mellman W. Mosaic mongolism. II. Cytogenetic studies. J Pediat 1970; 76:880–885.

23. Kohn G, Yarkoni S, Cohen MM. Two conceptions in a 45,X woman. Am J Med Genet 1980; 5:339–343.

24. Goldenberg RC, Grodin JM, Rodbard D, Ross GT. Gonadotropins in women with amenorrhea. Am J Obstet Gynecol 1973; 116:1003–1009.

25. Krauss CM, Turksoy N, Atkins L, McLaughlin C, Brown LG, Page DC. Familial premature ovarian failure due to an interstitial deletion of the long arm of the X chromosome. N Engl J Med 1987; 317:125–131.

26. Nakashima I, Robinson A. Fertility in a 45,X female. Pediatrics 1971; 47:770–772.

27. Groll M, Cooper M. Menstrual function in Turner's syndrome. Obstet Gynecol 1976; 47:225–226.

28. Ross GT. Disorders of the ovary and female reproductive tract. In Wilson JD, Foster DW, eds. William's Textbook of Endocrinology, 7th ed. Philadelphia: W.B. Saunders, 1985:206–258.

29. Sherman BM, Korenman SG. Hormonal characteristics of the human menstrual cycle throughout reproductive life. J Clin Invest 1975; 55:699–706.

30. Donald RA, Espiner EA. The plasma gonadotropin response to gonadotropin-releasing hormone in patients with primary hypogonadism. J Clin Endocrinol Metab 1974; 39:364–369.

31. Hsueh AJW, Adashi EY, Jones PBC, Welsh Jr TH. Hormonal regulation of the differentiation of cultured granulosa cells. Endocr Rev 1984; 5:76–127.

32. Baker HWG, Bremner WJ, Burger HG, DeKretser DM, Dulmanis A, Eddie LW, Hudson B, Keogh EJ, Lee VWK, Rennie GC. Testicular control of follicle-stimulating hormone secretion. Rec Progr Horm Res 1976; 32:429–469.

33. Grace HJ, Quinlan DK, Edge WEB. 45,X lymphocyte karyotype in a fertile woman. Am J Obstet Gynecol 1973; 115:279–282.

34. Johnson Jr TR, Peterson EP. Gonadotropin-induced pregnancy following "premature ovarian failure." Fertil Steril 1979; 31:351–352.

35. Zachmann M, Sobradillo B, Frank M, Frisch H, Prader A. Bayley-Pinneau, Roche-Wainer-Thissen and Tanner height predictions in normal children and in patients with pathological conditions. J Pediatr 1978; 93:749–755.

36. Shokier MHK. Pregnancy in five women with 45,X/46,XX and 45,X/47,XXX gonadal dysgenesis. Birth Defects: Original Article Series, 1978; 14(6c):171–184.

37. Rosenfield RL, Fang VS. The effects of prolonged physiologic estradiol therapy on the maturation of hypogonadal teenagers. J Pediatr 1974; 85:830–837.

38. Rosenfield RL. Low-dose testosterone effect on somatic growth. Pediatr 1986; 77:853–857.

DISCUSSION

DR. ARTHUR ROBINSON: In any of those cases where the Turner syndrome had a real ovum that you looked at, was it biopsied and was the karyotype checked?

DR. ROBERT ROSENFIELD: There are 11 cases in which the karyotype of 45,XO was shown in at least two tissues, and in 3 of the cases the karyotype was only done in blood, but they had chromatin-negative buccal smears.

DR. ROBINSON: But in those tissues was one of those tissues the ovary?

DR. ROSENFIELD: One of them was skin in most cases. I believe one of them or 2 had ovaries as well.

DR. GORDON CUTLER: I wondered if the reports in the literature on the adult height of these girls who had spontaneous puberty included the midparental heights.

DR. ROSENFIELD: There is very little information about that.

DR. CUTLER: It is potentially important if estrogen is harmful. On the other hand, when it is only a few centimeters, it is possible that if a girl were on the tall side and had relatively taller parents and went through puberty, then that group might be missed or might be less likely to ever come to diagnosis, because they went through puberty. So there is a possible ascertainment bias, and parental height might be helpful if the reports would include it.

DR. MELVIN GRUMBACH: We have had 5 patients, which Dr. Conte is going to discuss later, who went through spontaneous puberty and were short; their mean height was in the range of the untreated to a little bit lower.

Dr. Robinson is at the National Jewish Center and the University of Colorado Health Science Center, Denver, Colorado. Dr. Rosenfield is at the University of Chicago Pritzker School of Medicine, Chicago, Illinois. Dr. Cutler is at the National Institute of Child Health and Human Development, Bethesda, Maryland. Drs. Grumbach and Conte are at the University of California at San Francisco, San Francisco, California. Dr. Crowley is at Massachusetts General Hospital, Boston, Massachusetts. Dr. Lippe is at the University of California at Los Angeles School of Medicine. Dr. Simpson is at the University of Tennessee at Memphis, Memphis, Tennessee.

DR. ROSENFIELD: Do you know their midparental height?

DR. GRUMBACH: Mean parental height correlates just as it does in all the other instances of Turner's syndrome.

DR. ROSENFIELD: The only other thing I would say in response to Dr. Cutler, too, is that the 10 patients reported end up in size comparable to the other Turner's.

DR. GRUMBACH: It does correlate in those 5 patients; it correlates just as it would in the bigger group.

DR. BILL CROWLEY: Just a comment and a question: Patricia Donohoe at our institution has done a number of ovarian biopsies in children with Turner's with horseshoe kidneys and a variety of GU abnormalities and confirms the impression that you have in your 7 patients, that many of these have relatively normal ovarian complement of oocytes in their ovaries, particularly, the younger you are, the more normal the ovary looks. I wondered if you had taken your children and looked at them over the developmental spectrum to see if that correlated in your population, confirming your impression of basically menopause before menarche. Secondly, I wondered what was the database for the pregnancies in the Turner's, being, if I understood it, mosaics having a preponderance over 45,XO. Would you review the information on that?

DR. ROSENFIELD: The patients with the isochromosomes of X that I presented here constitute my total personal experience. The conclusions I reached were based on reading the literature that is available. So I cannot answer a lot of your questions. It is very theoretical.

DR. CROWLEY: But the database for your assertions.

DR. ROSENFIELD: The data about the outcome of pregnancies is from a paper by Reyes et al. (Am J Obstet Gynec 1976, 126:668) and another by Dewhurst (J Med Genetics 1978, 15:132). Something like 15% of the pregnancies result in 45,XO offspring; a similar number result in Down's syndrome. That is on the negative side if you talk about getting ova from these people. There is a high frequency of spontaneous abortions as well, but a number of the patients that are reported have normal offspring.

DR. BARBARA LIPPE: To add to Dr. Cutler's comment, or at least to comment on that, in the collaborative study that I am a part of in Turner syndrome, one of our 70 patients went into spontaneous puberty and is rapidly approaching final height, which will be less than the mean of the patients who are being treated in the study, and her midparental height is tall. So she, too, will be shorter.

DR. JOE L. SIMPSON: I think there is a major ascertainment bias in looking at the outcome, and it was pointed out in Dewhurst's paper and some reviews that I have done as well, and that is very often the abnormality in the mother is detected only after the child with a spontaneous abortion or a congenital anomaly is ascertained. So if you start with an abnormal population and you go back, it is very difficult to make a real statement one way or the other. In support of that, you can actually go back and look at the ascertainment. If patients are ascertained because of primary amenorrhea or secondary amenorrhea and then you follow the offspring, in my opinion there is no increase in congenital anomalies. But if the index case is abnormal and then you look at the parent, that is the one in which you very often find typically a mosaic in the mother and a congenital anomaly in the child. And I would submit that if the congenital anomaly in the child had not occurred, you never would have gone back and looked at the parent to begin with.

DR. FELIX CONTE: I sort of look at this a little differently. I think we all agree that girls with Turner syndrome have what we think is normal germ cell migration and normal function, from the studies of Carr and other people. Jerseck has shown very nicely in histologic studies that what happens apparently is that the oocytes do not get surrounded by granulosa cells, and so they do not get saved, as he calls it. They go through meiosis, and there is a tremendous atretic rate. And I do not believe that they are born with normal ovaries, even any percentage, because when we look at their gonadotrophins, they go up immediately. If you follow a series of girls with Turner syndrome, as we have done, they have a marked rise in FSH level as early as 10 days of age. I think that the number of oocytes that they have is markedly reduced. They may have ovaries, but they certainly do not have normal ovaries. You can follow that along through infancy and childhood, but I find it hard to accept that they have normal ovaries at birth.

DR. ROSENFIELD: I refer you to the paper of Conan and Glass in JCEM 1963. They have nice pictures and they say the ovary is normal size, and they show you pictures, and they describe preantral follicles. I am not claiming that the majority do. Carr also reported that his newborns had ovaries that were of normal size with a lot of empty follicles. They had a huge rate of atresia, but there were a few. I am not one to claim that it is all or none as a lot of us have been led to believe.

DR. CONTE: That is agreeable. The question is with the term "normalcy." We have also seen patients who are menstruating, who stopped menstruating, whose gonadotrophins go way up. And you say, well that is it. But no, they come back down again and they begin to menstruate again. I think they recruit a whole new set of follicles. As you know, you do not have to be afollicular to have high gonadotrophins. So there may be a few follicles, but I doubt whether that is normal.

DR. ROSENFIELD: Probably if you have less than 10,000 follicles when you should have a million, your gonadotrophins go up. In those patients who have 15,000, their gonadotrophins are going to be normal.

DR. CUTLER: I have often wondered whether these girls have any phenotypic consequence prepubertally of their presumed estrogen deficiency, and I wondered if the bone age has been looked at in those who go into spontaneous puberty and whether they have the bone age delay that is typical of the normal Turner patient.

DR. ROSENFIELD: There are no bone ages in the literature ascertained by gynecologists and obstetricians.

DR. PRADER: The few ones we have seen with spontaneous and abortive puberty had a markedly delayed bone age, similar to constitutional delay of growth in puberty.

12

Spontaneous Growth in Ullrich-Turner Syndrome

Michael B. Ranke and Jürgen R. Bierich

Children's Hospital, University of Tübingen, Tübingen, Federal Republic of Germany

Peter Stubbe

Children's Hospital, University of Göttingen, Göttingen, Federal Republic of Germany

Frank Majewski

University of Düsseldorf, Düsseldorf, Federal Republic of Germany

INTRODUCTION

Growth in Ullrich-Turner Syndrome (UTS) can be divided into four phases: (1) Intrauterine growth is retarded; (2) growth is normal up to a bone age of about 2 years, with a tendency to compensate for the loss in growth during intrauterine life; (3) stunting of growth is severe during childhood; (4) after a bone age of about 10 years—the time when puberty normally starts—the growth phase is prolonged, but total height gain is not essentially reduced. Based on 150 of our own cases, whose spontaneous growth was observed, standards of height and height velocity (means, standard deviations) were calculated, which may serve to mathematically analyze the spontaneous growth and growth during treatment in these patients. The auxological characteristics in UTS do not support the assumption that growth hormone deficiency plays a primary role in the pathogenesis of the growth disorder.

In 1938 H. H. Turner (1) gave a detailed description of a syndrome whose essential features had been reported by Ullrich in 1930 (2). In Ullrich's index case, a lady from Munich, the karyotype was later proven to be 45,X (3). Among the three main problem areas of the Ullrich-Turner Syndrome (UTS), namely dysmorphic feature, gonadal dysgenesis, and short stature, the affected patients often consider short stature to be the feature most disadvantageous in everyday life. Any attempt to influence growth in UTS has to begin with an analysis of the natural growth process. In recent years, several authors have reported about growth in larger series with UTS (4-8). We have published the German experience based on 150 cases who never received therapy for growth promotion or induction of sex characteristics (9,10) from three large centers located in the northern, western, and southern part of our country. The aim of this report is to discuss these data in conjunction with the findings of others and to emphasize a few aspects of auxology which are of importance for the analysis of the growth process in such patients.

PATIENTS AND METHODS

Detailed descriptions of the methods applied are given elsewhere (9,10). The analysis or our data is based on 150 patients of which 90 (60%) showed the "classical" karyotype—45,X—and the remaining either mosaicism of the 45,X/ 46,XX type and/or structural abnormalities of the second X chromosome. The data on height (length < 2 years of age), weight and bone age (determined by the TW2-RUS method (11)) were determined in a mixed longitudinal/cross-sectional fashion, while results on height velocity were based entirely on longitudinal data.

WEIGHT AND LENGTH AT BIRTH

It is a common observation that newborns with UTS are too small for gestational age. In our group of patients born near term (> 38th week of gestation) a mean weight of 2828 ± 573 g ($n = 57$) and a mean length of 48.3 ± 3.2 cm ($n = 49$) was observed. This represents a reduction of these parameters of about one SD below the mean of the normal population. These data are in the same order of magnitude as seen by other authors (4-6). As is illustrated in Fig. 1, weight and length are also reduced in prematurely born patients. In 25 of 71 (35%), newborn weight was below the 10th percentile, and in 18 of 69 (26%), newborn length was below the 10th percentile. Thus, smallness at birth is common but not obligatory. In addition, our data do not point to a difference between cases with the "classical" karyotype and with other characteristic chromosomal abnormalities.

HEIGHT (LENGTH)

Single height (length) measurements ($n = 348$) in relation to the normal ranges (12) are illustrated in Fig. 2. Means and standard deviations for height, which were derived by smoothing of the raw data (10), are given in Table 1. Up to a chronological age of 10 years, mean height remains at about two SD below the

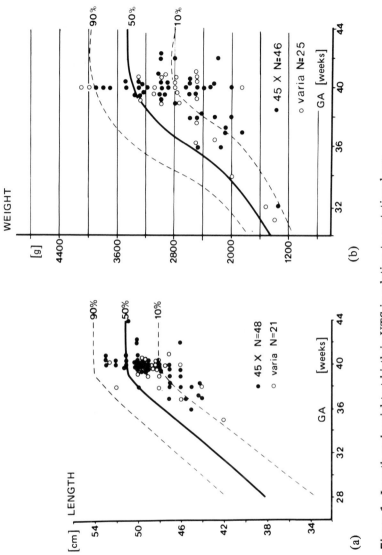

Figure 1 Length and weight at birth in UTS in relation to gestational age.

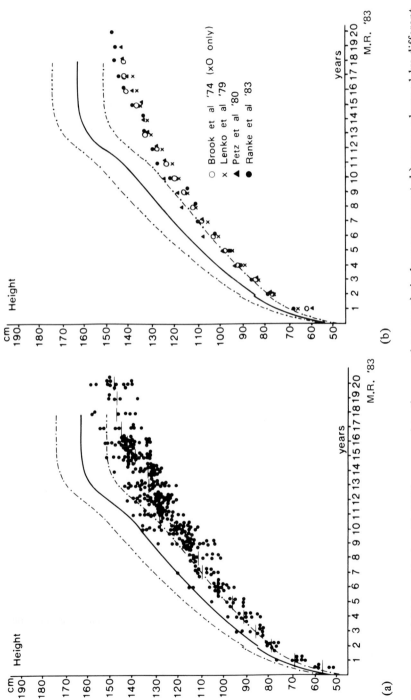

Figure 2 Height in patients with UTS compared to the normal range: a) single measurement; b) means observed by different investigators.

Table 1 Height, Bone Age, and Height Velocity in Ullrich-Turner Syndrome

Age (yr)	Height mean/SD (cm)	Bone age[a] mean (yr)	Height velocity[b] mean/SD (cm/yr)
2	77.30/2.60	1.10	7.80/1.95
3	85.10/3.50	1.90	6.45/1.61
4	91.55/3.75	2.90	5.70/1.43
5	97.25/4.00	3.90	5.25/1.31
6	102.50/4.20	4.90	4.85/1.21
7	107.35/4.40	5.90	4.55/1.14
8	111.90/4.60	6.90	4.30/1.08
9	116.20/4.75	7.90	4.10/1.03
10	120.30/4.95	8.90	3.90/0.98
11	124.20/5.10	9.90	3.75/0.94
12	127.95/5.25	10.85	3.50/0.88
13	131.45/5.40	11.75	3.20/0.80
14	134.65/5.50	12.55	2.90/0.73
15	137.55/5.65	13.25	2.55/0.64
16	140.10/5.75	13.80	2.10/0.54
17	142.20/5.85	14.30	1.70/0.43
18	143.90/5.90	14.70	1.10/0.28
19	145.00/5.95	15.00	
+19	146.30/6.10		

[a](TW2-RUS).
[b]Height velocity data are centered at chronological ages depicted 0.5 yr.

normal mean. Then height deviation increases further, reaching a nadir of about −4 SD at an approximate age of 14 years. Thereafter, growth is followed by a slow approach toward the normal centiles. Commonly, adult height appears not to be reached before the end of the second decade of life. In 14 adult patients, we observed an average height of 146.8 ± 5.8 cm, which corresponds to 2.6 SD below the mean of normal adult females (12). The data on height during childhood observed in some of the recent large series (4-6,13,14) are remarkably similar. There is some variance, however, in the assumption of what the mean adult height in UTS is (9). While the mean adult height observed in our series of about 146 cm is similar to the figure reported by Sybert (13) and Nielsen (14), the summarized figure calculated by Lyon et al. (8) on the basis of 138 cases was 142.9 ± 7.3 cm. There may be several reasons for the published differences. In addition to the obvious possibility of ethnic and environmental differences between populations, that may account for the observed variation, methodological problems may also be involved: One problem relates to the relatively small number of adult patients on which the given figures are mostly based. This also accounts for our sample. The second problem may be related to differences in age of the patients, when adult stature is assumed. It should be considered that in normals some growth may still be observed until the early twenties. There is also some indication for a secular growth trend (approx. 1.5 cm per decade) existing for the patients with UTS. Since the spontaneous height of UTS reached in a given population is of utmost importance for the interpretation of results obtained through the various modes of treatment under investigation, every effort must be made to collect more data in individuals so far untreated.

Similar to other reports (8), in our sample the coefficient of variation of mean height at a given age averaged $4.66 \pm 0.88\%$, a figure only slightly higher than the one seen in the normal population. This observation appears to suggest that the yet unknown factors causing short stature in UTS do not completely derange the normal structures of growth regulation. There is also another line of evidence supporting such an argument. Brook et al. (4) have shown that final height in "classical" UTS is positively correlated with midparental height. Our own data ($n = 21; r = 0.375; p < 0.05$) give equivalent results.

One of the areas of ongoing discussion relates to the question of whether or not patients with the "classical" karyotype reach a different adult stature in comparison to those with other chromosomal abnormalities (7,9). Our data are in favor of the view that there is no difference, and the data from the literature in our view make no strong case for the existence of such a difference. However, this controversy needs to be settled on the basis of further empirical evidence.

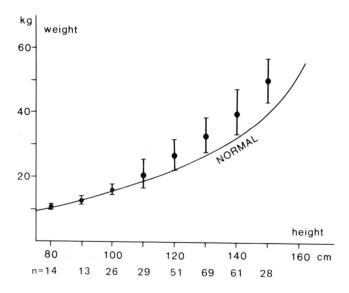

Figure 3   Weight to height ratio in UTS.

WEIGHT

It is the general impression from clinical experience that patients with UTS are somewhat compact and less lean than normal girls. This impression is substantiated by the finding that the weight to height ratio (Fig. 3) ascends with increasing age, reaching a level of significance at about an age of 10 years, when these girls average 120 cm in height. As far as we can say today, this relative increase in weight is caused by an increase in subcutaneous fat. We do not know what the reason for this developmental change in body shape is. However, obesity must be considered whenever data on growth hormone secretion are discussed, since, on one hand, growth hormone deficiency is accompanied by obesity and, on the other hand, obesity itself causes an impairment of growth hormone secretion.

HEIGHT VELOCITY

Single measurements of height (length) velocity are depicted in Figure 4. Means and standard deviations of smoothed data are given in Table 1. During postnatal growth until an age of about 3 years, length (height) velocities are in the normal range. Thereafter height velocity continuously deviates from the normal mean, and at about the age of 10 years falls short of the lowest limit of normal. Due to the failure of puberty to occur, there is no adolescent growth spurt, but growth continues over a longer span of time at low rates. Our data show striking similarities to those of other groups which are based on longitudinal data (4,5).

BONE AGE

Bone age (BA) determinations in UTS pose particular difficulties, since there are always structural abnormalities of the bone. In addition, there is a subjective element of the investigator influencing the ratings. Moreover, presently there are not many systematic investigations on bone age in UTS, and most investigators tend to apply the Greulich and Pyle system. Since we believe that the TW2 system allows a more accurate reading, we decided to apply this method. Based on our data and those published by Brook et al. (4), which were found to be almost identical, postnatal bone age development can be divided into three phases (Fig. 5). (Mean bone age levels compared to chronological age (CA) are given in Table 1.) After birth, up to an age of about 3 years, there is a decline in bone age. The ratio of BA versus CA stays below unity. From a chronological age (CA) of 3 years to about 12 years BA progresses normally at a rate of one year per year CA. After a CA of 12 years there is a continuous decline in bone age progression over CA with epiphyseal closure generally not reached before the end of the teens.

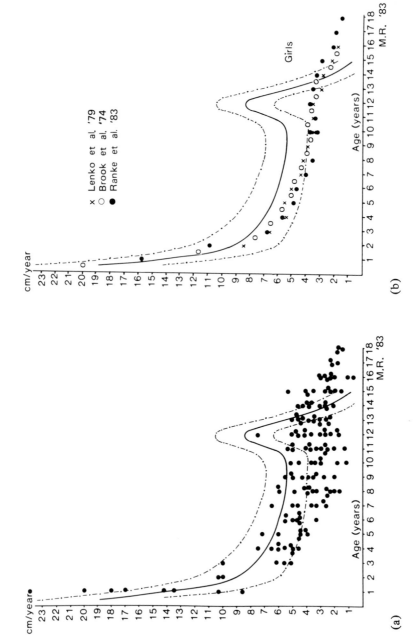

Figure 4 Height velocity in patients with UTS compared to the normal range: a) single measurements; b) means observed by different investigators.

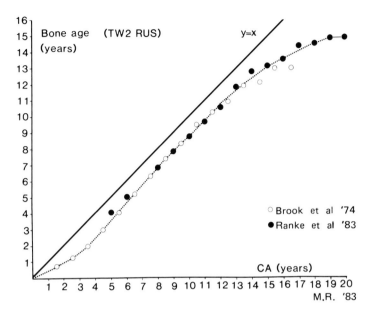

Figure 5 Bone age (TW2-RUS) (smoothed means) compared to chronological age (CA) in patients with UTS.

Since bone age is the most relevant parameter for growth development, growth parameters have to be analyzed in respect to this parameter and not only in respect to CA. By calculating data on height (length) and height (length) velocity per year bone age rather than CA, a somewhat different picture emerges (Fig. 6): During the first two bone age years, height (length) and its velocity stay within the upper normal range. From a bone age 2 (ca. 3 years CA) years to a bone age of 10 years (ca. 12 years CA) the dramatic decrease of these parameters becomes apparent. However, after the BA of 10 years the pattern of the height curve resembles normality, since an apparent height velocity spurt emerges. This apparent growth spurt is low in magnitude and appears to be somewhat delayed. Thus, it is different from a normal pubertal growth spurt, which is usually more pronounced and occurs—in contrast to boys—in girls early in puberty, peaking at a bone age of 11 to 12 years.

DISCUSSION

The establishment of standards of essential auxological parameters in UTS, as we have attempted to do on the basis of our data, is probably useful for the medical community. The application of such standards allows one to analyze

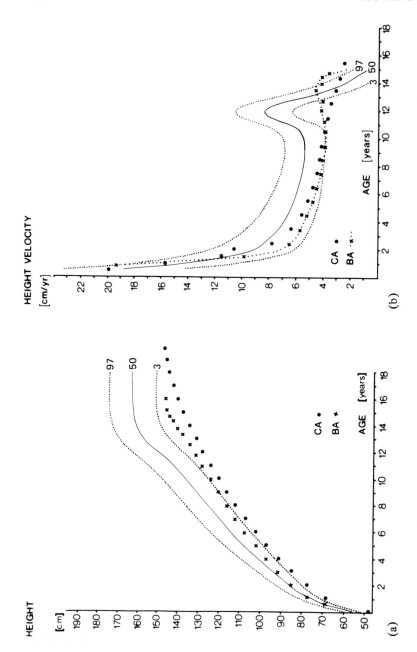

Figure 6 Mean height a) and height velocity b) in patients with UTS based on chronological age (CA) and bone age (BA) compared to normal ranges.

growth data of an individual patient in a mode more meaningful than if standards of normally growing females are used for comparison. In particular, standard deviation scores can be calculated, which allow the handling of data from an individual patient or from a group of patients at different ages and during treatment trials with growth-promoting agents. Nevertheless, one should keep in mind that such "standards" are derived from still too small a sample. We certainly need more data on the essential parameters, such as height, weight, height velocity, and bone age, but we also need information on other parameters, such as head circumference, size of hands and feet, sitting height etc., although it is increasingly difficult to collect data from untreated patients.

In addition to just describing the natural growth in patients with UTS, we also need to ask what such data may possibly add to our understanding of the pathogenesis of the underlying growth disorder. In order to make an attempt towards this problem, the essential features of growth in UTS can be divided into four phases of growth (Table 2): (1) intra-uterine growth retardation; (2) a phase of postnatal growth up to the age of 3 years, when growth rate is normal—during this phase there is a delay in bone maturation; (3) a phase of decreasing height velocities between the ages of 3 and 12 years, when bone age progression is normal; and (4) after an age of 12 years (BA 10 years) the growth phase is prolonged with low growth rates, decelerating bone age progression, and a relative increase in weight.

We know very little about intrauterine growth, except that it is certainly diminished during the third trimester of pregnancy, that length and weight are approximately equally effected, and that bone age maturation is probably not impaired. During postnatal life there are two phases with a concomitant retardation of bone age: one during early childhood and another during the absence of puberty. We know that during both phases gonadotropins are higher than normal, which allows one to speculate whether the phenomenon of delay in osseous maturation is caused by inappropriately low secretion of ovarian steroids. Despite the similarities of the two phases, there are essential differences. These differences are more obvious by looking at the gain in height at

Table 2 Auxological Characteristics in Ullrich-Turner Syndrome During Different Phases of Life

Phase of life	Height velocity	Weight/ height	Bone age progression	Total height gain
Intrauterine	low	normal	normal (?)	low
Infancy–3 years	normal	normal	low	high/normal
Childhood	low	normal	normal	low
"Adolescence"	low	high	low	low/normal

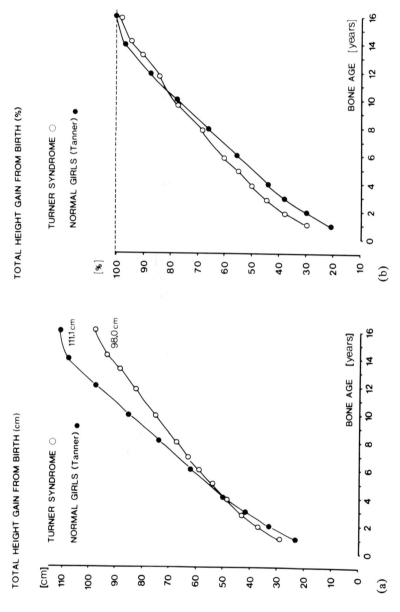

Figure 7 Mean height gain after birth in patients with UTS and in normal girls during development. a) In terms of centimeters; b) in terms of percentage of total postnatal height gain.

different phases of development: On the average, normal girls grow 111.1 cm from birth to adulthood (12), while patients with UTS grow only 98 cm. The difference in total growth is, thus, 13 cm, while the mean difference in final height is 16 cm in UTS. The total mean height gain after birth in UTS is higher than normal (Fig. 7) up to a bone age of 3 years but smaller thereafter. Mean height gain during development expressed as the percentage of total height gain (Fig. 7) is higher up to a bone age of 10 years, but thereafter it is similar to the normal figures. This suggests that in UTS during early postnatal life there is a tendency to compensate for intrauterine loss of growth. After a bone age of about 10 years the percentage of mean total height gain (Fig. 8) and the relative gain in height (Fig. 7) are approximately identical in normal girls and in UTS. The difference of 16 cm between adult height in normal girls and in UTS is already reached at a bone age of about 9 years. This shows that, while there is a relative gain in height during the second phase of growth (childhood), during the phase of absence of puberty there is only a minor loss in height. Similar results will be obtained if such an analysis is made using other standards for normal girls. Thus, height is essentially lost before birth and during childhood. It is not

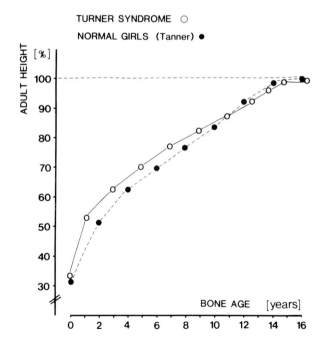

Figure 8 Percentage of adult height reached during development in patients with UTS and in normal girls.

clear which other growth disorders, whose pathogenesis is firmly established, show a similar growth pattern. Certainly, the pattern of growth in children with congenital growth hormone deficiency is different during all of the mentioned four phases of growth. Only if growth hormone deficiency is accompanied by gonadotropin deficiency do there appear to be similarities during the phase of absence of puberty. During this phase, however, total growth is not essentially reduced in UTS, as it is in untreated growth hormone deficiency. In summarizing, it seems fair to state that the growth pattern in UTS shows no resemblance to growth hormone deficiency. This statement, however, does not exclude that in UTS appropriate doses of exogenous growth hormone will improve final height.

REFERENCES

1. Turner HH. A syndrome of infantilism, congenital webbed neck, and cubitus valgus. Endocrinology 1938; 23:566–574.
2. Ullrich O. Über typische Kombinationsbilder multipler Abartung. Z Kinderheilk 1930; 49:271–276.
3. Butenandt O. Personal communication.
4. Brook CGD. Mürset G, Zachmann M, Prader A. Growth in children with 45,XO Turner's syndrome. Arch Dis Child 1974; 49:789–795.
5. Lenko HL, Peerhentupa J, Söderholm A. Growth in Turner's syndrome: spontaneous and fluoxymesterone stimulated. Acta Paediatr Scand (Suppl) 1979; 277:57–63.
6. Pelz L, Timm D, Eyermann E, Hinkel GK, Kirchner M, Verron G. Body height in Turner's syndrome. Clin Genet 1982; 22:62–66.
7. Park E, Bailey JD, Cowell CA. Growth and maturation of patients with Turner's syndrome. Pediatr Res 1983; 17:1–7.
8. Lyon AJ, Preece MA, Grant DB. Growth curve for girls with Turner Syndrome. Arch Dis Childhood 1985; 60:932–935.
9. Ranke MB, Pflüger H, Rosendahl W, Stubbe P, Enders H, Bierich JR, Majewski F. Turner syndrome: Spontaneous growth in 150 cases and review of the literature. Eur J Pediatr 1983; 141:81–88.
10. Ranke MB. Spontanes Wachstum beim Turner-Syndrom. Normalwerte und Somatogramme nach dem 2. Lebensjahr. der kinderarzt 1985; 16: 1205–1208.
11. Tanner JM, Whitehouse RH, Marshall WM, Healy MJR, Goldstein. Assessment of skeletal maturity and prediction of adult height (TW2 method). Academic Press, New York, 1975.
12. Tanner JM, Whitehouse RH, Takaishi M. Standards from birth to maturity for height, weight, height velocity and weight velocity, British children. Arch Dis Child 1966; 41:454–471, 613–635.
13. Nielsen J, Nyborg H, Dahl G. Turner's syndrome. Acta Jutlandica XLV, Medicine Series 21, 1977.
14. Sybert VP. Adult height in Turner syndrome with and without androgen therapy. J Pediatr 1984; 104:365–369.

13

Final Height in Turner Syndrome With and Without Gonadal Function

Itsuro Hibi and Ayako Tanae

National Children's Hospital, Tokyo, Japan

INTRODUCTION

In a series of 123 patients with Turner syndrome, 48 patients born in or prior to 1970 lacked gonadal function, 26 patients entered puberty spontaneously, and the remaining 49 patients were too young for gonadal function to be assessed. As 13 patients with spontaneous puberty were born in or prior to 1970, the incidence of spontaneous puberty in Turner syndrome was calculated to be 21.3%. Mean final height was 135.4 + 4.2 cm in 17 patients with spontaneous puberty, significantly shorter than the 141.9 + 3.6 cm in 45 patients without gonadal function. Of 17 patients with spontaneous puberty, 6 with a history of prepubertal anabolic steroid use had a final height significantly shorter and were significantly younger on average at menarche than 11 patients without such a history. It was concluded that the therapeutic use of anabolic steroids may decrease final height in approximately 20% of Turner syndrome patients. The percentage of the presence of the normal 46,XX cell line in karyotype was almost identical in patients with and without gonadal function, though 45,X monosomy was less frequently found in patients with spontaneous puberty. Serum FSH and LH and their responses to gonadotropin releasing hormone studied in the prepubertal period had very limited value in predicting gonadal function at puberty.

The influences of such factors as birth weight, parental heights, karyotype, estrogen treatment and the timing of its introduction, androgen treatment, and even secular trends (1-8) on the final height of girls with Turner syndrome have been discussed. Although it is uncertain whether androgen treatment is beneficial or not in increasing final height, it is believed generally that it has at least no adverse effect on final height (1,4). However, it is not known whether this belief also holds true in patients with Turner syndrome whose gonadal function has been preserved, nor whether the presence of gonadal function itself can influence final height, nor has it been reported what percentage of patients with Turner syndrome enter puberty spontaneously, although it is known that there exists a very wide spectrum in Turner syndrome, from complete failure of gonadal function to fertility. Lippe et al. and Lyon et al. separately reported patients who experienced menarche spontaneously (1-3), but the exact incidence of spontaneous puberty in Turner syndrome cannot be calculated from these reports because the age distribution of all subjects was not noted in these studies.

The present study was undertaken to clarify the exact incidence of spontaneous puberty in Turner syndrome, the influence of gonadal function on final height, and the effect of an anabolic steroid use on final height in patients with Turner syndrome whose gonadal function was preserved.

SUBJECTS AND METHODS

Subjects

The subjects were 123 patients for whom a diagnosis of Turner syndrome had been given between 1966 and 1987 after clinical and cytogenetic examinations at the National Children's Hospital, Tokyo, Japan. Most patients came to our clinic because of their short stature; a very limited number came to our clinic complaining of marked lymphedema on neck and/or extremities in the neonatal period. The 123 subjects were divided into three groups.

Group A consisted of 48 patients with proven total gonadal dysfunction. They were born in or prior to 1970 and failed to show any sign of puberty at or after age 17 years. In this group, 41 out of 48 patients had a history of anabolic steroid treatment, which started at age 12.3 ± 3.6 years and was continued for 7.5 ± 3.9 years on average. The anabolic steroid was Stanozolol at a daily dose of 1.0 mg. Thirty-six out of 48 patients were on estrogen and progesterone replacement, which was introduced at age 19.2 ± 2.3 years.

Group B consisted of 26 patients who experienced spontaneous puberty. In this group 23 out of 26 patients spontaneously experienced menarche at age 12.7 ± 1.8 years. Six out of 26 patients had a history of anabolic steroid treatment, which started in the prepubertal period and was continued for at least one year prior to the appearance of menarche. The anabolic steroid and dose was the same as mentioned above. Thirteen out of 26 patients of this group were born in or prior to 1970 and had reached age 17 years or more at the last examination. These 13 patients were designated as group B'.

Group C consisted of 49 patients who lacked pubertal signs at the last examination but were too young to permit evaluation of their gonadal function.

Cytogenetic Examination

Peripheral blood lymphocytes were used for chromosome analysis. The number of mitoses examined per subject ranged from 30 to 50.

Endocrinological Studies

Serum FSH and LH levels were measured using an ordinary radioimmunoassay. Gonadotropin releasing hormone (GnRH) loading tests used an intravenous dose of 100 $\mu g/m^2$.

Evaluation of Final Height

Examining the individual growth records of the subjects, the measured height was interpreted as the final height when the annual gain in the preceding year was known to be less than one cm. The SD score of the final height was calculated based on data presented in 1980 school statistics, Ministry of Education of Japan (9).

RESULTS

Incidence of Spontaneous Puberty

As shown in Table 1, age-matched comparison between the subjects in group A and group B indicated the incidence of spontaneous puberty to be 21.3% in Turner syndrome.

Influence of Gonadal Function on Final Height

The final height was obtained in 45 patients in group A and 17 patients in group B (Table 2). The final height differed markedly according to the presence or absence of gonadal function in Turner syndrome. Preserved gonadal function decreased final height by 6.5 cm or 1.2 SD score on average. The mean final height of 11 patients who showed spontaneous puberty and had no history of anabolic steroid treatment in their prepubertal period was significantly higher than that of the remaining 6 patients of group B with such a history (Table 3), but still shorter than that of group A, proving that the presence of gonadal function itself could have an influence on the final height when anabolic steroid treatment is not given.

Table 1 Incidence of Spontaneous Puberty in Girls with Turner Syndrome

Group	Gonadal function	Number of patients	Age (yr)	Year of birth	%
A	Proven to lack spontaneous puberty	48	≥17	≤1970	78.7
B	Proven to manifest spontaneous puberty	26 { 13 (group B')	≥17	≤1970	21.3
		13	<17	>1970	
C	Too young to be assessed	49	<17	>1970	
	Total	123			

Table 2 Influence of Gonadal Function on Final Height in Turner Syndrome

Spontaneous puberty	n	Final height (cm)	SD	
Absent	45	141.9 ± 3.6	−3.0 ± 0.7	$\Delta = 1.2 \ (p < 0.001)$
Present	17	135.4 ± 4.2	−4.2 ± 1.1	

Correlation Between Age at Menarche and Final Height in Group B

This was assessed in 17 patients of group B. As shown in Figure 1, the final height correlated positively with the age at menarche.

Influence of Anabolic Steroid Treatment in Prepubertal Period on Final Height in Turner Syndrome

This could be assessed only in group B, because only 4 out of 45 patients in group A did not have a history of anabolic steroid treatment. As mentioned, 6 girls in group B had a history of anabolic steroid use, which started in pre-puberty and was continued for at least one year prior to the appearance of menarche. The average final height of these 6 patients was shorter than that of the remaining 11 patients (Table 3). Because the mean age at menarche was significantly lower in patients with a history of anabolic steroid use, this disadvantageous effect of anabolic steroid use is thought to arise from triggering by the anabolic steroid of earlier onset of puberty when gonadal function is not fully impaired.

Table 3 Influence of Previous Treatment with Anabolic Steroid on Final Height in Girls with Turner Syndrome with Spontaneous Puberty

Previous treatment with anabolic steroid[a]	n	Final height (cm)		Age at menarche (yr)	
+	6	131.6 ± 6.8	$p < 0.05$	11.7 ± 1.4	$p < 0.05$
−	11	137.5 ± 3.7		13.7 ± 1.6	

[a]Anabolic steroid was administered during over 1 year before the appearance of menarche.

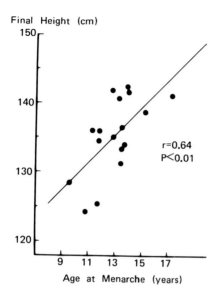

Figure 1 Correlation between age at menarche and final height in Turner syndrome with spontaneous puberty.

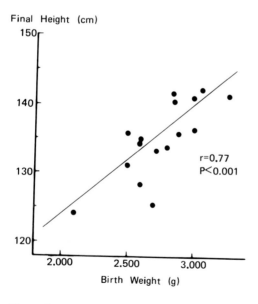

Figure 2 Correlation between birth weight and final height in Turner syndrome with spontaneous puberty.

Table 4 Summary of the Cytogenetic Findings in 123 Turner Syndrome Patients[a]

Karyotype	Group A	Group B	Group C	Total
Karyotype including no 46,XX cell line				
45,X	20 (41.7%)	6 (23.1%)	20 (40.8%)	46 (37.4%)
45,X/46,Xi(Xq)	5	3	4	12
45,X/46,XXp-	1	1	0	2
45,X/46,XYq-	0	0	1	1
45,X/46,Xr(X)	1	2	3	6
45,X/46,Xr(Y)	1	0	1	2
45,X/47,XXX	1	2	1	4
45,X/46,X+mar	2	1	5	8
45,X/46,X+mar/46,X+mar'	0	1	1	1
46,Xi(Xq)	5	3	5	13
46,XXp-	0	1	0	1
Karyotype including 46,XX cell line				
45,X/46,XX	10 ⎫	5 ⎫	6 ⎫	21 ⎫
45,X/46,XX/47,XXX	1 ⎬ 12 (25.0%)	2 ⎬ 7 (26.9%)	1 ⎬ 8 (16.3%)	4 ⎬ 27 (22.0%)
46,Xi(Xq)/46,XX	1 ⎭	0 ⎭	1 ⎭	2 ⎭
Total	48	26	49	123

[a]Comparison of percentage of presence of normal 46,XX cell line in karyotype by groups.

Correlation Between Birth Weight and Final Height in Turner Syndrome

This was separately assessed in 16 patients from group B and in 40 patients from group A. In patients who experienced spontaneous puberty, the final height correlated positively with the birth weight as shown in Figure 2. However, the final height did not correlate significantly with the birth weight in patients who lacked gonadal function, though there was slight tendency toward a positive relationship ($p < 0.1$).

Presence of Normal 46,XX Cell Line and Incidence of Spontaneous Puberty

The normal 46,XX cell line was observed in 12 out of 48 patients in group A (25.0%) and in 7 out of 26 patients in group B (26.9%) as shown in Table 4. These two percentages were quite similar to each other. Thus, the presence or

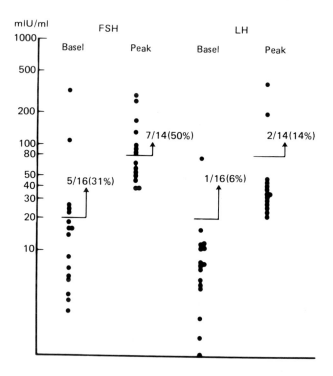

Figure 3 Serum FSH and LH and their response to GnRH in P-1 stage of girls with Turner syndrome who manifested spontaneous puberty later.

absence of normal 46,XX cell line is not very useful in predicting the future appearance of spontaneous puberty in girls with Turner syndrome. However, 45,X monosomy was less frequently found in group B compared to group A.

Serum FSH and LH and Responses to GnRH and Future Appearance of Spontaneous Puberty

Reviewing case records of 26 patients of group B, we found the basal serum FSH and LH levels in 16 patients and their responses to GnRH in 14 patients who were studied in prepuberty (Fig. 3). The serum basal FSH level was at least 20 mIU/ml in 5 (31%) and at least 40 mIU/ml in 2 (12.5%) out of 16 prepubertal patients. The serum basal LH level was at least 20 mIU/ml in 1 (6.3%) and at least 40 mIU/ml in 1 (6.3%) out of 16 patients. The peak serum FSH level in response to GnRH was at least 80 mIU/ml in 7 (50%) out of 14 patients. The peak serum LH level in response to GnRH was at least 80 mIU/ml in 2 (14%) out of 14 patients. Thus, both elevated serum basal gonadotropin levels and the exaggerated response of serum gonadotropins to GnRH were found not to exclude the possibility of eventual spontaneous puberty.

DISCUSSION

Incidence of Spontaneous Puberty in Turner Syndrome

Lippe et al. and Lyon et al. reported separately finding spontaneous menarche in 3 out of 80 patients, 13 out of 116 patients, and 8 out of 93 patients, respectively (1-3). However, they did not mention the age distribution of their subjects. To our best knowledge, therefore, the exact incidence of spontaneous puberty in Turner syndrome has been assessed for the first time in the present study. The incidence of 21.3% was so high as to be neglected in any discussion on the growth of Turner syndrome.

Influence of Gonadal Function on Final Height in Turner Syndrome

Many studies (1-8) deal with final height in Turner syndrome without making any distinction as to gonadal function. Park et al. (2) reported that 13 patients in whom menarche occurred spontaneously were not taller as adults than those without spontaneous puberty, but they did not mention their exact height in cm. Our findings disagree with those of Park et al. We found the presence of gonadal function to have an unfavorable effect on final height, even when an anabolic steroid was not used. A similar effect of gonadal function on final height was observed in growth-hormone-treated growth-hormone-deficient children (10,11). Furthermore, it was found in the present study that the earlier puberty began in patients with Turner syndrome, the shorter the final height attained. Such a correlation between the timing of onset of puberty and the final height is claimed to be present in normal males (12) and in normal females (13), though this relationship is very weak. It has also been reported that obese children begin puberty approximately one year earlier and reach a final height shorter by 2 cm on the average than nonobese children (14). It is also known that most sexual precocious children become shorter adults and children with untreated gonadal failure become taller adults. Accordingly, it is not surprising to find a correlation between age at menarche and final height in patients with Turner syndrome with gonadal function, but no reasonable explanation explains why a very marked correlation occurs in Turner syndrome with spontaneous puberty. In normal early maturing girls the total height gain after the onset of puberty is known to exceed that of normal late maturing girls and to offset the shorter growing period (13). Therefore, the final height is only very weakly related to time of onset of puberty in normal girls. However, in girls with Turner syndrome with spontaneous puberty, the total height gain after the onset of puberty was very small, as shown by the very small peak height velocity (2), and could not fully offset the shorter growing period in the early maturing patients.

Influence of Treatment with Anabolic Steroid on Final Height in Turner Syndrome

We know that excess androgens in prepuberty can frequently induce true sexual precocity ("androgen induced true sexual precocity"). In a nationwide etiological survey of 268 patients with central sexual precocity (15), we found such true sexual precocity in 5 patients with untreated 21-hydroxylase deficiency, in 21 patients with treated 21-hydroxylase deficiency, in 2 patients after removal of virilizing adrenal tumor, and in 2 patients with a history of anabolic steroid treatment (15). This effect of excess androgens on sexual maturation becomes manifest only when the hypothalamo-pituitary-gonadal axis remains normal. It is therefore not strange that prepubertal anabolic steroid treatment was found in the present study to decrease the final height in Turner syndrome patients whose gonadal function was not completely lost, though treatment has been reported elsewhere to have a harmless effect, at worst, on final height in Turner syndrome without gonadal function (1,4). Because a considerable percentage of patients with Turner syndrome retains gonadal function, every discussion on the utility and efficacy of anabolic steroid treatment to increase final height in Turner syndrome should include data on gonadal function.

Predictability of the Future Appearance of Spontaneous Puberty in Turner Syndrome

It is known that the presence of primary gonadal failure cannot always be predicted from elevated basal serum FSH and LH levels or their exaggerated response to GnRH (16), but this inability is partly due to changes in hypothalamic gonadostat sensitivity with children's age (17). Furthermore, the limitations of these endocrinological tools in predicting the appearance of spontaneous puberty result from the widely varying severity of primary gonadal failure. In Turner syndrome, also, there is known to be a wide variation in gonadal function, from complete absence to fertility.

Karyotyping was also found to be useless in predicting gonadal function in puberty, though there was an apparent tendency for patients with 45,X monosomy to lack gonadal function. Several authors reported individuals who were mosaic with a normal 46,XX cell line to be taller than those with single cell line 45,X monosomy. The former findings have been controverted recently by many studies (2-6). Our findings offer further proof that the presence of a normal 46,XX cell line in the karyotype has very limited significance in the manifestation of the clinical features of Turner syndrome.

Influence of Birth Weight on Final Height in Turner Syndrome

Park et al. (2) report a very close positive correlation between the birth weight and final height in Turner syndrome. We confirmed their findings in patients with spontaneous puberty but could not clearly confirm such a correlation in patients with gonadal failure. The discrepancy appears to be inexplicable at our present stage of knowledge.

REFERENCES

1. Lippe BM. Primary ovarian failure. In Kaplan SA (ed) Clinical Pediatric and Adolescent Endocrinology. Philadelphia, WB Saunders Co, 1982:269.
2. Park E, Bailey JD, Cowell CA. Growth and maturation of patients with Turner syndrome. Pediatr Res 1983; 17:1.
3. Lyon AJ, Preece MA, Grant DB. Growth curve for girls with Turner syndrome. Arch Dis Child 1983; 60:932.
4. Sybert VP. Adult height in Turner syndrome with and without androgen therapy. J Pediatr 1984; 104:365.
5. Ranke MB, Pfluger H, Rosendahl W, Enders H, Bierich JR, Majewski F. Turner syndrome: Spontaneous growth in 150 cases and review of the literature. Eur J Pediatr 1983; 141:81.

6. Pelz L, Timm D, Eyermann E, Hinkel GK, Kirchner M, Verron G. Body height in Turner's syndrome. Clin Genet 1982; 22:62.
7. Brook CGD, Murset G, Zachmann M, Prader A. Growth in children with 45,xo Turner's syndrome. Arch Dis Child 1974; 49:789.
8. Urban MD, Lee PA, Migeon CJ. Reply (to Letter). J Pediatr 1980; 96:168.
9. Ministry of Education, Government of Japan. Report on School Statistics, 1980.
10. Burns EC, Tanner JM, Preece MA, Cameron W. Final height and pubertal development in 55 children with idiopathic growth hormone deficiency, treated for 2 to 15 years with human growth hormone. Eur J Pediatr 1981; 137:155.
11. Hibi I, Tanae A, Kagawa J, Hashimoto N. Studies on usefulness of gonadal suppressive therapy with cyproterone acetaed and medroxyprogesterone acetate in increasing the matured height of boys with idiopathic pituitary dwarfism who manifested spontaneous sexual development during human growth hormone therapy. Japanische-Deutsche Medizinische Berichte 1986; 27:275.
12. Tanner JM. Growth at adolescence. Blackwell, Oxford, 1955.
13. Tanaka T, Suwa S, Yokoya S, Hibi I. Analysis of linear growth during puberty. Acta Paediatr Scand [Suppl] 1988; 347:25.
14. Lloyd JK, Wolff OH. Childhood obesity. A long-term study of height and weight. Brit Med J 1961; 3:145.
15. Hibi I. Diagnostic criteria and etiological classification of central sexual precocity. Int Med 1985; 55:1527.
16. Razdan AK, Rosenfidld RL, Kim MH. Endocrinologic characteristics of partial ovarian failure. J Clin Endocrinol Metab 1976; 43:449.
17. Conte FA, Grumbach MM, Kaplan SL. A diphasic pattern of gonadotropin secretion in patients with the syndrome of gonadal dysgenesis. J Clin Endocrinol 1975; 40:670.

DISCUSSION

DR. ROBERT BLIZZARD: I have a couple of questions for Dr. Hibi and one for Dr. Ranke as well. For Dr. Hibi first, in respect to the use of anabolic steroids, can you tell us what anabolic steroid and what were the limitations of starting the anabolic steroid in relation to the bone age of the children. In other words, did children who had bone ages less than nine get anabolic steroids, and what was the dosage used?

DR. ITSURO HIBI: We usually used stanozolol in very low dose, 1 mg per day. We are now very careful on the use of anabolic steroids.

DR. BLIZZARD: What were the bone ages of your patients when you started? Were their bone ages ever less than nine?

DR. HIBI: About the age of the start of anabolic steroids, around 10. My patients who have shown spontaneous puberty had a history of anabolic steroids given at another hospital.

DR. BLIZZARD: The comment would be that I do not know anything about the anabolic steroid that you use. I am not certain that it would be the same finding that one might have with Anavar, but we would need data to demonstrate whether that was or was not the case, of course.

DR. HIBI: I suppose it was identical to the oxandrolone.

DR. BLIZZARD: I am not sure that it can be said to be the case, because in my opinion, Anavar is the only one of the steroids that really has any dissociation between growth promotion and virilization, so I am not sure. But very nice data, and thank you very much. For Dr. Ranke, I do not quite understand, this is my

Dr. Blizzard is at the University of Virginia at Charlottesville, Charlottesville, Virginia. Dr. Hibi is at the National Children's Hospital, Tokyo, Japan. Dr. Ranke is at Kinderklinik, Tubingen, Federal Republic of Germany. Dr. Crowley is at Massachusetts General Hospital, Boston, Massachusetts. Dr. Prader is at Kinderspital, Zürich, Switzerland. Dr. Grumbach is at the University of California at San Francisco, San Francisco, California. Dr. Lippe is at the University of California at Los Angeles School of Medicine, Los Angeles, California. Dr. Cutler is at the National Institute of Child Health and Human Development, Bethesda, Maryland. Dr. Rosenwaks was at the Jones Institute for Reproductive Medicine, Eastern Virginia Medical School, Norfolk, Virginia. He is currently at Cornell University Medical Center–The New York Hospital, New York, New York.

ignorance, you talk about total height gain at adolescence of the patients with Turner syndrome being normal, if I understood the last column on your slide.

DR. MICHAEL RANKE: Relative height gain in relation to their final height was the last slide. The point I want to make is that from a certain bone age that would mark the initiation of party in a normal child, you are not very likely to gain anything in height. And in conjunction with Dr. Hibi and what was discussed is that the likelihood is that if you induce puberty in these patients, you either do not change anything in height prediction or you do harm to them because you might not do it appropriately.

DR. BLIZZARD: Are you saying that if these patients are not given estrogens or if they do not produce estrogens, that they grow for a longer period of time?

DR. RANKE: Yes.

DR. BLIZZARD: And even though they do not have an adolescent growth spurt, the total increment is the same?

DR. RANKE: Yes, that is what I am saying. You see, the point is that in that respect Turner do not behave differently from normals. And I must say, I am a little bit at variance with the growth hormone deficiency data that Dr. Hibi presented as such, since our observation is that patients with growth hormone deficiency and gonadotropin deficiency that are not substituted will reach the same adult stature as those that are substituted. So what I am saying is puberty in itself, whether it is there or it is not, does not influence final height. I mean, that is the general message.

DR. WILLIAM CROWLEY: Yes, first of all I think the presentations are both terrific. I would really like to think about these a little longer. I am not sure I can absorb it that quickly. But some of the things which struck me to be very, very similar to some of the data we are seeing in children with central precocious puberty receiving the GnRH analog are quite noteworthy and certainly worth underscoring. And that is that the children that are completely suppressed with sufficient GnRH analog. . . . I am switching models now to central mediated precocious puberty, early introduction of gonadal steroids, and then their termination with the GnRH analog . . . you have data which strikes me as very, very similar when you stand far enough back and look at the growth data after you remove gonadal steroids. And the conclusions, which are similar, are as follows: Number one, if you suppress completely gonadal steroids, that is, that you have a complete pituitary suppression, your response to exogenous LHRH is totally oblated, your gonadal steroids, vaginal maturation indices are completely reduced to prepubertal levels, you have the best improvements in predicted height, and you have the greatest gains that are being made. On the other hand, if you have patients who are incompletely suppressed due to poor compliance, due to an inappropriate selection of LHRH analog dosage or not having a potent enough analog or for a variety of reasons, such that there is incomplete suppression of gonadal steroids, that almost invariably reduces the increases in predicted height that you see, very similar to a little bit of steroids in your models being worse off than complete suppression of steroids. The second line of evidence from that same group of patients is that those children who are on the analog with complete suppression and who remain completely preadrenarchal during the course of the study, that is, are as devoid of gonadal steroids as we can make them, have also the greatest height gains, the greatest increase in predicted height, and I might add now we are seeing some final heights to fulfill the predictions. On the other hand, those patients who go into and have adrenarche during the course of this study have advancements of skeletal maturation over chronological age which are slightly greater and that erodes their height predictions in final height. All three of those now when put end to end suggest that a little bit of gonadal steroids, perhaps not totally the physiologic levels of puberty, may in fact reduce the growth patterns at puberty, as opposed to a complete deficiency of gonadal steroids in which the extended period of time and sort of alleviation of epiphyseal fusion permits you a greater length of time to grow, and albeit at a stronger growth velocity, achieve a final height. Therefore, the question I have, particularly of Dr. Ranke, is have you been able to look at the weight versus height profile and the ultimate height and velocities of the children in relation to adrenarche across the Turner's population? And what impact does that have as a variable?

DR. RANKE: I have not.

DR. ANDREA PRADER: As concerns precocious puberty, we have done a study on the growth of untreated patients. Quite many reach normal adult stature.

DR. HIBI: Yes, I agree with you. Anabolic steroids used frequently brings precocious puberty, not only in Turner's syndrome with reserved gonadal function, but in the normal short-stature children. But in our series the earliest menarche was 11.4 years, and not so early.

DR. CROWLEY: Forget for a moment the predicted heights or whether or not they reached tall heights. I am talking about the auxologic data during complete gonadal suppression. I am looking at this now as a physiologic model. I mean, you and I agree about that. I am addressing Dr. Prader here, that the growth velocities and the patterns of the growth here have a similarity, with a little bit of gonadal steroids here, resulting in not an increase in height velocity and final height in this, but actually having an adverse effect. It is quite similar to what we are seeing in incompletely suppressed patients or patients who are in adrenarche. That is all.

DR. RANKE: If I may say something, there are data about treatment of Turner's with low, really low doses, and most probably we will discuss this more in the session. For these data indicate that you shorten the growth process by these lower doses, but you presumably are not impairing final height.

DR. CROWLEY: All of those look very short too.

DR. RANKE: May I ask a question too? I would like to ask a question to Dr. Hibi, because I have not addressed this question, but he has, i.e., the relation between birth weight and final height that has been discussed by many of the authors. I think that one of the problems about these data, in principle, is that one should use an analysis of variance between mothers' height and birth parameters and ultimate height in order to separate the two influences from each other, and I think nobody has really done it. I think that is something that is needed to finally elucidate what the impact of intrauterine growth failure on final stature is.

DR. HIBI: You could easily do it. You have the data.

DR. MELVIN GRUMBACH: I would like to ask Professor Hibi a question, because I have been struck by the prevalence of spontaneous pubertal signs, much less menarche. What I was not clear about, Professor Hibi, is how many of your patients were 45,X versus how many were XO mosaics or structural abnormalities, because you really need to separate those two out. If you are talking about the pure XOs, that would be an extraordinary group of patients.

DR. HIBI: In my series of 123 patients, X monosomy was found in 38% only.

DR. GRUMBACH: What percent of that 38% had spontaneous puberty?

DR. HIBI: The percentage of X monosomy in patients with spontaneous puberty is equal, not different by gonadal function frequency. A very big percent of patients who manifested spontaneous puberty had X monosomy. We have only done the peripheral blood lymphocyte stimulation, and it is my rule to count 30 mitoses per patient, and if a small number of abnormal karyotypes are found, the number will be extended to 50. That is in my policy.

DR. FELIX CONTE: I just want to make a comment to Dr. Ranke. We had the opportunity of looking at American data over the last 20 years, from the literature and some of our own data, and we calculated final heights as you did with the European data. And there is some suggestion, among treated and untreated patients, that there may be a secular trend. And we agree that it may be 1 cm per decade looking like 141.5 before 1969, and between 1969 and 1980, maybe 142.5 and maybe 143 after that, but these are both estrogen- and anabolic-treated patients. One of the things that has perplexed me is the discrepancy between your final heights plus Sybert's final heights and final heights from the rest of the world. When we add in Sybert's final heights to United States data, it comes out at 143, which is exactly what it is in Europe. It may be related, as you said, to midparental height. Did you look at midparental height in your socioeconomic group and is it different, since there is a correlation between midparental height and final height in Turner's? Is it different from Brook's data, and is it different from the data from the United States? Are you dealing with a much taller population of parents than we are dealing with to explain this 4-cm discrepancy that you are seeing between what we are giving as final heights and Sybert and you are getting?

DR. RANKE: The midparental height of our population was not, on the average, higher than the mean of the population. I do not feel that it is me and Sybert against the rest of the world. There is Nielsen from Denmark, who also gives something like 146 cm, but really I must say this is one of the problems that, on final height we have too little data. So I think what it really is, I think the fact that you see patients at an older age may contribute a little bit, and that is I think perhaps one of the differences. What the real mean height is, I do not know, but I know that is one of the most important figures if we talk about treatment effects. I agree, it is different whether you think it is 143 or whether it is 146; it is an essential difference.

DR. PRADER: I would like to make another comment to Dr. Hibi. You demonstrated that there is a correlation between the age of menarche and final height. The later the menarche occurs, the shorter is final height. This is perhaps a point which many of us would expect to be so. But in fact, in normal children it is not so. In our longitudinal study of normal children we found absolutely no correlation between final height and the timing of puberty or the extent of the pubertal growth spurt. It is hard to believe that patients with Turner's syndrome behave differently.

DR. HIBI: Yes, I would agree with you. But in the patients with idiopathic pituitary growth hormone deficiency, also the age of the start of puberty is correlated with the final height, when the growth hormone treatment is started at the same age.

DR. BARBARA LIPPE: Inversely?

DR. GORDON B. CUTLER: Dr. Conte's comment made me just want to re-numerate the various factors, some of which I think were mentioned, between ethnic factors, historical and secular trends, the possibility of selection, whether these series are truly unselected or there may be a reason why shorter children disproportionately get into them. When you put all these factors together, it is not, I think, surprising that the historical series differ a lot. And the one conclusion that I have drawn from this, when we have been thinking about how we ought to try to design studies to produce valid answers about whether we are influencing final height, is that we need to do well-controlled studies, because there is no way, I think, that we can know which historical series to pick as the baseline when they differ by 7 cm.

DR. RANKE: Basically I agree, but if you take the highest levels, and then the final heights of the treated are still higher, you are surely on the right side.

DR. ZEV ROSENWAKS: But they are historical, you know. With each generation it depends how old they are. You do not know that they would not have been higher in an untreated control group, either.

DR. ROBERT ROSENFIELD: Dr. Hibi, in the patients with spontaneous puberty, could you tell us whether there might be some other explanation for the seemingly poor growth of those who went into puberty earlier. For example, did you look at how closely they came to reaching the height predictions in the group that went through puberty and the group that did not? And did you look at the correlations with midparental height between those who did and did not?

DR. HIBI: I am very sorry, I have not studied this point, but almost all the parents and the patients are living, and we will study your suggestion.

DR. ROSENFIELD: And, Dr. Ranke, I am bothered by your claim that there is very little growth loss during puberty, because that just is not our experience, and I wonder if this is not a semantic discussion. At what bone age did you decide to consider puberty? If you picked a bone age of 13, nobody grows very much after that.

DR. RANKE: Ten, which was close to, but, in fact, puberty is earlier, we know. Taking ten is most probably not bad. But if you want to, I think it is a little bit a matter of semantics. I think the main point is that during childhood you lose at least three-quarters of what you finally lose. And so any approach to improve height at an age when puberty usually should start will have to fail. It will not bring very much growth, probably, and it may well be that it means that to induce puberty makes things worse.

DR. ROSENFIELD: You are including in your analysis patients in whom you have induced puberty, I presume?

DR. RANKE: No, no. Not at all.

DR. ROSENFIELD: May I underline what Michael Ranke has just said. You can easily understand that this growth deficit has been accumulating through prepubertal childhood if you think of the mean growth velocity. You cannot have a mean growth velocity at the 25th centile and not end up very small. Growth velocities are not like growth distances where you stay on your centile. If you start off one year with a growth velocity over one year at the 25th centile, the next year you have got to be at, roughly speaking, the 75th, or you lose height centiles as in Turner syndrome. A second brief underlining comment, and that is that the adolescent spurt of puberty does do one thing for you. It gives you relatively shorter legs, besides shutting down growth earlier, so that all this business of it actually not affecting your final height is true, but it affects your final shape quite a bit.

DR. PRADER: Well that is true in other types of growth disorders, but not in the Turner's. They do not get longer legs.

DR. ROSENFIELD: Just one last comment about this. You would be interested that we have just finished a study of growth in 20 children who have reached adult height with isolated gonadotropin deficiency. And they are smack at the mean, 50th height percentile. They are not taller; they started their testosterone no earlier than 15 years, between 15 and 18 years, and they are right smack at the mean. So in order to get tall with eunuchoidism, you really have to keep growing for a long time before your epiphyses shut down. It is not just two or three years.

14

Physical and Anatomical Abnormalities in Turner Syndrome

Barbara M. Lippe

University of California at Los Angeles School of Medicine, Los Angeles, California

In the 51 years since Henry Turner (1) first described the seven young women with the phenotype which bears his name, much has been learned about the etiology of this syndrome. While short stature remains an almost invariant phenotypic finding, the spectrum of anatomical, organic, and physiological abnormalities which affect these women is wide. That the precise mechanism whereby complete or partial X monosomy results in such a miriad of abnormalities is still unknown reflects the complexity of the genetic control of development. Nevertheless, if one views the multiple abnormalities in Turner syndrome not as a list of numerous unconnected anomalies but instead as the consequence of a fewer number of primary pathogenetic mechanisms, then the abnormalities become more comprehensible if not yet completely defined. This report will focus on some of the physical and anatomical abnormalities found in these patients and attempt to develop a strategy to understand them based on the author's classification of the possible pathogenetic mechanisms.

This approach to classification of the most common physical findings in Turner syndrome is illustrated by the data presented in Table 1. The incidence findings are derived from personal assessment of over 140 patients with Turner syndrome seen in our clinic in the last 18 years and are consistent with other reported series (2,3). The classification implies that two mechanisms, one being disordered skeletal growth and the other being a disturbance of intrauterine (and consequent postnatal) lymphatic development, accounts for the majority

Table 1 Physical Findings in Patients with Turner Syndrome

Primary defect	Secondary defect	Incidence (%)
Chromosomal aneuploidy	Short stature	100.0
Skeletal growth disturbance	Short neck	40.0
	Abnormal US/LS	97.0
	Cubitus valgus	47.0
	Short metacarpals	37.0
	Madelung deformity	7.5
	Scoliosis	12.5
	Genu valgus	35.0
	Micrognathia	60.0
	High arched palate	36.0
	Irregularities of the knees	common
Lymphatic obstruction/	Webbed neck	27.0
edema	Low posterior hairline	42.0
	Rotated ears	common
	Edema of hands/feet	25.0
	Severe nail dysplasia	13.0
	Ptosis	11.0
	Shield chest	26.0
	Hypoplastic nipples/? damaged breast primordia	<10.0
Vascular dysplasia	Cardiovascular	35.0
Unknown	Renal	33.0
	Multiple pigmented nevi	26.0
	Strabismus	17.5

of the physical findings exhibited by the individual with Turner syndrome. When one extends the assessment of these patients to include anatomical abnormalities of nonosseous organ systems, namely the cardiovascular and renal systems, then a third mechanism, involving vascular development, may be operative. In addition, there are clearly as yet unknown mechanisms. However, I will discuss evidence that some of the cardiovascular and renal defects may also be secondary to the lymphatic abnormality. Finally, it is clear that almost all of the abnormalities involve mesenchymal tissue. Therefore, I propose a hypothesis to explain most of the anomalies, specifically, that *a major defect in Turner syndrome is disordered mesenchymal tissue growth.*

Short stature is the most common physical finding in Turner syndrome. It appears to result from a degree of primary impairment of intrauterine growth coupled with postnatal growth failure which is most marked after the second year of life (4). The concept that the statural defect is a reflection of chromosomal aneuploidy per se and not specific to the X monosomy is discussed in Chapter 23 and included as a separate mechanism in the classification system in Table 1. If, as he further suggests, the skeletal abnormalities represent disordered growth of some but not all bones and are not a distinct skeletal dysplasia, then a single mechanism resulting in differential disruption or disordered control of bone growth satisfactorily explains the multiple osseous findings.

The hypothesis that fetal lymphedema, arising as a consequence of disrupted development of the fetal lymphatic system, results in many of the features of Turner syndrome is not unique to this author. In 1949, the German physician, O. Ullrich, recognized that the patients he had described with lymphedema, webbed neck, gonadal dysgenesis, and dwarfism were likely to have the same condition as Turner's patients. He called attention to the work of Kristin Bonnevie, who described similar findings in mice in association with distention of the subcutaneous tissues by fluid and proposed the eponym Status Bonnevie-Ullrich to describe the set of specific anomalies arising from a single mechanism (lymphangiectasia) (5). It is now recognized that the nuchal hygromas arise from a lag in the formation of the communication between the developing jugular lymph sac and the internal jugular vein (6). This lag results in fetal lymphatic obstruction and distension of nuchal soft tissues with fluid (Fig. 1). If the obstruction improves and the fetus survives, the fluid tends to disappear, leaving behind either loose skin in the neck area or cicatrized skinfolds (pterygium coli). That an obstruction to lymphatic drainage is the primary abnormality has been questioned by one group (7), who find hypoalbuminemia in fetuses with 45,X karyotype and nuchal hygroma and believe that the hypoalbuminemia is primary, the edema secondary, and the lymphatic abnormalities result thereafter. Nevertheless, they, too, concur that the physical abnormalities listed in the table are secondary to the edema.

The relationship of the lymphatic abnormalities to the cardiac defects is discussed by Clark (8). He elegantly reviews the embryology of lymphatic sac drainage into the venous system and believes that it is this event which may not occur appropriately in many affected Turner fetuses. He notes that, while not studied in the human embryo, in the chick disordered drainage corresponds to a mechanism that would distend the cardiac lymphatics. He proposes that this would encroach upon the ascending aorta and alter intracardiac blood flow. Finally, in a detailed discussion he relates the pathogenesis of aortic coarctation, and other aortic abnormalities, to the lymphatic obstruction and thereby to the webbed neck phenotype. This relationship, of webbed neck and coarctation being phenotypically linked, is supported by the literature and by our own data. That this relationship may also be associated with the degree of X monosomy is also suggested. Engle and Forbes (9) reported the association only in 45,X patients, while Palmer and Reichmann (2) found it in some mosaic patients as well

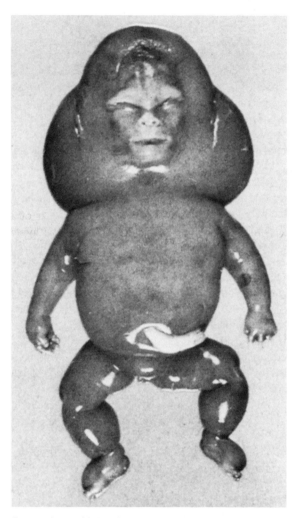

Figure 1 A 45,X abortus demonstrating generalized edema. The distension of the nuchal soft tissue and the pronounced swelling of the dorsal aspects of the extremities are evident. (From AJDC 1978; 132:417. Reproduced with the permission from the publisher. Copyright 1978, American Medical Association.)

(although they had one 45,X cell line) but not in patients with an isochromosome X or a ring X. In our series, Table 2, we noted that coarctation, which was present in 10.4% of 134 patients examined, was almost invariably found among the patients with a 45,X karyotype [13 of the 14 patients with coarctation were 45,X (93%) although this karyotype constituted only 55% of the group (74/134 = 55%)]. Eleven of the 14 patients with coarctation were clinically described as having a webbed neck (79%), while only 34 of the 134 patients (25%) were so described. Thus, there is strong clinical evidence to support the hypothesis that the lymphatic defect could be responsible for both the webbed neck phenotype and coarctation of the aorta.

The pathogenesis of the other cardiovascular abnormalities found in Turner syndrome does not have as clear a potential etiological mechanism. We have described a high incidence of aortic root dilation (10) and have now experienced three patients with dissection and rupture. We reviewed (10) case reports of at least 15 Turner patients with dissection and note that risk factors such as hypertension and aortic valve disease are associated in most, but not all, cases. That aortic root diameters are greater in 45,X patients than matched controls (11) suggests a degree of intrinsic primary abnormality. Pathological evidence of cystic medial necrosis is reported in some cases and suggests that the intrinsic disorder might represent another possible example of a mesenchymal defect. Alternatively, the tendency toward significant dilation might be secondary to intrauterine hemodynamic events which are also secondary to the lymphatic disorder. Our clinical data that the six patients we have identified with significant dilation have a 45,X karyotype and five of the six have the webbed neck phenotype support this hypothesis.

Table 2 Cardiovascular Abnormalities Observed in Turner Syndrome: Relationship to Karyotype and Phenotype

Abnormality	Positive/ examined[a]	%	45,X (74/134)	Webbed neck (34/134)
Coarctation	14/134	10.4	13/14	11[b]/14
Dilated aorta	6/67	8.9	6/6	5/6
Bicuspid aortic valve without coarctation	20/67	29.9	12/20	6[c]/20
Mitral valve prolapse	6/67	8.9	4/6	3/6

[a]All patients had chest X-rays; recently, patients have routine echocardiography, $n = 67$.
[b]All 45,X.
[c]4 were 45,X.

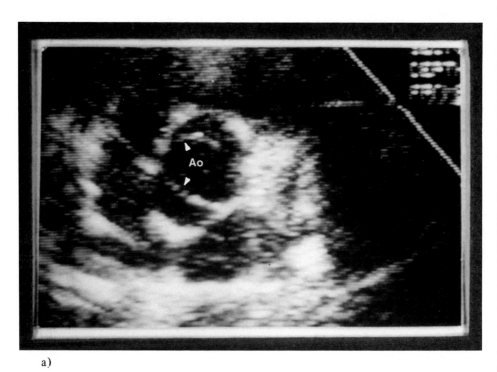

a)

Figure 2 a) A parasternal ultrasonographic scan through the aorta (Ao) showing the configuration of an open bicuspid aortic valve (the arrows point to the two cusps). b) In the same patient, the arrow points to the closure of the two aortic cusps. c) This scan is essentially indistinguishable from Fig. 2a, indicating an open bicuspid aortic valve. d) This midclosure scan still appears to demonstrate only two cusps. e) This image of aortic valve closure in the Turner syndrome patient depicted in c and d demonstrates three cusps (arrows) consistent with a functionally bicuspid but anatomically tricuspid aortic valve. The 2-D echocardiographic images were obtained using a ATL-UM 8 scanner with a 5 mHz transducer or an ATL-Mark 600 scanner with a 5 mHz transducer. (Reproduced with the permission of Dr. Thomas Santulli, Jr., Department of Pediatrics, Division of Cardiology, UCLA School of Medicine.)

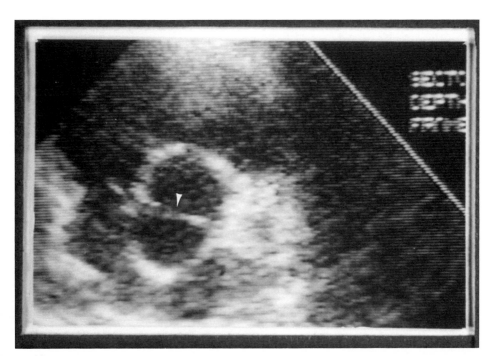

b)

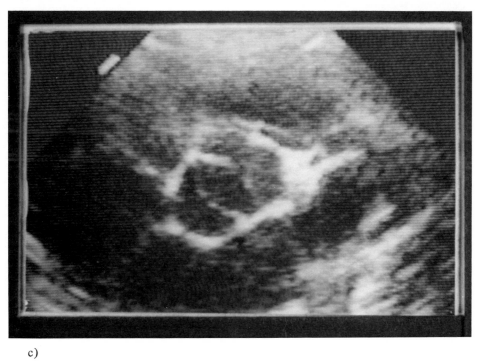

c)

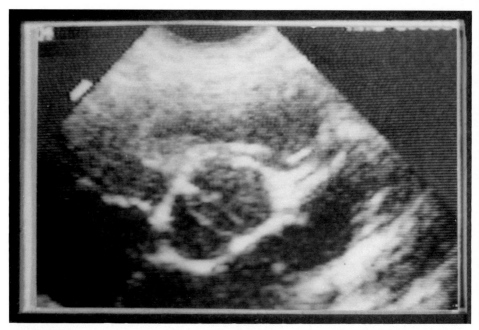

d)

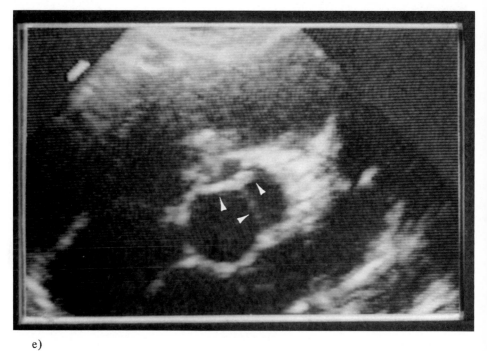

e)

Figure 2 (continued)

We have also noted an increased incidence of aortic valve pathology in Turner syndrome (12). In our initial study we identified echocardiographic evidence of bicuspid aortic valve in 35% of patients studied prospectively. We currently find abnormalities in 30% (Fig. 2a,b). However, newer echocardiographic techniques suggests that some of these valves are anatomically tricuspid (Fig. 2c,d,e), but have eccentric closure and are functionally "bicuspid," while others are actually bicuspid. When taken together there does not appear to be an association between the "bicuspid" valve and the 45,X karyotype or webbed neck phenotype. However, we are currently evaluating the data to determine if there are differences between the functional and the anatomic bicuspid valve and the karyotype or phenotype. In either case, "bicuspid" valves are predisposed to the same secondary pathology (stenosis, insufficiency, calcification, and infection) and subject the patients to the risks of endocarditis, cardiac dysfunction, and aortic dilation.

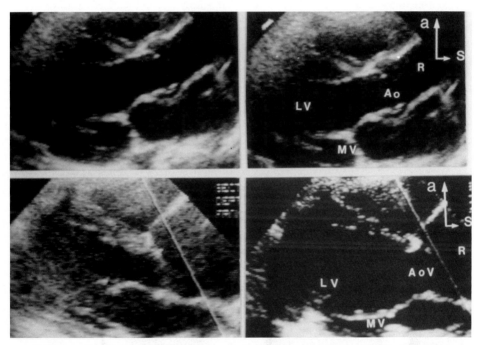

Figure 3 Ultrasonographic parasternal long axis views of the left ventricle outflow tract and the ascending aorta in two patients with Turner syndrome. The top left image shows normal anatomy. LV = left ventricle, Ao = aorta, R = aortic root, MV = mitral valve. The bottom left image shows a dilated proximal aortic root and dilated left ventricle. LV = left ventricle, AoV = aortic valve, R = aortic root, MV = mitral valve.

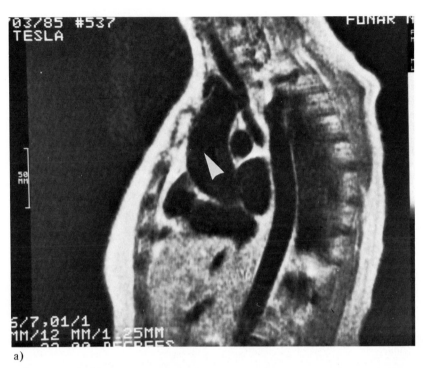

a)

Figure 4 a) MRI scan of the thoracic aorta in a patient with Turner syndrome and a dilated aortic root. The arrow lies in the dilated aortic root. b) MRI scan of the thoracic aorta in a Turner syndrome patient with a dilated sinus of Valsalva (sv). Both sagittal scans were obtained with a 0.3 Telsa permanent magnet imaging system (Fonar Corp., Melville, NY) by methods previously described (10).

The report that death from aortic dissection was greatly in excess of the expected in a large prospective study of Turner syndrome patients registered with a karyotype registry (13), coupled with our own experiences, has prompted us to adopt an aggressive approach to cardiovascular surveillance in these patients. We recommend that all patients with Turner syndrome be referred to a pediatric cardiologist for an initial evaluation, to include a cardiac ultrasound. Follow-up imaging of the aortic root with either ultrasound or, if indicated, magnetic resonance imaging (MRI) should be performed if significant aortic valve pathology is found or if dilation of the aortic root is suspected. Figures 3 and 4 illustrate the utility of ultrasound and MRI in demonstrating aortic root dilation. Patients with functional or true bicuspid aortic valves should be given standard subacute bacterial endocarditis (SBE) prophylaxis. Hypertension should be treated aggressively if aortic valve or root pathology is present.

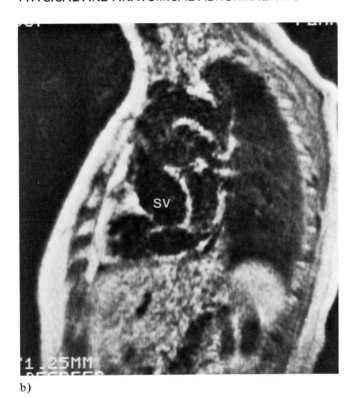

b)

If aortic root dilation progresses or sudden aortic regurgitation occurs, then guidelines for elective surgical therapy similar to those for the patient with Marfan syndrome should be considered (14).

Renal malformations are also found with increased frequency in Turner syndrome (15-17). We prospectively study all Turner patients, regardless of symptoms, and therefore have data obtained without ascertainment bias on 141 patients. Prior to 1980 the intravenous pyelogram (IVP) was used as the initial imaging technique. Subsequently, we have used ultrasonography. Since ultrasonography detects all but the most subtle of rotational abnormalities, we can combine the data. In so doing we found abnormalities in 47 patients (33%). These are listed in Table 3, classified according to their morphological type. In addition, we have suggested several proposed embryological mechanisms to explain the diversity of findings.

Using this approach, we have proposed that the 16 patients with malformations of number (11% of patients studied) have defects which can be explained by abnormalities in ureteric or metanephric budding (double collecting systems, absent kidneys, and extra renal pelvic development). We have categorized

Table 3 Renal Malformations in 141 Turner Syndrome Patients

Type	# (%)	Proposed mechanism
Malformations of number:		
Double collecting system	11 (7.8)	
Absent kidney	4 (2.8)	Disordered ureteric or
Extra renal pelvis	1 (0.7)	metanephric budding
Malformations in position/form:		
Horseshoe kidney	10 (7.1)	
Rotated kidneys	8 (5.7)	Vascular dysplasia
Ectopia	4 (2.8)	
Other malformations:		
UPJ obstruction	3 (2.1)	?Vascular dysplasia
Partial obstructed calyx	3 (2.1)	Vascular dysplasia
Multiple vessels	1[a]	Vascular dysplasia
UVJ obstruction	2 (1.4)	??

[a]Only one patient studied with renal arteriography, therefore percent of patients with abnormality unknown.

the 22 patients (15.6% of the total number of patients) with malformations of renal position or form (horseshoe kidneys, rotated kidneys, and ectopia) as having vascular dysplasia as their basic etiology. This etiologic mechanism is suggested because the blood supply is an intrinsic determinant of the migrational path of the developing kidney. In the case of the horseshoe kidney, for example, it is likely that it arises from the union of the two nephrogenic blastemas brought together by the developing umbilical arteries and that the malposition is then due to vascular obstruction in the path of ascent. The other malformations, numbering 8 (5.6% of the group), can also be accounted for, in large part, by abnormal vasculature. Partial calyceal obstruction is believed to be secondary to an aberrant vessel crossing the upper pole of the kidney, while UPJ obstruction is proposed to be secondary to extrinsic compression on a vascular basis (18). Only one of our patients underwent renal arteriography for the evaluation of hypertension, and she was noted to have multiple renal arteries and veins. Therefore, the incidence of this abnormality is unknown. Uretero-vesical junction (UVJ) obstruction was found in two patients, both of whom required corrective surgery. The mechanism responsible for this abnormality is unknown but the frequency (1.4%) is not dissimilar to the normal population and may, therefore, be unrelated to the condition. Thus, while there appear to be numerous renal malformations in Turner syndrome, their etiology may be secondary to a limited number of embryological mechanisms. Since ultrasonography is a noninvasive imaging technique, we recommend that all Turner patients have an initial renal ultrasound to define their basic anatomy and that follow-up studies be performed according to clinical indications.

In summary, this report attempts to provide a pathogenetic approach to the multiplicity of physical and anatomical anomalies which occur in the patient with Turner syndrome. While such a framework might assist the clinician in understanding the anomalies, it in no way lessens the need for the comprehensive evaluation of these patients. Instead, it should provide a framework for the systematic approach to the elucidation and correction of those anomalies which might lead to morbidity or mortality.

REFERENCES

1. Turner HH. A syndrome of infantilism, congenital webbed neck and cubitus valgus. Endocrinology 1938; 23:566-74.
2. Palmer CG, Reichmann A. Chromosomal and clinical findings in 110 females with Turner syndrome. Hum. Genet 1976; 35:35-49.
3. Hall JG, Sybert VP, Williamson RA, Fisher NL, Reed SD. Turner's syndrome. West J Med 1982; 137:32-44.
4. Ranke MD, Pfluger H, Rosendahl W, Stubbe P, Enders H, Bierich JR, Majewski F. Turner syndrome: Spontaneous growth in 150 cases and review of the literature. Eur J Pediatr 1983; 141:81.
5. Ullrich P. Turner's syndrome and status Bonnevie-Ullrich. Am J Human Genet 1949; 1:179-202.
6. Smith DW. Recognizable Patterns of Human Deformation. WB Saunders, New York, 1981.
7. Shepard TH, Fantel AG. Pathogenesis of congenital defects associated with Turner's syndrome: The role of hypoalbuminemia and edama. Acta Endo [suppl 279] 986; 113:440-7.
8. Clark EB. Neck web and congenital heart defects: A pathogenic association in 45 X-O Turner syndrome? Teratology 1984; 29:355-61.
9. Engle E, Forbes AP. Cytogenetic and clinical findings in 48 patients with congenitally defective or absent ovaries. Medicine 1965; 44:135-63.
10. Lin AE, Lippe BM, Geffner ME, Gomes A, Lois JF, Barton CW, Rosenthal A, Friedman WF. Aortic dilation, dissection, and rupture in patients with Turner syndrome. J Pediatr 1986; 109:820-6.
11. Allen DB, Hendricks SA, Levy JM. Aortic dilation in Turner syndrome. J Pediatr 1986; 109:302-5.
12. Miller MJ, Geffner ME, Lippe BM, Itami RM, Kaplan SA, DiSessa TG, Isabel-Jones JB, Friedman WF. Echocardiography reveals a high incidence of bicuspid aortic valve in Turner syndrome. J Pediatr 1983; 102:47-50.
13. Price WH, Clayton JF, Collyer S, De Mey R, Wilson J. Mortality ratios, life expectancy, and cause of death in patients with Turner's syndrome. J of Epidemiology and Community Health 1986; 40:97-102.
14. Pyeritz RE, McKusick VA. The Marfan syndrome: diagnosis and management. N Engl J Med 1979; 300:772-7.

15. Reveno JS, Palubinskas AJ. Congenital renal abnormalities in gonadal dys-genesis. Radiology 1966; 86:49-51.
16. Matthies A, Macdiarmid WD, Rallison ML, Tyler FH. Renal anomalies in Turner's syndrome. Clin Pediatr 1971; 10:561-5.
17. Litvak AS, Rousseau TG, Wrede LD, Mabry CC, McRoberts JW. The association of significant renal anomalies with Turner's syndrome. J Urol 1978; 120:671-2.
18. Kelalis PP. Ureteropelvic junction. In Clinical Pediatric Urology, vol 1, PP Kelalis, LR King, AB Belman (ed). WB Saunders Co, Philadelphia, 1985; pp 450-86.

15

Natural History and Associated Abnormalities
An Echocardiographic Perspective of Cardiac Abnormalities in Turner Syndrome

Norman H. Silverman

University of California at San Francisco, San Francisco, California

We have examined 25 patients with Turner syndrome by echocardiography: 5 had aortic coarctation (Table 1). Isolated aortic valve abnormalities in the presence of aortic coarctation have only been found in 1 of these 25 patients. Several miscellaneous cardiac abnormalities have been present. We have 1 patient with a left superior vena cava coronary to sinus connection, one partial anomalous pulmonary venous return, and one atrial septal defect. These defects are present at the same frequency as isolated aortic valve abnormalities in the absence of aortic coarctation. I believe we should not try to explain these findings as part of the Turner syndrome. Experience would suggest that an isolated bicuspid aortic valve is not as common as some would have us believe. With regard to isolated aortic root dilatation, this has not been found in our series without the presence of aortic valve abnormalities. With new technology, such as Doppler or color flow mapping, it is possible that many of those with supposed idiopathic dilatation of the aortic root may be recognized to have an explainable cause.

Let us consider the anatomy of the aortic valve. The three cusps can be identified. The cusps are the right, the left, and the noncoronary cusps, and they are of approximately equal size in the normal heart.

It is well known that 60-90% of patients with coarctation have bicuspid aortic valves. The variability relates to differences in defining the presence of the aortic abnormality by angiography or by pathological inspection.

Table 1 25 Patients with Turner Syndrome at UCSF

Diagnosis	Number of patients with diagnosis	Percentage of patients with diagnosis
Aortic coarctation	5	20%
Aortic valve abnormalities	1	4%
Left superior vena cava to coronary sinus	1	4%
Partial anomalous pulmonary venous return	1	4%
Atrial septal defect	1	4%
Isolated aortic root dilatation	0	0%

The morphology of a bicuspid aortic valve is extremely variable. In most valves said to be bicuspid, a raphe is present, representing the fusion between two cusps. This raphe is most frequently between the left and right cusps, making the bicuspid aortic valve extremely difficult to recognize echocardiographically. In an earlier attempt to define aortic valve abnormalities by echocardiography, when compared with the surgical description, we were only able to identify a bicuspid valve correctly by M-mode or two-dimensional echocardiography in 50% of cases. It should be noted that we used the same criteria as Dr. Lippe and colleagues in their study in Chapter 14. If the sensitivity for the diagnosis of bicuspid aortic valve were only 50%, that would lead us to infer a 50% too high or too low incidence of diagnosis. What is really important is that it seems that the echocardiographic technique may not be as sensitive as one would like in order to screen a population for bicuspid or tricuspid aortic valves. The reasons for the M-mode finding of a bicuspid aortic valve relate to the position of the orifice. When the valve leaflets are opposed in diastole and they run from relatively anterior to posterior direction, the closure line can be eccentric. When the closure line runs from side to side, this eccentric closure echocardiogram does not occur on the M-mode. If the beam is directed away from the central position of the valve, it is possible that eccentricity may be created artifactually. The high sensitivity and low specificity of this M-mode echocardiographic method for looking at bicuspid aortic valves may account for the findings of an excessive number of bicuspid aortic valves reported by the UCLA group.

With regard to the two-dimensional technique, there are also problems. The raphe may be defined echocardiographically and, therefore, a bicuspid valve with a raphe may look like a tricuspid valve, unless the valve is observed in the open position where a restricted orifice is observed. If the leaflets are deformed, it may not be possible to observe them clearly, or if the equipment used is substandard by current criteria, aortic valves may be considered bicuspid when they are, in fact, tricuspid. Using the same equipment as that in the UCLA series, our accuracy, when confirmed by surgical inspection, was also 50%, that is, no better than M-mode and of really quite substandard accuracy. I believe that the high frequency of bicuspid valves in the UCLA series is explicable on the basis of a technique which is too sensitive.

To increase the specificity of ultrasound in determining an aortic valve abnormality, it is currently our practice to use Doppler ultrasound, including color Doppler flow mapping, in the diagnosis of aortic valve abnormalities. I think this provides a much greater sensitivity and specificity than has been possible, even with this improved imaging spawned from an improved technology.

To compound this problem of diagnosis, aortic stenosis can occur with tricuspid aortic valves as well. In reviewing the cardiac literature on Turner syndrome, it is not clear whether the abnormal aortic valves were tricuspid and stenotic or bicuspid and stenotic. The term stenotic aortic valve appears to be a more suitable one.

A further problem that makes the issue murky is the diagnosis of coarctation. It is relatively easy to diagnose severe coarctation. Mild coarctation or pseudocoarctation can be quite a different issue. One of our Turner patients with severe aortic stenosis had a mild coarctation of the aorta defined by angiography which did not require any surgery. Mild coarctation may be difficult to define by any noninvasive procedure, including magnetic resonance imaging. An unanswered question, therefore, in the patient with Turner syndrome and bicuspid aortic valve, is how does one assure that a mild coarctation is not present? Both echocardiography and magnetic resonance imaging are likely to lead to errors in the diagnosis of mild coarctation.

With regard to aortic root dilatation, it is not clear that dilatation occurs in Turner syndrome without an aortic valve abnormality. In Dr. Lippe's series, published in *Pediatrics*, none of the patients with dilated aortic roots had bicuspid aortic valves or, at least, some form of aortic valve abnormality, including aortic regurgitation. In many of the patients that we have examined who have dilated aortic roots, ultrasound, including the use of Doppler and color Doppler mapping techniques, has shown minor aortic valve abnormalities. Doppler and color flow mapping shows the jet extending out into the ascending aorta and hitting one of the aortic walls. The jet directed in that direction over the years causes trauma to the media of the aorta, which responds by dilating and, frequently, may develop atherosclerosis or dissection.

It is also interesting to note that the other lesions frequently associated with marked dilatation of the aortic root, namely mitral and tricuspid prolapse, are not common in Turner syndrome. The aortic valve lesions, the coarctation, and the dilated root are, in our experience, no different from other patients with these abnormalities. There certainly is a statistically increased incidence of coarctation, and a higher association with the coarctation of aortic valve abnormality in Turner syndrome; isolated aortic valve abnormalities are, in our experience, not as common as Dr. Lippe has stated. Dilatation of the aortic root, especially the ascending aorta, has not been common in our experience without associated aortic valve abnormalities.

One question of some concern remains. How should patients with Turner syndrome be investigated for cardiac abnormalities? Clinical examination with blood pressure and pulse character difference between the upper and lower extremities remains the cornerstone for the diagnosis of coarctation. The aortic valve should be examined by ultrasound, including Doppler and color flow mapping, early in infancy and then again if found to be normal or minimal after the first decade. Aortic root measurement can be made and compared against standards for body size. After childhood, aortic size may be assessed by X-ray or ultrasound. I would resort to magnetic resonance imaging only if ultrasound imaging proved inadequate, because of the expense of using the latter technique.

DISCUSSION

DR. ROBERT L. ROSENFIELD: I would like to know whether these two speakers are trying to tell us that we should do ultrasounds or echoes on all Turner's or are we supposed to do this on those that we hear clicks or what-not on?

DR. ANDREA PRADER: I think that is a clear message, wasn't it.

DR. BARBARA M. LIPPE: I am not sure. I know what my message is and that is to say I think these patients are at high risk for primary or secondary aortic disease, and that if one believes that prophylaxis, at least for those with functional aortic abnormalities, might prevent consequent events later, we put our patients on the same SBE prophylaxis that anybody with an abnormal aortic valve has. So if we find them, we treat them. And then, if we see the dilation

Dr. Rosenfield is at the University of Chicago Pretzker School of Medicine, Chicago, Illinois. Dr. Prader is at Kinderspital, Zürich, Switzerland. Dr. Lippe is at the University of California at Los Angeles School of Medicine, Los Angeles, California. Dr. Silverman is at the University of California at San Francisco, San Francisco, California. Dr. Robinson is at the National Jewish Center and the University of Colorado Health Science Center, Denver, Colorado. Dr. Hall is at the University of British Colombia, Vancouver, Canada. Dr. Saenger is at Montefiore Medical Center/Albert Einstein College of Medicine, Bronx, New York. Dr. Page is at Whitehead Institute, Cambridge, Massachusetts.

which we have seen in 5 patients now, these patients are going to start to be looked at by our cardiothoracic people. So I do not know where my 5 came from, but they are above 35 mm, and for the small Turner girls, they are approaching, relatively, the size of 50 mm Marfan roots.

DR. NORMAN H. SILVERMAN: Do they have abnormalities of the aortic valve or not?

DR. LIPPE: Two do and three do not. Well, I do not think they do. I do not know until we get in there, since you are right or wrong 50% of the time.

DR. SILVERMAN: You are wrong 50% of the time.

DR. LIPPE: Oh no. No, no, no.

DR. SILVERMAN: I do think that an echocardiogram is a very benign and non-invasive test and I mean if you are really bothered by it, it is probably reasonable to obtain an echocardiogram. But I think that the thrust of my presentation should be that it is very difficult sometimes to tell when there is an aortic valve abnormality. So I think that this is a problem and I do not know that there is really a simple answer to this question as to what to do. This is obviously something that you would want to discuss. I think echocardiography is practiced with varying levels of skill throughout the world, and I think that one has to have some idea of the quality, I should not say quality, the skill of the people who are interpreting these studies before you would refer everybody. In our experience, all the patients that have passed through our laboratory, none of them have had any cardiac findings suggestive of a bicuspid aortic valve. So I think that auscultation in the hands of those that can do it well probably would be enough to decide. Obviously one would not prophylaxis anybody who did not have an aortic valve abnormality, but then as it is so difficult to define what the abnormality is, I think it becomes more difficult to decide who you are going to prophylaxis and who you are not.

DR. ARTHUR ROBINSON: I was just wondering, is the aortic lesion progressive, when should it be looked for, and how often should it be looked for?

DR. LIPPE: If you are talking about dilation of the aortic root, which is the thing that I am most concerned about, because that is what I think will ultimately be associated with dissection in some of these patients, there are measurements that one can make from either the echo or the MRI and our cardiologists have set up a schema much like they have done for Marfan's syndrome. If we have a patient with an aortic root that is dilated greater than two times the size of the descending aorta, on measurement with MRI, we treat that patient right now, with propranolol. So we have 2 patients on propranolol.

DR. ROBINSON: But when do you look for it?

DR. LIPPE: Well, I look for it when we do the echo. If we see a dilated root, then we do the MRI.

DR. ROBINSON: Yes, but when do you do the echo?

UNIDENTIFIED: Routinely?

DR. LIPPE: What I have chosen to do, to be perfectly frank with you, is to refer our patients to a cardiologist and let them decide. Sometimes they will auscultate the patient once or twice and when the patient gets a little older, they will do their first echo and then look at the size of the root. So I am not making that decision alone. But in answer to the question, there have been patients who have ruptured their aorta in the first decade; the majority of the patients reported have been in the second and third decade.

DR. SILVERMAN: With regard to the aortic valve lesion, there is no question that this is a progressive lesion, so that we have many patients in our series who presented in childhood with nothing more than a bicuspid aortic valve with a click and who at puberty or around about that period of time, have presented with significant aortic stenosis requiring surgical or now catheter treatment for their aortic stenosis. And I believe that that really is a thing that is most important: that one should be aware that the aortic root lesion, especially the degree of stenosis, becomes progressive as the valve becomes more and more distorted and calcifies. So I think that that would be one answer. Together with that, the aortic root will dilate obviously as the jet becomes more and more accelerated, due to the fact that as the orifice of the valve becomes more and more stenotic and trauma is exerted on the wall of the aorta, the aortic root will dilate. I personally have not seen young children with markedly dilated aortic roots with aortic stenosis, that this is usually something that occurs in late childhood and early adolescence.

DR. PRADER: I wonder whether there is any more comment on pathogenesis? Dr. Hall, do you want to underline what Dr. Lippe said?

DR. JUDITH G. HALL: I wanted to ask Barbara what she thought about keloids, because I think they are one of the interesting phenomena that are seen in Turner's that is not necessarily explained by edema?

DR. LIPPE: Oh, I do not agree. The worst place they keloid is their earlobes. And that is the area that is the most likely to have been distended and damaged if they have nuchal abnormalities. They pierce their ears and they get these terrible keloids on their ears.

DR. HALL: So you think it is due to having had edema?

DR. LIPPE: That is right. And the repair of the webbed neck.

DR. HALL: Actually if you take keloids from normal people, they have chromosomal abnormalities so it may be related to the chromosomes.

DR. LIPPE: Or mesenchymal tissue growth and repair.

DR. PRADER: Tell me, if it is a defect of connective tissue, then a study of connective tissue or fibroblast cultures should perhaps give a result.

DR. PAUL SAENGER: A very brief question, and I hope it does not engender that much controversy. Barbara, why do they have problems doing a good backstroke?

DR. LIPPE: That is the skeletal abnormality. They have dysplasia of the head of the radius.

DR. SAENGER: So it has nothing to do with the Madelung deformity?

DR. LIPPE: No I do not think so. Very few have Madelung deformities, but a lot of them have the increased carrying angle which is dysplasia, and they do not do well on the violin either.

DR. DAVID PAGE: Barbara, does the mesenchymal theory in any way account for in utero lethality?

DR. LIPPE: I am not a geneticist and I had a very simplistic view of in utero lethality which is the total opposite of everybody else's here. So thank you for the chance of letting me try it out. How do you know that other monosomic states are not more lethal and you never know about them? Is it not possible that because X monosomy is one of the few monosomies that is not lethal, it allows itself to be seen and that if you lose a chromosome 1 after fertilization or prior to or chromosome 2 or chromosome 8 you would never know about it. So, I wonder if maybe that rather than arguing that X monosomy is so lethal, I would argue that a lot of these survive better than any other monosomies.

DR. PAGE: I think it may not be true, Barbara. I think they do. There is just a recent report from Paris in which 32% of unfertilized oocytes had chromosomal abnormalities. They were either monosomics or disomics, so that what you are seeing is that you take the ovum and you look at the oocyte, which they have done, and they are finding a very high proportion, I think, that never make it. I think the XOs are less lethal.

DR. LIPPE: That is exactly what I said.

DR. PRADER: All right, you agree.

DR. LIPPE: So, I was answering David's question where he asked me why I thought they are so lethal and I think they are very unlethal. That was just what I was saying.

DR. PAGE: But 98% get wiped out and that's prohibitive.

16

Autoimmunity in Turner Syndrome

Desmond A. Schatz and Noel K. Maclaren

University of Florida College of Medicine, Gainesville, Florida

Barbara M. Lippe

*University of California at Los Angeles School of Medicine,
Los Angeles, California*

INTRODUCTION

There are a number of reports suggesting that patients with Turner syndrome as well as members of their families are unusually afflicted by autoimmunities. This chapter is a review of the literature and a report of our own experience of autoimmunity in Turner syndrome probands and their families.

THYROID AUTOIMMUNITY

Although Hashimoto's (chronic lymphocytic) thyroiditis was first described in 1912, it was not until 1961 that Engel and Forbes (1) first described the occurrence of thyroiditis in a patient with gonadal dysgenesis. The first well-documented report of autoimmunity in Turner syndrome was published by Williams et al. in 1964, who found thyroid antibodies in 13 out of 25 patients (2). Subsequently, several other studies have confirmed that Hashimoto's thyroiditis is the most common autoimmune disorder in persons with Turner syndrome (3-5). A high incidence of thyroid antibodies has been described in both adults (2,6,7) and children (5,8) with Turner syndrome when compared to age- and sex-matched general populations (9,10). Estimates of the incidence of thyroid antibodies have ranged from 12 to 87% (with a mean of 30%) in such patients, depending on the methods used in their measurement and the ages of the patients studied. The frequencies of thyroid autoantibodies in Turner syndrome patients is age dependent, increasing to about 16 years of age (8,9), and approximate those frequencies seen in the general population of females beyond five decades of life (10).

THYROID AUTOIMMUNE DISEASE

Most patients with Turner syndrome have few clinical signs or symptoms of thyroid disease when their thyroid antibodies are first detected. Alterations of thyroid functions are most often reflected in compensated hypothyroidism, diagnosed on the basis of a normal T4 associated with goiter, high basal plasma TSH, or exaggerated TSH response to TRH in an asymptomatic individual. Overt hypothyroidism characterized by classical symptoms and low T4 and high TSH levels is found less frequently. Although Germain and Plotnick found that the presence of thyroid antibodies was highly predictive for the subsequent development of thyroid abnormalities (9), thyroid dysfunction has been described in several patients with negative antibody titers, a finding previously reported in patients with biopsy-proven Hashimoto's thyroiditis (11,12). It is estimated that approximately 20% of patients with Turner syndrome develop a documentable functional thyroid abnormality by mid-adolescence, with the highest incidence of hypothyroidism near 15 years of age (8). Failure to identify thyroid insufficiency may further diminish growth velocity in already growth-compromised Turner patients.

OTHER AUTOIMMUNITIES

Although a higher incidence of carbohydrate intolerance and even rarely frank diabetes (13-18) has been reported in 15-60% of patients with Turner syndrome, insulin-dependent diabetes (IDD) or type I diabetes has not been shown to be associated. Rather, metabolic profiles (high plasma insulin levels to an oral glucose load suggesting insulin resistance) similar to those seen in patients with mild non–insulin-dependent diabetes (NIDD) have been reported. Relative obesity is common and may account for the insulin resistance in young and old patients alike. The lack of diabetes in the majority of the parents of these patients with Turner syndrome argues strongly that classic NIDD is not present (19).

Whereas autoimmune ovarian failure is associated with Addison's disease (20), the specific concurrence of Addison's disease with gonadal dysgenesis and Turner syndrome is rare and consistent with the very low incidence of adrenal antibodies. Similarily, pernicious anemia has not been associated with Turner syndrome. The latter is surprising considering the previously reported findings of an increased incidence of parietal cell autoantibodies and pernicious anemia in the presence of thyroid autoimmunity in non-Turner patients (10,11). This

Table 1 Autoantibodies in Turner Syndrome

		Autoantibodies			
n	Thyroid TMA/IGA	Parietal cell (PCA)	Islet cell (ICA)	Adreno-cortical (AA)	Reference
24	87.5%	0%	0%	0%	Bright et al. (1982)
100	50.0%	1.3% (1/76)	ND	2.6% (1/76)	Germain and Plotnik (1986)
20	35.0%	0%	5.0%	5.0%	Schatz, Maclaren and Lippe (1987)
Totals 144	57.5%	0.8%	0.8%	2.5%	

could be due in part to the fact that thyroid autoimmunity characteristically appears long before pernicious anemia in individual patients affected by both disorders. Notwithstanding, parietal cell autoantibodies have previously been reported in 20% of control (9) children and 25–30% of control adults (21,22) with autoimmune thyroiditis. Other autoimmune disorders reported in Turner syndrome include Graves disease (23), vitiligo and alopecia totalis (24), and ulcerative colitis (25). There have been no reported instances as yet of the classical autoimmune polyglandular syndrome.

A summary of several of the more comprehensive studies of autoimmunity in Turner syndrome is shown in Table 1.

AUTOIMMUNITY AND CHROMOSOMAL ABNORMALITIES

Although originally described in association with the X isochrome X karyotype (4), thyroid autoantibodies are also reported in both 45,XO individuals, the most common karyotypic abnormality (approximately 60%) of all Turner patients (26,27), and those with mosaic karyotypes (2,8). Several authors have reported the highest incidence of thyroid autoantibodies and thyroid dysfunction in patients with the 46,Xi(Xq), or the long arm isochrome X variant (2,4, 28,29) (13–20% of patients with Turner syndrome). Other chromosomal syndromes, particularly Down syndrome (trisomy 21) and Klinefelter syndrome (XXY) (4), are also associated with an increased incidence of autoimmune disorders. Chronic lymphocytic thyroiditis (30–32), IDD, Graves disease, Addison's disease, celiac disease (33), alopecia areata and vitiligo (34) have also been described in patients with Down syndrome. The presence of thyroid antibodies has been noted in both young individuals and adults with Down syndrome with reported incidences between 10 and 39% (31,32), a finding similar to that seen in Turner syndrome. These findings suggest that autoimmunity may be a feature of several chromosomal disorders, possibly the result of nondysjunctional events. As in Turner syndrome, mothers of patients with Down syndrome have an increased frequency of thyroid autoimmunity, with as many as 28% of mothers with Down syndrome having thyroid antibodies compared to 14% of age-matched controls (35,36).

AUTHORS' STUDY

We examined the sera of 20 patients with Turner syndrome and their family members for a variety of organ-specific antibodies (see Table 2). Fourteen had the XO karyotype, 4 the 45X,46Xi(Xq), and 2 the 46,Xi(Xq) karyotypes. Thyroid autoantibodies (antimicrosomal antibody titer of $\geqslant 1:100$ by hemagglutination inhibition or positive by indirect immunofluorescence and/or anti-

Table 2 Characteristics of Patients with Turner Syndrome and Their Families with Positive Thyroid Antibodies

	Age (yr)	Karyotype	TMA		TGA	PCA	ICA	AA	TSH	T4
			IF	HI						
EB	14	XO	3.0+	1:25600	1:1600	–	–	–	↑	→
Mother	49		2.5+	2:1600	–	–	–	–	N	N
Father	49								N	N
Sister	21		2.5+	1:400	–	–	–	–	N	N
Brother	24									
KM	13	XO	3.0+	1:1600	–	–	–	–	N	
Mother	42		3.0+	1:6400	1:1600	–	–	–	N	
Father	41									
JR	23	XO	3.0+	1:102400	–	–	1+	2+	↑	→
Mother	51		3.0+	1:1600	–	–	–	–	N	N
Father	51									
Sister	24		3.0+	1:400	–	–	–	–	N	N
Brother	26									
Maternal Grandmother	74		2.5+	1:1600	1:100	–	–	–		
KS	16	XO	3.0+	1:400	–	–	–	–	N	N
Mother	49		2.5+	1:100	–	–	–	–	N	N
Father	48		–	–	–	–	–	–	N	N

Table 2 (Continued)

	Age (yr)	Karyotype	TMA		TGA	PCA	ICA	AA	TSH	T4
			IF	HI						
Sister	14		–	–	–	–	–	–	N	N
Sister	22		–	–	–	–	–	–	N	N
Brother	24		–	–	–	–	–	–	N	N
SR	20	45X 46Xi(Xq)	–	[a]	–	–	–	–	N	N
Mother	52		–	1:100	–	–	–	–	N	N
Father	52									
Sister	29		3+	1:25600	–	–	–	–	N	N
Sister	22		3+	1:6400	–	–	–	–	N	N
Sister	17		1+	1:6400	–	–	–	–	N	N
Sister	27									
Brother	25									
FI	14	46X Xi(Xq)	–	1:100	1:100	–	–	–	N	N
Mother	39		2.0+	1:1600	–	–	–	–	N	N
Father	45									
Brother	12									

[a] 1:100 2 yr previously.

Abbreviations: TMA = thyroid microsomal antibodies; IF = indirect immunofluorescence; HI = hemagglutination inhibition; TGA = thyroglobulin antibodies; PCA = parietal cell antibodies; ICA = islet cell antibodies; AA = adrenocortical antibodies.

Table 3 Autoantibodies in Turner Pedigrees

	Autoantibodies				
	TMA	TGA.	PCA	ICA	AA
Patients (20)	6	2	0	1	1
	(30%)	(10%)	–	(5%)	(5%)
Relatives (71)	13[a]	5[a]	1	1	0
	(18.3%)	(7%)	(1.4%)	(1.4%)	–

[a]All female.

thyroglobulin antibodies titer $\geqslant 1:32$) were present in 6 of these patients. All 6 patients were over the age of 10 years, with 4 having the XO karyotype, one a 45X,46Xi(Xq) mosaic and the other a 45,Xi(Xq) isochrome defect. Two of these 6 patients had overt hypothyroidism, requiring thyroid hormone replacement. One patient had an asymptomatic goiter with an elevated TSH and normal T4 and was not on any treatment. One patient had classical Graves disease and was on appropriate medical therapy. Other organ-specific autoantibodies (specifically islet cell, adrenocortical, and parietal cell types) were also studied with a single patient having positive islet cell and adrenocortical antibody titers without any apparent clinical disease. These results are thus consistent with the previous studies reported.

Thyroid autoantibodies were also detected in the 6 mothers of the antibody-positive Turner girls (Table 3). Four of the 6 probands with thyroid autoantibodies had 1 or more sisters. In 3 out of these 4 families, 5 out of a total of 8 sisters had detectable thyroid autoantibodies. None of the brothers or fathers had positive antibody titers. These findings are consistent with the data of Vallotton and Forbes (4), who initially suggested that thyroid autoimmunity was dominantly inherited and would also support a linkage to the X chromosome.

DISCUSSION

The data reported here document that thyroid autoimmunity is clearly increased in patients with Turner syndrome, whereas frequencies of other organ-specific autoimmunities of the gastric mucosa, pancreatic islets, and adrenal cortex are normal or only slightly more than expected. Further, thyroid autoimmunity is also abnormally frequent among mothers and female siblings of probands with Turner syndrome. These findings could contribute to the understanding of the inherited predisposition to thyroid autoimmunity.

Thyroid autoimmunity in the women could give rise to events leading to chromosomal anomalies in their offspring by as yet unknown mechanisms or, conversely, could provide a gestational environment which could lead to the preservation of the Turner conceptus.

Evidence in support of the concept that thyroid autoimmunity in mothers is protective to the Turner conceptus is supported by incidence data. The incidence of Turner syndrome has variably been reported to be between 1 in 2,000 and 1 in 10,000 of live births (26,27). The number of live births with the disorder, however, reflect only a small number of the conceptii with abnormalities of the X chromosome. It has been suggested that the 45X karyotype occurs in as many as 1 in 15 spontaneous abortions, and that less than 1% of all of these XO fetuses survive past 28 weeks gestation (37). Why so few fetuses with Turner syndrome survive to term is not known. Our findings of an increased incidence of maternal and maternally transmitted thyroid autoimmunity in Turner families suggest that thyroid autoimmunity in pregnant women may somehow alter the maternal fetal environment, enhancing the viability of the chromosomally abnormal conceptus.

The findings of elevated titers of autoantibodies in parents giving rise to chromosomal aberrations could also be explained by study of the HLA region. Immune response genes within the HLA complex located on chromosome 6 have been associated with a wide variety of autoimmune disease. For example, insulin-dependent diabetes mellitus is strongly linked to HLA DR3 and/or DR4 haplotypes (38). Although thyroid autoimmunity has been suggested to be HLA associated as well, only a relatively small number of patients have been studied to date, and the results remain controversial. Increased frequencies of HLA DR5 have been reported in patients with goitrous autoimmune thyroiditis (39), and DR3 with atrophic thyroiditis (40). Our own unpublished recent studies in the disease document slight increases in DR3 and DR4. If specific HLA-DR types are found more commonly in probands with Turner syndrome who have autoimmune thyroiditis and their mothers, one might hypothesize that abnormal gametogenesis might be a consequence of immunological dysfunction associated with the HLA region. Such studies are currently in progress.

Other studies to determine possible autoimmune and genetic differences between families with a history of an abortus bearing a Turner karyotype and families with a viable Turner individual are also underway.

The increased frequency of autoimmune thyroiditis in women in general, and in patients with Turner syndrome in particular, suggests that the X chromosome may harbor the gene or genes responsible. Williams initially proposed that thyroiditis may be due to a recessive gene located on the short arm of the X chromosome, the expression of which may be limited by genes on the accompanying Y chromosome (2). The findings of an even greater incidence of thyroiditis in Turner syndrome patients with X isochrome defects suggests that is the long arm of the X chromosome, in fact, which may carry such a gene or genes for thyroid autoimmunity. In a recent study (41) using restriction fragment length polymorphisms (RFLP) to determine the parental origin of sex chromosomal monosomy, Hassold et al. found that the retained X in six out of nine spontaneously aborted XO fetuses was maternal in origin, with the other three being parental. With this technology, X chromosome RFLPs can then be traced through affected families in an attempt to determine if thyroid autoimmunity segregates in positive linkage and a transmitted X chromosomal segment.

SUMMARY

Thyroid autoimmunity, but not other autoimmunities, is increased in patients with Turner syndrome, as well as other females in the pedigrees if the patient is so affected. It is important, therefore, to screen all Turner patients for thyroid antibodies and follow thyroid function closely, especially from the commencement of adolescence. First-degree relatives should also be checked for the presence of thyroid autoimmunity.

An as yet undetermined gene or genes on the X chromosome (possibly the long arm) may be involved. It is now important to perform molecular genetic studies to show that long arm RFLPs of the X chromosome abnormally segregate with thyroiditis in the Turner patient, her mother, and affected sisters in pedigree studies. The coincident influence of other immune response genes such as HLA-D (Class II MHC), T cell receptor genes, immunoglobulin allotypes, and complement allotypes, if any, might also be worthy of investigation.

If the X chromosome can be shown to harbor thyroiditis genes, it would then be important to reconcile why other chromosomal abnormalities such as Trisomy 21 also predispose to the disorder. The answer is probably that multiple common genes are involved.

It is important to screen all Turner patients for thyroid antibodies and to follow those found positive for thyroid function tests on an annual basis or more frequently, especially during their adolescent period.

REFERENCES

1. Engel E, Forbes AP. Abnormal medium sized metacentric chromosome in a woman with primary gonadal failure. Lancet 1961; 2:1004.
2. Williams ED, Engel E, Forbes AP. Thyroiditis and gonadal dysgenesis. N Eng J Med 1964; 270:804–810.
3. Doniach D, Roitt JM, Polan PE. Thyroid antibodies and sex chromosome anomalies. Proc Roy Soc Med 1968; 61:278–280.
4. Vallotton MB, Forbes AP. Autoimmunity in gonadal dysgenesis and Klinefelter's syndrome. Lancet 1967; 1:648–651.
5. Bright GM, Robert M, Blizzard RD, Kaiser DL, Clark WL. Organ-specific autoantibodies in children with common endocrine diseases. J Pediatr 1982; 100:8–14.
6. Sparkes RS, Motulsky AB. Hashimoto's disease in Turner's syndrome with isochromosome X. Lancet 1963; 1:947.

7. Engel E, Forbes AP. Cytogenetic and clinical findings in 48 patients with congenitally defective or absent ovaries. Medicine 1965; 44:135–164.
8. Pai GS, Leach DC, Weiss L, Wolf CH, Van Dyke DL. Thyroid abnormalities in 20 children with Turner's syndrome. J Pediatr 1977; 91:267–269.
9. Germain EL, Plotnick LP. Age-related anti-thyroid antibodies and thyroid abnormalities in Turner syndrome. Acta Paediatr Scan 1986; 75:750–755.
10. Maclaren NK, Riley WJ. Thyroid, gastric and adrenal autoimmunities associated with insulin-dependent diabetes mellitus. Diabetes Care 1985; 8(1):34–38.
11. Loeb PB, Drash AL, Kenny FM. Prevalence of low titre and "negative" antithyroglobulin antibodies in biopsy proved juvenile Hashimoto's thyroiditis. J Pediatr 1973; 82:17–21.
12. Rallison ML, Dobyns BM, Keating FR, Rall JE, Tyler FH. Occurrence and natural history of chronic lymphocytic thyroiditis in childhood. J Pediatr 1975; 86:675–682.
13. Forbes AP, Engel E. The high incidence of diabetes mellitus in 41 patients with gonadal dysgenesis, and their close relatives. Metabolism 1963; 12: 428–439.
14. Polychronakos C, Letarte J, Collu R, Ducharme JR. Carbohydrate intolerance in children and adolescents with Turner's syndrome. J Ped 1980; 96:1009–1014.
15. Van Campenhout J, Antaki A, Rasio E. Dioabetes mellitus and thyroid autoimmunity in gonadal dysgenesis. Fertility & Sterility 1973; 24:1–9.
16. Nielsen J, JOhansen K, Yde H. The frequency of diabetes mellitus in patients with Turner's syndrome and pure gonadal dysgenesis. Acta Endo 1969; 62:251–269.
17. AvRuskin TW, Crigler JF, Soeldner JS. Turner's syndrome and carbohydrate metabolism. 1. Impaired insulin secretion after tolbutamide and glucagon stimulation tests: evidence of insulin deficiency. Am J Med Sci 1979; 277:145–152.
18. Neufeld ND, Lippe B, Sperling MA. Carbohydrate (CHO) intolerance in gonadal dysgenesis. A new model of insulin resistance. Diabetes 1980; 25: Suppl. 1:379.
19. Rimoin DL, Harder E, Whitehead B, Packman S, Peake GT, Sly WS. Abnormal glucose tolerance in patients with gonadal dysgenesis and their parents. Clin Res 1970; 18:395.
20. Irvine WJ, Chan MM, Scarth L, Kolb FO, Hartog M, Bayliss RIS, Drury MI. Immunological aspects of premature ovarian failure associated with idiopathic Addison's disease. Lancet 1968; 2:883.
21. Markson JL, Moore JM. "Autoimmunity" in pernicious anemia and iron deficiency anemia. Lancet 1962; 2:1240–1243.
22. Irvine WJ, Davies SH, Teitelbaum S, Delamore IW, Williams AW. The clinical and pathological significance of gastric parietal cell antibody. Ann NY Acad Sci 1965; 124:657–691.
23. Brooks WH, Meek JC, Schimke RN. Gonadal dysgenesis with Graves' disease. J Med Genet 1977; 14:128–129.

24. Blumberg B, Rotter J, Lippe B, Aleck K, Sparkes R, Mohandas T. Alopecia totalis in Turner syndrome. Proceedings of the San Diego Birth Defects Meeting 1980; p. 42.

25. Nishimura H, Kino M, Kubo S, Kawamura K. Hashimoto's thyroiditis and ulcerative colitis in a patient with Turner syndrome. JAMA 1985; 254:357.

26. Gerald PS. Sex chromosome disorders. N Engl J Med 1976; 294:706–708.

27. Hook EB, Hamerton JL. The frequency of chromosome abnormalities detected in consecutive newborn studies. In Hooke B, Porter IH, eds. Population Cytogenetics. New York: Academic Press, 1977; 63–79.

28. Sparkes RS, Motulsky G. The Turner syndrome with isochrome X and Hashimoto's thyroiditis. Ann Int Med 1967; 67:132–144.

29. Fialkow PJ. Genetic aspects of autoimmunity. In Steinberg AG, Bearn AG, eds. Progress in Medical Genetics. Vol. VI. New York: Grune & Stratton, 1969; 117–67.

30. Baxter RG, Larkins RG, Martin FR, Heyma P, Myles K, Ryan L. Down's syndrome and thyroid function in adults. Lancet 1975; 2:794–795.

31. Sare L, Ruvalcaba RHA, Kelley VC. Prevalence of thyroid disorder in Down's syndrome. Clin Genet 1978; 14:154–158.

32. Lobo E de H, Khan M, Tew J. Community study of hypothyroidism in Down's syndrome. Br Med J 1980; 1:1253.

33. Ruch W, Schurmann K, Gordon P, Burgin-Wolff A, Girard J. Coexistant celiac disease, Graves disease and diabetes mellitus type I in a patient with Down's syndrome. Eur J Pediatr 1985; 144:89–90.

34. Du Vivier A, Munro DD. Alopecia areata, auto-immunity and Down's syndrome. Br Med J. 1975; 1:191–192.

35. Faialkow PJ, Hecht F, Uchida IA, Motulsky AG. Increased frequency of thyroid autoantibodies in mothers of patients with Down's syndrome. Lancet 1965; 2:868–870.

36. Doniach D, Nilsson LR, Roitt IM. Autoimmune thyroiditis in children and adolescents: II. Immunological correlations and parent study. Acta Paediatr Scand 1965; 54:260–274.

37. Carr DH, Gredeon M. Population cytogenetics in human abortuses. In Hook EB, Porter IH, eds. Population Cytogenetics. New York: Academic Press, 1977; 1–9.

38. Platz P, Jakobsen BD, Morling N, Ryder LP, Svejgaard A, Thomsen M, Kromonn H, Benn J, Nerup J, Green A, Hauge M. HLA-D and DR-antigens in genetic analysis of insulin-dependent diabetes mellitus. Diabetologia 1981; 21:108–115.

39. Farid NR, Sampson L. Moens H, Barnard JM. The association of goitrous autoimmune thyroiditis with HLA-DR5. Tissue Antigens 1985; 17:265–268.

40. Moens H, Farid NR. Hashimoto's thyroiditis is associated with HLA-DRw3. N Engl J Med 1978; 299:133–134.

41. Hassold T, Kumlin E, Takaesu N, Leppert M. Determination of the parental origin of sex-chromosome monosomy using restriction fragment length polymorphisms. Am J Hum Genet 1985; 37:965–972.

DISCUSSION

DR. ANDREA PRADER: Does anyone want to discuss the problem of the X chromosome?

DR. DAVID L. RIMOIN: I wonder if you have looked at the origin of the X chromosome that persists in your Turner patients whose mothers were thyroid positive, because if they were missing their maternal X then you wouldn't expect the X to have anything to do with it.

DR. BARBARA LIPPE: Funny that you should ask. We are doing that now. We are using simple X markers and RFLPs. We are making DNA from the parents and trying to answer that. I have only done two so far. They are both maternal X-derived. But, again, in 70% or more the monosomic X will be maternal and perhaps much higher than that is going to be my prejudice. So I have a feeling that it is not going to be informative, although that is one of the first things we are doing.

DR. RIMOIN: The other thing is that if it were the mother's X that was producing both things, then half of the sons should have gotten that same X chromosome and had thyroiditis probably.

DR. LIPPE: But that is a very good point. It would be interesting if they didn't, and we are going to be able to do that, too.

DR. ROBERT BLIZZARD: This phenomenon about chromosomes and thyroid autoimmunities are not new to you, Noel, and you must have thought about this a lot through the years. I am a little bit perplexed by your proposition that the X may be the predisposing factor because we are talking about Turner's having

---

Dr. Praeder is at Kinderspital, Zürich, Switzerland. Dr. Rimoin is at Cedars-Sinai Medical Center, Los Angeles, California. Dr. Lippe is at the University of California at Los Angeles School of Medicine, Los Angeles, California. Dr. Blizzard is at the University of Virginia at Charlottesville, Charlottesville, Virginia. Dr. Tanner is at the University of Texas Health Center, Houston, Texas. Dr. MacLaren is at the University of Florida College of Medicine, Gainesville, Florida. Dr. Hall is at the University of British Colombia, Vancouver, Canada. Dr. Rosenwaks was at the Jones Institute for Reproductive Medicine, Eastern Virginia Medical School, Norfolk, Virginia. He is currently at Cornell University Medical Center–The New York Hospital, New York, New York. Dr. Golbus is at the University of California at San Francisco, San Francisco, California. Dr. Sotos is at Children's Hospital of Columbus, Columbus, Ohio. Dr. Becker is at Children's Hospital, Pittsburgh, Pennsylvania. Dr. Robinson is at the University of Colorado, Denver, Colorado. Dr. Hibi is at National Children's Hospital, Tokyo, Japan.

one X versus two Xs. We know that females have an increased incidence of thyroiditis over males, and they have two Xs. On that thesis, Turner patients who have one X should have half as much thyroiditis. Maybe the place we should be looking is to the Y in some way being a suppressor for people who are predisposed in some way. If you look at the incidence of thyroid autoimmunity in the patients with Klinefelter's who have two Xs and two Ys, you do not find an increased incidence of autoimmunity of the thyroid. You find the same as you do in the male population. And then just to take it a step further to . . .

DR. JAMES TANNER: I agree perfectly with this line of logic to this point.

DR. BLIZZARD: Well then, why didn't you say maybe the Y was responsible?

DR. TANNER: Well I am waiting for you to make that connection with the help of David Rimoin.

DR. BLIZZARD: Well, then if you talk about the patient with Down's who has an increased incidence of thyroid autoimmunity, you don't get the sex chromosomes involved at all, but you have an extra chromosome on the 21 or 22, and I guess I find it a little bit difficult to come up with any kind of better hypothesis than I have come up with in the last 18 years. Incidentally, a comment. It isn't just thyroiditis that patients with Turner's have, but they also have an increased incidence of thyrotoxicosis, and it is not as common as hypothyroidism or goiters. But we have three patients in our clinic with Turner's who have thyrotoxicosis.

DR. NOEL K. MACLAREN: That is a very good point. I should have said of the six patients with antibodies, three had thyroid abnormalities, one was a Graves, and two had hypothyroidism, one of which had been already recognized and being treated. No, the proposition with Down syndrome is a bother, but for insulin-dependent diabetes, certainly in mouse models, we have very clear evidence for four genes and I suppose for thyroid autoimmunity, we ought to have at least more than one. So one can say that maybe other genes are responsible for the Down's, but the Lippe hypothesis would make me also wonder whether thyroid autoimmunity in the mother in some way predisposes to nondysjunctional events or something of this sort or in fact affects the outcome in terms of survival. I don't have any answers either beyond that point.

DR. JUDITH HALL: Just to add potential hypotheses as long as they are being looked for. One could be that Turner who are mosaic having one of two cell lines basically react against the other cell line, so that one of the questions would be whether or not there seems to be more autoimmunity in obviously mosaic patients. Anyhow, those patients with X chromosomal abnormalities may become mosaic, at least in cells that we are not looking at. The other explanation which has been used in terms of diabetes is that there is a selection because of HLA typing apparently for those children who have inherited a particular HLA type that predisposes them to diabetes, and what that would mean is that there was selection for those fetuses that carry a particular immune system to be maintained, that is not to be aborted. If that were true, one of the explanations for why those Turner's children weren't miscarried is that they had a particular HLA type that allowed them to be maintained. And so, whatever it is about thyroid disease that predisposes that offspring to get thyroid disease also selects them for not being aborted.

DR. MACLAREN: We will settle that latter question when Barbara Lippe can get the specimens to do HLA typing on these six families. Rotter has raised in diabetes the problem of a transmission bias which is, I think, argued by many different groups of geneticists, whether in fact it is true or not. But what is clearly true in that disease is of course a male transmission bias, but I think we are getting off the Turner's path right now.

DR. ZEV ROSENWAKS: You have listed quite a bit of other autoimmune diseases not being present in an increased amount of these patients. Once I came across a girl with XO having alopecia totalis. And when I addressed the dermatologists, they said this is very frequent in 45 XO, and I wonder whether you have any similar experience or others have?

DR. LIPPE: Noel is laughing because I showed him a slide of one of my patients with alopecia. We have had three patients reported, in conjunction with Dave Rimoin's group. So there may be a somewhat increased incidence, I agree with you.

DR. MITCHELL S. GOLBUS: Do they have any other isolated alopecia or do they have thyroid antibodies?

DR. LIPPE: Two out of the three had positive antithyroid antibodies.

DR. ROSENWAKS: Mine not.

DR. JUAN SOTOS: Do you have any information now to immunity in Noonan's or definitely Turner's with normal chromosomes?

DR. MACLAREN: No, I don't. Does anybody else?

DR. HALL: We have actually collected a huge number of Noonan syndrome patients as a collaborative study, and it is reported in Noonan syndrome but it was not our observation in this large group of about 400 cases.

DR. DOROTHY BECKER: Noel, I am intrigued by your one patient or 5% with islet cell antibodies, and my bias was that there were actually going to be more. Do you know if anybody else has looked and do we know anything about the carbohydrate metabolism in that one patient?

DR. MACLAREN: I showed you a couple of the recent studies where others had looked. I think it is obvious that many of the Turner patients had a diabetic phenotype, but as far as I can determine, it is rare to get insulin-dependent diabetes clinically in the accepted sense. Is that your experience, too?

DR. BECKER: Yes, but maybe we are not going old enough yet and maybe there is something modulating it. What about the assays in some of the other studies. Do you know? I didn't see who they were. Would they be comparable?

DR. MACLAREN: This appears to be so for islet cell antibodies. I think it must be rare. This one patient we had had both adrenal antibodies and islet cell antibodies, and I suppose that that is just an unusual event. Of course these diseases are less common than thyroid autoimmunity, and maybe we need to enlarge the series somewhat.

DR. ARTHUR ROBINSON: I just would like to ask, Dr. MacLaren, why insulin-dependent diabetes really appears to be rare in patients with XO gonadal dysgenesis. If you look at the series that Ann Forbes reported of patients on up into their 50s, glucose intolerance is not at all uncommon as they get into adolescence. I don't remember whether she found a modest increase in diabetes, but it wasn't clear whether it was insulin-dependent or not at a very late age.

DR. MACLAREN: In my experience I haven't seen personally an insulin-dependent diabetic who has Turner, whereas glucose intolerance is pretty common. I think that it may be relatable to the relative obesity that we heard discussed before, so that seems to deal with that. Now, to answer your question, whether it be actually unusually infrequent, you would need to study a lot of patients, though. The frequency in the U.S. in a lifetime is about 1 in 300, and if we are talking about some people in their mid-20s, the frequency of insulin-dependent diabetes is about 1 in 500, so one would need a pretty big series to show that it is, in fact, abnormally frequent. But you might be right.

DR. ITSURO HIBI: I would like to comment on two points. One point is the positive titers of islet cell antibodies. In my series it is very rare, less than 10%, and I feel the disease is different. I have studied almost all patients with OGTT and found frequently intolerance only.

DR. MACLAREN: I wonder, Dr. Hibi, what the frequency of thyroid auto-immunity, in general, is in the Japanese population. I had a feeling that it was somewhat lower than we see in the U.S. and Europe probably.

DR. HIBI: I am sorry, I don't know the exact percentage in grown-up females. When I surveyed the Turner patients, the age of these patients was under 17.

DR. MACLAREN: I might comment that for the immunologists in the audience, if there are any, Turner syndrome would seem to be an obvious group of patients to study for immunological defects, and certainly I haven't yet, but do intend to.

DR. HIBI: And of course I have read a nice paper written by Dr. Barbara Lippe, and now we are following up antimicrosomal titer on the grown-up patients, but as yet the results have not derived, I am sorry.

DR. HALL: I just wanted to mention Sybert's data from the adult Turner Clinic that she has been following for many years. Five out of 120 women with Turner syndrome over 21 years of age do have true diabetes, but it is primarily adult onset.

DR. BECKER: Well, I was actually going to make this comment tomorrow, but our data on about 30 patients with Turner syndrome is slightly different from Dr. Hibi, in that the glucose intolerance and the hyperinsulinism could be due to obesity in the children under the age of 13. If one matched them for body mass index and matched the patients' glucose levels and insulin levels, they weren't that different. However, the glucose intolerance I think was more severe. Insulin levels were not that different, but glucose tolerance was abnormal. However, over the age of 13, they certainly had more glucose intolerance than body mass index-matched patients, and the insulin levels were relatively low. So, rather than having the insulin excess that you would expect with obesity, they tended to have lower insulin levels than you would expect for the degree of hyperglycemia, and that is why I was wondering about maybe a marginal degree of autoimmunity, maybe not quite as severe as you see in insulin-dependent diabetes. I would like to offer some more sera to you so that maybe we can look a little harder, especially in the older ones.

Summary of Part II

Dr. Andrea Prader

*Kinderspital
Zürich, Switzerland*

NATURAL HISTORY AND ASSOCIATE ABNORMALITIES

Many of us feel that the natural history and the associated abnormalities of Turner syndrome are well known. The papers and discussions of this session demonstrate that our knowledge is far from complete and that we do not understand at all the pathogenesis.

Dr. Arthur Robinson reviewed the *abnormal karyotypes*, the *prenatal mortality*, and the *postnatal prevalence*. Between 98 and 99% of all 46,X conceptuses end as spontaneous abortions. The cause is unknown. This very high prenatal mortality may be low compared with other monosomies, as discussed by Dr. Lippe. The prevalence at birth is about 1 in 3000 with large variations in different studies. Maternal age is not increased in contrast to other chromosomal abnormalities. The lacking X chromosome is predominantly of paternal origin. Among the problems raised are the hypothesis that the isochromosome for the long arm of the X (46,XXqi) may have a fetoprotective influence and the question whether and how often "normal" females have the mosaic karyotype 46,X/46X without short stature and without associated abnormalities.

Dr. Mitchell Golbus discussed the *prenatal diagnosis*. A 46,X karyotype in chorionic villus sampling at 9-12 weeks of gestation reflects only the placental tissue while the fetus may be normal. A reliable karyotype may be obtained from amniotic fluid at 12-16 weeks of gestation. In ultrasound at a later gestational age, a large cystic hygroma in the nuchal area is suggestive of Turner syndrome.

Dr. Zev Rosenwaks presented the possibility of *egg donation* and pregnancy maintenance. In the discussion, alternative solutions were mentioned: donation of an in vitro fertilized embryo and gamete (oocyte and sperm) intrafallopian transfer (GIFT). The technical and ethical problems involved in all these *reproductive technologies* are only partly resolved, and the success rate is still low.

Dr. Robert Rosenfield reviewed the *development of the ovaries* and the rare event of spontaneous puberty. At birth the ovaries may still look normal but the number of germ cells and follicles is decreasing. At this stage or later, typical streak ovaries are found. Patients with spontaneous puberty are not taller as adults than those without. Spontaneous puberty usually is followed by *premature menopause*.

Growth was discussed by *Dr. Michael Ranke*. At birth, weight and length is about -1 SD, at age 10 about -2 SD, and at age 14 about -4 SD. In the absence of spontaneous puberty there is no pubertal growth spurt, but the ratio weight/height begins to increase. Bone age is retarded, and adult height is reached only at the age of 20. Mean adult height is 146.8 cm. Others have found slightly lower values. Possibly there is a slight secular trend. Adult height is correlated with midparent height as in normal individuals.

Dr. Itsuro Hibi found that in *Japan* more girls with Turner syndrome develop spontaneous puberty (21%) than in U.S. and Europe even if in prepuberty they have increased FSH values and hyperresponsiveness to LHRH. In his experience spontaneous puberty and/or treatment with anabolic steroids are followed by decreased adult height. Different experiences and questions were voiced in the discussion.

Dr. Barbara Lippe presented a stimulating *pathogenetic concept of the many typical abnormalities*. In her opinion the basic defect is a growth disorder of the mesenchymal tissue. This leads to skeletal and vascular growth abnormalities. The latter is followed by lymphatic obstructions which easily explain most of the dysmorphic features as secondary abnormalities. So far there are no experimental data to support this concept.

Dr. Noel Maclaren discussed the *high incidence of thyroid autoimmunity* (30%) in the presence of a low incidence of other forms of autoimmunity. The regular concordance of thyroid autoimmunity in the patient and her mother and the higher incidence of thyroid autoimmunity in females in general stimulated speculations about an X chromosomal gene predisposing to thyroid autoimmunity or a Y chromosomal gene protecting from it. The incidence of *diabetes mellitus* is increased in adult patients and probably normal in children with Turner syndrome.

Dr. Norman Silverman confirmed the *high frequency of aortic valve lesions* (bicuspid valves due to secondary fusion of tricuspid valves) progressing in adolescence and adulthood to general aortic root lesions. There was no uniform opinion whether expert auscultation is sufficient to identify those patients who need prophylactic treatment with antibiotics or whether additional echocardiography and/or magnetic resonance imaging (MRI) should be recommended.

Part III

Growth Hormone Secretion and Bone/Cartilage Development

INTRODUCTION

Dr. Robert M. Blizzard, University of Virginia at Charlottesville, Charlottesville, Virginia.

The goal here is to focus on the growth retardation and the growth potential of patients with Turner syndrome. Do they have a skeletal defect? Do they have a hormone deficiency? Do they have both?

How do we treat to overcome the short stature? When do we treat with estrogens, and how much? When do we treat or do we treat with anabolic steroids? If so, which ones? Do we treat with growth hormone? If we change the growth velocity, does that mean that we are changing the ultimate height?

Historically, growth hormone was first used to treat patients with Turner syndrome 20 years ago, and some of you may be surprised to know that growth hormone did work at that point in time. There were about three patients that were treated in Baltimore. We reported that it did not work, but that was because it did not work in a relative way compared to treatment of hypopituitary children. Those patients did have some increase in growth, but for the investment of the material it was certainly a failure, and therefore it was discarded as a potential therapeutic agent.

Then halotestin was utilized by Dr. Johanson and myself in patients with Turner syndrome, and from that, eventually, oxandrolone, a better anabolic agent for that purpose, was utilized. We are going to hear more about that, particularly, in this part.

These are the questions that will be addressed. Dr. Cutler and Dr. Albertsson-Wikland will be talking about the possibility that these patients have growth hormone deficiency: relative, absolute, or none. That will be followed by discussions by Drs. Horton, Baylink, Rimoin, Rubin, and others regarding the bone and cartilage in Turner syndrome.

17

Are Girls with Turner Syndrome Growth Hormone-Deficient?

Gordon B. Cutler, Jr., and Susan R. Rose

National Institute of Child Health and Human Development,
Bethesda, Maryland

Judith L. Ross

Hahnemann University, Philadelphia, Pennsylvania

INTRODUCTION

The question of whether girls with Turner syndrome are growth hormone-deficient encompasses three questions. First, what test(s) is most sensitive and specific for the diagnosis of growth hormone (GH) deficiency? Second, what are the actual criteria for the diagnosis? And third, do girls with Turner syndrome meet these criteria?

TESTS FOR GROWTH HORMONE DEFICIENCY

Before 1963 the diagnosis of GH deficiency rested entirely on clinical criteria. Development of the GH radioimmunoassay led to laboratory approaches to diagnosis. However, single measurements of serum GH were not adequate to evaluate GH secretion because of the intermittent, pulsatile secretion of this hormone (1,2). To circumvent this difficulty, GH stimulation tests were developed (3-11). Such tests became the gold standard for the diagnosis of GH deficiency.

The adequacy of these conventional GH stimulation tests, however, has recently been challenged (12-14). A substantial proportion of short children who have normal responses to GH stimulation tests have been reported to have decreased spontaneous GH secretion with low mean 24-hr GH levels. It was concluded from these observations that measurement of spontaneous GH secretion is a more sensitive test of GH deficiency than the standard GH stimulation tests.

To reexamine this issue, we have been measuring both stimulated and spontaneous GH secretion in prepubertal short children (15). Stimulated GH levels have been determined every 15 min for 2 hr during a combined arginine-insulin tolerance test (arginine, 0.5 g/kg, administered intravenously over 30 min, followed 30 min later by insulin 0.1 units/kg, administered as an intravenous bolus (7)) and every 30 min for 2 hr during a levo-dopa stimulation test (125 mg orally for body weight less than 15 kg, 250 mg for body weight 15 to 30 kg, and 500 mg for body weight above 30 kg (11)).

Short children with peak GH levels less than or equal to 7 μg/liter after all three stimuli have been given the diagnosis of GH deficiency. The remaining short patients who have had no identifiable endocrine, genetic, systemic, or psychosocial cause of short stature have been given the diagnosis of idiopathic short stature.

Spontaneous GH levels (the mean of measurements on samples obtained every 20 minutes) have also been measured in these short children and in normal, prepubertal controls. However, the mean 24-hr spontaneous GH level has been a relatively insensitive test for GH deficiency. It has detected less than 60% of the GH-deficient children who were identified by the GH stimulation tests. The mean 24-hr GH levels of the remaining GH-deficient children have been within the normal range for prepubertal children (1.0–6.5 μg/liter). No child with normal stimulated GH levels (idiopathic short stature) has had low spontaneous GH secretion.

The above data differ from those of two earlier studies of spontaneous GH secretion (12,13). Both of the earlier studies found high sensitivity of the mean 24-hr GH level for the diagnosis of GH deficiency and a substantial incidence of low spontaneous GH levels in short children who had normal responses to GH stimulation tests. These earlier studies, however, did not match patients and controls for pubertal stage, and the number of prepubertal control subjects was small. Thus, these studies compared mean 24-hr GH level between short, predominantly prepubertal patients and normal, predominantly pubertal controls. The difference between patients and controls in mean 24-hr GH levels may therefore have resulted primarily from the difference in pubertal status.

We conclude from the available data that conventional GH stimulation tests are the most sensitive means to detect growth hormone deficiency.

LABORATORY CRITERIA FOR THE DIAGNOSIS
OF GROWTH HORMONE DEFICIENCY

Our operational criterion for the diagnosis of GH deficiency has been a peak level of ≤7 μg/liter after the arginine-insulin and levo-dopa tests. Unfortunately, this criterion is based upon limited data from normal subjects (7,11). These published normal data are too scanty to establish reliable 95% confidence limits or to indicate how the criterion for a normal response should be adjusted for age, sex, or pubertal status. A further problem is the possibility of a systematic difference between our current radioimmunoassay measurement of GH and that of the published studies. Thus, there are not yet adequately validated criteria for the interpretation of GH stimulation tests.

Despite this unfortunate circumstance, most investigators would agree that a GH response > 10 μg/liter represents a normal response, since it is not uncommon for normally growing children to have responses that do not exceed this level.

Although measurement of the spontaneous mean 24-hr GH level is less sensitive than stimulation tests for the detection of GH deficiency, the normal range for spontaneous GH secretion by prepubertal children has been determined with greater precision. The 95% confidence limits (after logarithmic transformation) were 1.0-6.5 μg/liter for 4-12-year-old normal volunteers (equally divided between boys and girls) who were between the 10th and 90th height percentiles for age (updated data from Ref. 15). Among these prepubertal children there was no significant effect of age or sex on the mean 24-hr GH level.

INCIDENCE OF GROWTH HORMONE DEFICIENCY IN TURNER SYNDROME

All 21 of our patients with Turner syndrome (ages 2-20 years) who underwent arginine-insulin and levo-dopa tests had peak GH concentrations > 10 μg/liter (16). Thus, none of our patients were GH-deficient by conventional GH stimulation tests.

All 15 prepubertal-aged girls (ages 2-8) with Turner syndrome who underwent measurement of spontaneous GH secretion had mean 24-hr levels within the normal range (15,16). The average of the mean 24-hr levels for these 15 girls with Turner syndrome did not differ from that of the prepubertal normal volunteers. Thus, none of our patients were GH-deficient, relative to normal prepubertal children, by measurement of spontaneous GH secretion.

SPONTANEOUS GROWTH HORMONE SECRETION IN UNTREATED PUBERTAL-AGED GIRLS WITH TURNER SYNDROME

Patients with Turner syndrome 9-20 years old had significantly lower mean 24-hr GH levels as a group than age-matched normal girls (2.4 ± 0.2 SEM vs. 5.6 ± 0.8 μg/liter, $p < 0.005$ (16)). However, the mean 24-hr GH levels of these untreated pubertal-aged girls remained within the normal prepubertal range of 1.0-6.5 μg/liter in 13 of the 15 girls. The other 2 girls had mean 24-hr GH levels just below the normal range for prepubertal girls. Since puberty has been shown to increase the mean 24-hr GH level (17–23), the simplest explanation for decreased 24-hr GH level compared to age-matched normal girls would be the failure of girls with Turner syndrome to enter puberty. If this hypothesis is correct, this age-related difference in spontaneous GH secretion between normal girls and girls with Turner syndrome should be correctable by administration of exogenous estrogen to induce puberty.

SUMMARY

Measurement of spontaneous GH secretion over 24 hr was a less sensitive test for GH deficiency in prepubertal children than the conventional GH stimulation tests.

None of our prepubertal-aged patients with Turner syndrome had GH deficiency by either spontaneous or stimulated GH measurements.

Pubertal-aged patients with Turner syndrome who were not receiving estrogen had mean 24-hr GH levels that were similar to the levels of normal prepubertal girls and significantly less than the levels of age-matched normal girls. Since puberty appears to cause increased spontaneous GH secretion, we hypothesize that the decreased GH secretion of untreated pubertal-aged girls with Turner syndrome is due to their failure to enter puberty.

In conclusion, girls with Turner syndrome have not yet been shown to have an intrinsic abnormality in the neuroendocrine regulation of GH secretion. Whether supplemental GH will increase the adult height of girls with Turner syndrome is a question that will require long-term clinical trials such as are in progress at the NIH and other centers.

REFERENCES

1. Greenwood FC, Hunter WM, Marrian VJ. Growth hormone levels in children and adolescents. Brit Med J 1964; 1:25.
2. Takahashi Y, Kipnis DM, Daughaday WH. Growth hormone secretion during sleep. J Clin Invest 1968; 47:2079–90.
3. Fass B, Lippe BM, Kaplan SA. Relative usefulness of three growth hormone stimulation screening tests. Am J Dis Child 1979; 133:931–3.
4. Buckler JMH. Exercise as a screening test for growth hormone release. Acta Endocrinol 1972; 69:219–29.
5. Merimee TJ, Lillicrap DA, Rabinowitz D. Effect of arginine on serum levels of human growth hormone. Lancet 1965; 2:668–70.
6. Glick SM, Roth J, Yalow RS, Berson SA. The regulation of growth hormone secretion. Rec Progr Horm Res 1965; 21:241–83.
7. Penny R, Blizzard RM, Davis WR. Sequential arginine and insulin tolerance tests on the same day. J Clin Endocrinol Metab 1969; 29:1499–1501.
8. Weber B, Helge H, Quabbe H-J. Glucagon-induced growth hormone release in children. Acta Endocrinol 1970; 65:323–41.

9. Boyd AE, Lebovitz HE, Pfeiffer JB. Stimulation of human-growth hormone secretion by L-DOPA. N Engl J Med 1970; 283:1425.

10. Gil-Ad I, Topper E, Laron Z. Oral clonidine as a growth hormone stimulation test. Lancet 1979; 2:278-9.

11. Frasier SD. A review of growth hormone stimulation tests in children. Pediatrics 1974; 53:929-37.

12. Spiliotis BE, August GP, Hung W, Sonis W, Mendelson W, Bercu BB. Growth hormone neurosecretory dysfunction: a treatable cause of short stature. J Am Med Assoc 1984; 251:2223-30.

13. Zadik Z, Chalew SA, Raiti S, Kowarski AA. Do short children secrete insufficient growth hormone? Pediatrics 1985; 76:355-60.

14. Bercu BB, Shulman D, Root AW, Spiliotis BE. Growth hormone (GH) provocative testing frequently does not reflect endogenous GH secretion. J Clin Endocrinol Metab 1986; 63:709-16.

15. Ross JL, Radke JL, Rose S, Cutler GB Jr. Frequent growth hormone sampling offers little diagnostic advantage over classic growth hormone provocative testing. 68th annual meeting of the Endocrine Society, Anaheim, CA, June 25-27, 1986. Abstract.

16. Ross JL, Long LM, Loriaux DL, Cutler GB Jr. Growth hormone secretory dynamics in Turner syndrome. J Pediatr 1985; 106:202-206.

17. Finkelstein JW, Roffwarg HP, Boyar RM, Kream J, Hellman L. Age related change in the twenty-four hour spontaneous secretion of growth hormone. J Clin Endocrinol Metab 1972; 35:665-70.

18. Miller JD, Tannenbaum GS, Colle E, Guyda HJ. Daytime pulsatile growth hormone secretion during childhood and adolescence. J Clin Endocrinol Metab 1982; 55:989-994.

19. Mauras N, Blizzard RM, Link K, Johnson ML, Rogol AD, Veldhuis JD. Augmentation of growth hormone secretion during puberty: Evidence for a pulse amplitude-modulated phenomenon. J Clin Endocrinol Metab 1987; 64:596-601.

20. Ross JL, Pescovitz OH, Barnes K, Loriaux DL, Cutler GB Jr. Growth hormone secretory dynamics in children with precocious puberty. J Pediatr 1987; 110:369-72.

21. Costin G, Kaufman FR. Growth hormone secretory patterns in children with short stature. J Pediatr 1987; 110:362-8.

22. Liu L, Merriam GR, Sherins RJ. Chronic sex steroid exposure increases mean plasma growth hormone concentration and pulse amplitude in men with isolated hypogonadotropic hypogonadism. J Clin Endocrinol Metab 1987; 64:651-6.

23. Rose SR, Kibarian M, Gelato M, Ross JL, Muellner J, Gay K, Cutler GB Jr, Cassorla FG. Brief administration of sex steroid increases the mean 24-hour level of growth hormone in children with idiopathic short stature. J Pediatr Endocrinol 1988; 3:1-5.

DISCUSSION

DR. ROBERT M. BLIZZARD: Gordon, did you change your assay procedures in the last four or five years?

DR. GORDON B. CUTLER: The last change in the assay was about 4 to 5 years ago. It was a relatively minor change, and when the change was made, there was extensive cross-checking to insure that we were within a few percent of the answers that were obtained before. The method is the Hazelton Biotechnologies assay, which was originally identical to the National Pituitary Agency assay and now has a couple of minor modifications. Hazelton Biotechnologies is considering a change to a biosynthetic GH standard. There has been no change in the assay, though, for about four or five years.

DR. BLIZZARD: That is a polyclonal antibody, I think.

DR. CUTLER: Yes.

DR. BLIZZARD: Well, for the audience who may not know, there is a lot of confusion these days about what growth hormone values mean when reported from one laboratory versus another laboratory because the IRMA kits are not giving the same values when supplied by different commercial groups. For example, the Hybritech versus the Nichols kit assay: The Hybritech will measure 30 to 35% of the growth hormone that the Nichols assay measures, so there is a dilemma when we try to interpret that and we do not know what assay has been done. That is why I asked the question.

Dr. Blizzard is at the University of Virginia at Charlottesville, Charlottesville, Virginia. Dr. Cutler is at the National Institute of Child Health and Human Development, Bethesda, Maryland.

18

Dynamics of Growth Hormone Secretion in Girls with Turner Syndrome

Kerstin Albertsson-Wikland and Sten Rosberg

Göteborg University, Göteborg, Sweden

INTRODUCTION

Turner described in 1938 (1) girls with short stature and delayed skeletal and sexual maturation. These girls, with so-called Turner syndrome, have either one abnormal or one missing sex chromosome (2). Turner syndrome is one of the most common chromosomal aberrations, with an incidence of 1 out of 2500 female births (3,4). The most constant symptom is short stature; the girls are small at birth with an average length of 48 cm, corresponding to -1.2 SD of the mean for the age group, whereafter the growth rate falls to -2 SD up to the age of 8 to 9 years. Later on, the growth rate falls even more when compared to normal females, since no pubertal growth spurt occurs. An average adult height of about 145 cm is reached (5). However, the etiology of this growth disorder is still not known. The underlying cause can be an abnormal hormonal regulation, an altered peripheral responsiveness, or, most probably, both. Whether these girls have an altered growth hormone (GH) secretion has been the subject of many investigations. Some investigators have found normal or elevated GH serum concentrations after different GH provocation tests (6-10), whereas others found decreased GH concentrations (11,12). However, GH stimulatory tests do not necessarily reflect endogenous GH secretion (13). So far, the best way to estimate the spontaneous GH secretion is by measuring the blood GH levels over an extended period. Ross et al. (14) performed a study in Turner girls aged 2-20 years, where they collected serum GH samples over a 24-hr period. They found that the GH secretion in these girls below the age of 9 did not differ from that of age-matched control girls, whereas in older Turner girls, the mean GH level, mean peak amplitude, and mean peak frequency were found to be lower than that of the age-matched control girls. The unlimited supply of biosynthetic GH has made it possible to treat with exogenous GH in order to try to improve the tempo of growth and ultimately the final height. The preliminary results are so far very promising (15–17), even if the growth response of these girls is very heterogeneous.

We have investigated Turner girls in Sweden, who were willing to participate in a multicenter GH trial. Spontaneous GH secretion as well as the GH response to an arginine-insuline test were estimated. The plasma concentrations of GH were assessed with two radioimmunoassays, using either polyclonal or monoclonal antibodies.

CASE REPORT

Study Group

Thirty-eight patients with Turner syndrome participated. The diagnose was based on chromosome analysis of peripheral lymphocytes, and the karyotypes were 45,XO in 25 girls and mosaicism in the rest. None of the girls had ever been treated with any hormone. They were all willing to participate in a Swedish multicenter study with treatment of different combinations of GH, estrogen, and androgen (Nilsson et al., to be published). The age of the girls ranged from 9 to 15 years, and their bone ages were retarded. Before start of therapy, their GH secretion was estimated.

Control Group

Thirty healthy girls with normal karyotypes comprised a control group for the 24-hr GH profiles. These girls were of normal height (within ± 2 SD), and their ages were between 9.5 and 15.8 years at the time of investigation. Fourteen girls were prepubertal and 16 were in puberty.

Study Protocol

Arginine-Insulin Test

The standardized test was performed in 29 patients. Arginine was given as an infusion of 0.5 g/kg from time 0 to +30 min, and insulin (4 IU/m^2) was given as a bolus at time +90 min. Blood samples were drawn at 30-min intervals from −30 min to +180 min.

24-hr GH Profiles

The spontaneous secretion of GH was measured during a 24-hr period (48 sampling periods of 30 min each) in 28 of the Turner girls, and during a 8- to 12-

hour period in the remaining 10. In the control girls, 72 sampling periods of 20 min each were taken. The girls stayed at hospital for at least 2 days. They received a normal diet, with breakfast at 08.00, lunch at 12.00, dinner at 17.00, and they were allowed normal activity and sleep. A heparinized needle (Viggo AB, Helsingborg, Sweden) was inserted the first evening. The following morning at 08.00–09.00 hr, the blood withdrawal began with a now-thrombogenic catheter (Viggo AB, Helsingborg, Sweden) inserted through the needle. A constant withdrawal pump was used according to the Cormed-Kowarski method (18). The heparinized tubes were changed every 30 min for 24 hr in the Turner girls and every 20 min for 24 hr in the control girls. Integrated blood samples over 30 min were taken in 22 of the 28 girls in whom a 24-hr GH profile was performed. In the remaining girls, blood samples were drawn through an indwelling i.v. needle every 30 min.

In a few patients we drew discrete samples parallel to integrated samples. The results from these different ways of sampling did not differ per se, regarding AUC, AUC_b, number of peaks, or even the peak amplitude. Nor could we find any difference regarding these parameters when integrated samples over 20 min were compared with samples over 30 min (Albertsson-Wikland et al., to be published).

Growth Hormone Analyses

Polyclonal Antibodies

Measurements of GH with this radioimmunoassay were performed with a double antibody technique using polyclonal antibodies and with the WHO First IRP hGH 66217 as standard. All samples from a child were analyzed in the same assay. The GH levels are expressed in milliunits per liter (2 mU/liter = 1 ng/ml). The intraassay coefficient of variation was 24% below 5 mU/liter and 10% above 5 mU/liter. The interassay coefficient of variation was 31% below 5 mU/liter and 10% above 5 mU/liter.

Monoclonal Antibodies

The Tandem-R Immuno-radiometric kit by Hybritech Europe was used. This assay uses two monoclonal antibodies as previously described (19). The interassay coefficient of variation was 12% and the intraassay variations were 9.9%, 5.6%, 3.7%, and 3.1% at GH levels of 2, 5, 15, and 50 mU/liter, respectively.

Analysis of 24-hr GH Profiles

The GH curves obtained were analyzed with the Pulsar program (20) where a peak is strictly defined. The parameters G(1) to G(5) of the Pulsar program were set to: G(1) = 3.98; G(2) = 2.4; G(3) = 1.7; G(4) = 1.2, and G(5) = 0.9. The smoothing time was set to half of the total profile time, i.e., 12 hr (36 points) for the 24-hr GH profiles. The splitting parameter was set to 2.7, and the weight assigned to peaks was 0.05. The following values were extracted: the overall mean, the maximum value, the mean of the calculated baseline, the number of peaks, the peak amplitude, and the peak area. The area under the curve (AUC) was also estimated above the zero level as well as above the baseline (AUC_b).

The study was approved by the Ethical Committee of the Medical Faculty, University of Göteborg. Informed consent was obtained from patients and parents.

RESULTS

Arginine-Insulin Test

Figure 1 shows the peak serum concentration of GH obtained after the arginine-insulin test in Turner girls. When the serum concentrations of GH were analyzed with the RIA with polyclonal antibodies, the mean peak serum concentration of GH was 54.4 ± 7.6 mU/liter for these girls. One of the girls had a max GH level below 14 mU/liter, a commonly used cut-off limit for a subnormal response. In 21 out of the 29 girls, a GH response below 14 mU/liter was estimated when the serum concentrations of GH were analyzed with the other RIA with monoclonal antibodies. The mean peak serum concentration of GH was 13.7 ± 1.3 mU/liter with this assay. No difference between serum GH concentration in Turner with a karyotype of 45,XO or mosaicism was found with either assay.

Spontaneous GH Secretion

Figure 2 shows the heterogeneity of 24-hr GH profiles of Turner girls. As can be seen, a range from a substantially blunted (top) to normal (bottom) secretion is observed with assays. Some of the Turner girls showed a high basal level or had a serum interference in the assay with polyclonal antibodies (middle).

Spontaneous GH secretion, expressed as AUC_b/h, for all investigated Turner girls is shown in Figure 3. The correlation between the serum concentrations of GH obtained with polyclonal versus monoclonal antibodies is illustrated in Figure 4. In most girls, much higher values were observed with the polyclonal antibodies. Also in normal girls much higher plasma GH concentration was assessed with the RIA with polyclonal than the RIA with monoclonal antibodies (Fig. 5). However, higher amounts of GH were found in the pubertal girls than in the prepubertal girl with either assay.

The spontaneous GH secretion in the control group of 30 girls, assessed by polyclonal antibodies, is shown in Figure 6. When compared with the spontaneous GH secretion in Turner girls, it is obvious that the GH secretion in Turner girls is much lower compared with that of age-matched controls (Fig. 3 bottom, Fig. 6). The mean GH secretion expressed as AUC_b/h was 9.3 ± 1.8 for the Turner girls. This concentration is markedly lower than that of the

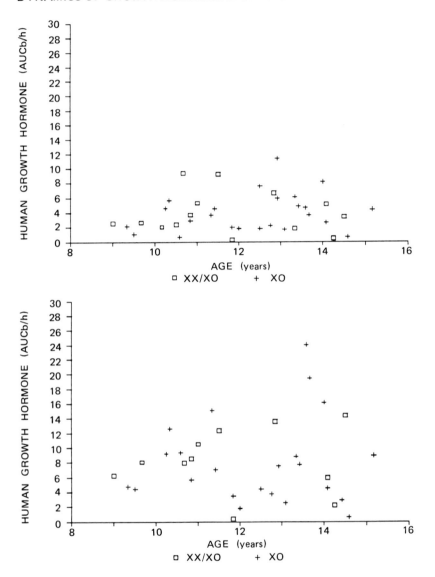

Figure 3 Spontaneous GH secretion in 38 Turner girls, expressed as area under the curve above the calculated baseline per hour (AUC$_b$/hr). The GH concentrations were assessed by radioimmunoassays using either polyclonal antibodies (bottom) or monoclonal antibodies (top).

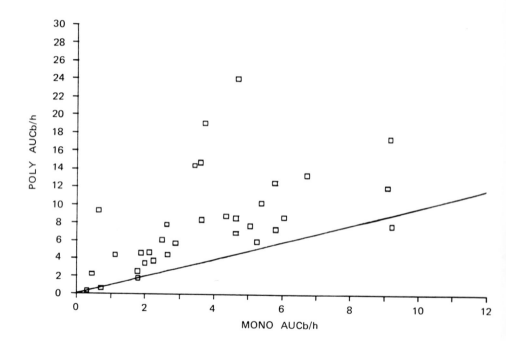

Figure 4 Relationship between GH concentrations assessed by radioimmuno-assays using polyclonal versus monoclonal antibodies. For help, the one-to-one correlation line is drawn in the figure.

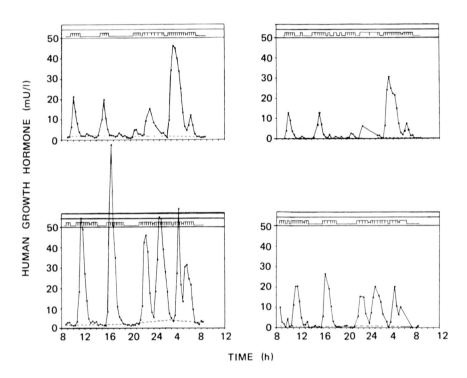

Figure 5 24-hr GH profiles of two normal girls—one prepubertal (top) and one pubertal (bottom). The plasma GH concentrations were assessed with two different radioimmunoassays, using either polyclonal antibodies (left) or monoclonal antibodies (right).

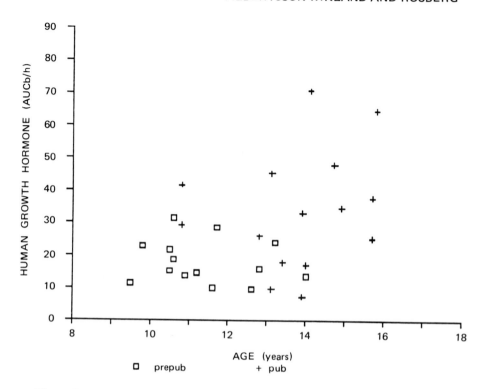

Figure 6 Spontaneous GH secretion in 30 healthy control girls, expressed as area under the curve above the calculated baseline per hour (AUC_b/hr). The GH plasma concentrations were assessed by radioimmunoassays using polyclonal antibodies.

age-matched control girls, both the prepubertal ones (mean AUC_b/h 17.9 ± 1.8) and especially the pubertal girls (mean AUC_b/h 34 ± 4.6).

DISCUSSION

The results of this study of Turner girls clearly shows that their spontaneous GH secretion is very heterogeneous. No difference was found between a karyotype of 45,XO or mosaicism. However, when compared with age-matched controls, the average GH secretion of the Turner girls is markedly reduced. Even if the average secretion of GH in the Turner girls was lower than that of control girls, a "normal" pulsatile secretory pattern was observed. The lower GH secretion in Turner girls is in agreement with previous reports (10,14). We found the GH secretion in 9-15-year-old Turner girls to be only half of that in prepubertal age-matched control girls and only one fourth of that in pubertal girls. This discrepancy can be explained by the abnormal gonadal function in Turner girls. In normal children, an increased spontaneous GH secretion is found in puberty (21-23), probably due to the increased secretion of estrogen (24). In Turner girls, no increase in serum androgens are observed, which normally occurs from the age of 9 (25), and only exceptionally are serum concentrations of estrogens measurable in Turner girls. It may be speculated that these hormones influence the GH secretion normally in girls above the age of 9. In younger girls, no difference in GH secretion has been observed between Turner and control girls (10, 14). In this study no girl below the age of 9 participated.

As previously described (11), GH-deficient patients in classical terms can be found among girls with Turner syndrome, maybe with an even higher incidence (12).

However, the danger in using a rigid cut-off limit between normal and subnormal GH response to provocative tests must be stressed. We assessed GH serum concentrations with two different radioimmunoassays: one with polyclonal and the other with monoclonal antibodies. With use of a cut-off limit of 14 mU/liter, one of the Turner girls had a low GH response to AITT assessed by polyclonal antibodies, while in contrast 21 had a low response assessed with monoclonal antibodies. Thus, when choosing the GH levels to be used as criteria for diagnosing GH insufficiency, one also has to take the characterizatics of the actual radioimmunoassay into account. The reason for the different results between different types of radioimmunoassays is at present unclear. However, one reason may be that one assay does not detect all forms of GH, e.g., the 20K form (19), and another reason may be different sensitivities to interfering substances in the plasma or serum.

In conclusion, in Turner girls above the age of 9 the spontaneous GH secretion is heterogeneous but in average markedly reduced compared to normal girls, both prepubertal and pubertal. Such comparisons have to be performed within the same radioimmunoassay, since remarkable differences in estimated GH levels are found with different assays. The low secretion of GH in Turner girls above 9 years of age, may, at least partly, explain the low growth rate observed in these girls. However, many other factors, such as defects in the target organs, may also play a role in the poor growth in girls with this syndrome.

ACKNOWLEDGMENTS

We would like to thank all collaborators in the Swedish Multicenter Study of Turner girls: Karl Olof Nilsson, Otto Westphal, Martin Ritzén, Anders Häger, Jan Gustavsson. Ms. Ann-Soffi Pettersson is gratefully acknowledged for excellent technical help.

This work was supported by grants from the Medical Research Council (27, 6465, 7509), Lundgren Foundation, KabiVitrum AB, and Hybritech.

REFERENCES

1. Turner HH. A syndrome of infantilism, congenital webbed neck and cubitus valgus. Endocrinology 1938; 23:566–578.
2. Ford CE, Jones KW, Polani PE, de Almeida JC, Briggs JH. A sex chromosomal anomaly in a case of gonadal dysgenesis (Turner's syndrome). Lancet 1959; 1:711–713.
3. Ferguson-Smith M. Karyotype-phenotype correlations in gonadal dysgenesis and their bearing on the pathogenesis of malformations. J Med Genet 1965; 2:142–154.
4. Kajii T, Ferrier A, Niikawa N, et al. Anatomic and chromosomal anomalies in 639 spontaneous abortuses. Hum Genet 1980; 55(1):87–98.
5. Ranke MB, Pflüger H, Rosendahl W, Stubbe P, Enders H, Bierich JR, Majewski F. Turner syndrome: Spontaneous growth in 150 cases and review of the literature. Eur J Pediatr 1983; 141:81–88.
6. Lindsten JE, Cerasi E, Luft R, Hultquist G. The occurrence of abnormal insulin and growth hormone (HGH) responses to sustained hyperglycaemia in a disease with sex chromosome aberration (Turner's syndrome). Acta Endocrinol (Copenh) 1967; 56:107–131.
7. Kaplan SL, Abrams CAL, Bell JJ, Conte FA, Grumbach MM. Growth and growth hormone. I. Changes in serum level of growth hormone following hypoglycemia in 134 children with growth retardation. Pediatr Res 1968; 2:43–63.
8. Donaldson CL, Wegienka LC, Miller D, Forsham PH. Growth hormone studies in Turner's syndrome. J Clin Endocrinol 1969; 28:383–385.
9. Saenger P, Schwartz E, Wiedemann E, Levine LS, Tsai M, New M. The interaction of growth hormone, somatomedin and oestrogen in patients with Turner's syndrome. Acta Endocrinol (Copenh) 1976; 81:9–18.
10. Ranke MB, Blum WF, Haug F, Rosendahl W, Attanasio A, Enders H, Gupta D, Bierich JR. Growth hormone, somatomedin levels and growth regulation in Turner's syndrome. Acta Endocrinol (Copenh) 1987; 116:305–313.
11. Brook CGD. Growth hormone deficiency in Turner's syndrome. N Engl J Med 1978; 298:1203.
12. Duke EM, Hussein DM, Hamilton W. Turner's syndrome associated with growth hormone deficiency. Scott Med J 1981; 26:240–244.
13. Bercu BB, Shulman D, Root AW, Spiliotis BE. Growth hormone (GH) provocative testing frequently does not reflect endogenous GH secretion. J Clin Endocrinol Metab 1986; 63:709–716.
14. Ross JL, Long LM, Loriaux DL, Cutler Jr GB. Growth hormone secretory dynamics in Turner syndrome. J Pediatr 1985; 106:202–206.
15. Rosenfeld RG, Hintz RL, Johanson AJ, et al. Methionyl human growth hormone and oxandrolone in Turner syndrome. Preliminary results of a prospective randomized trial. J Pediatr 1986; 109:936–943.

16. Takano K, Hizuka N, Shizume K. Growth hormone treatment of Turner's syndrome. Acta Paediatr Scand 1986 Suppl; 325:58–63.
17. Wilton P. Growth hormone treatment in girls with Turner's syndrome. A review of the literature. Acta Paediatr Scand 1987; 76:193–200.
18. Kowarski A, Thompson RG, Migeon CJ, Blizzard RM. Determination of integrated concentration of true secretion rate of human growth hormone. J Clin Endocrinol Metab 1971; 32:356.
19. Blethan SL, Chasalow FI. Use of a two-site immunoradiometric assay for growth hormone (GH) in identifying children with GH dependent growth failure. J Clin Endocrinol Metab 1983; 57:1031–1035.
20. Merriam GR, Wachter KW. Algorithms for the study of episodic hormone secretion. Am J Physiol 1982; 243:E310.
21. Finkelstein JW, Roffwarg HP, Boyar RM, Kream J, Hellman L. Age-related changes in twenty-four-hour spontaneous secretion of growth hormone. J Clin Endocrinol Metab 1972; 35:665–670.
22. Bierich JR. Untersuchungen zur Genese des Wachstumsschubs. Monatsschr Kinderheilkd 1981; 129:393–399.
23. Albertsson-Wikland K, Rosberg S, Hall K. Spontaneous secretion of growth hormone and serum levels of insulin like growth factor I and somatomedin binding protein in children of different growth rates. In: O. Isaksson et al. (Eds.) Growth hormone—Basic and clinical aspects. Elsevier Science Publishers B.V. 1987. International Congress Series 748. Nordisk Insulin Symposium No. 1.
24. Copeland KC, Johnson DM, Kuehl TJ, Castracane VD. Estrogen stimulates growth hormone and somatomedin-C in castrate and intact female baboons. J Clin Endocrinol Metab 1983; 58:698.
25. Apter D, Lenko HL, Perheentupa J, Söderholm A, Wihko R. Subnormal pubertal increases of serum androgens in Turner's syndrome. Hormone Res 1982; 16:164–173.

DISCUSSION

DR. ROBERT M. BLIZZARD: One or two comments and first a question: Dr. Albertsson-Wikland, I think you mentioned that the Hybritech assay system does not measure the 22K, you really mean the 20K. Right? The Hybritech does not measure the 20K, it does the 22 and a statement for clarification is that Dr. Albertsson-Wikland was talking about polyclonal versus monoclonal, and it is important for the discrepancies as she found them. It is important to state that you get the same discrepancies by using different monoclonal antibodies as well,

---

Dr. Blizzard is at the University of Virginia at Charlottesville, Charlottesville, Virginia.

as I said before, the Nichols versus the Hybritech, for example. Each of these assays has its own characteristics and, as she emphasized, we need to know what those characteristics are when we try to interpret data.

19

Spontaneous Nocturnal GH Secretion in Ullrich-Turner Syndrome

Jurgen R. Bierich

Children's Hospital, University of Tübingen,
Tübingen, Federal Republic of Germany

The pubertal growth spurt of normal adolescents rests upon (a) the increased production of growth hormone (GH), stimulated by the sexual hormones, and (b) the synergistic effect of GH and sexual hormones on the growing skeleton. During the last 10 years we have contributed investigations with respect to the first point, measuring the spontaneous GH secretion by night in the various stages of puberty. The sleep-associated GH secretion was determined through 5½ hours of deep sleep, taking blood samples every 30 minutes. The values (±1 SD) obtained are shown in Table 1. Patients with Ullrich-Turner Syndrome (UTS) who have the classical XO constellation possess no ovaries and, therefore, show no pubertal growth spurt.

We have measured the sleep-associated GH output in 40 girls with UTS. Seven were younger (group I), 33 were older (group II) than 9 years. One girl with a XO/XX mosaic had run a normal pubertal development and experienced regular menses. The results of the investigations—with the exception of those of the latter patient—are depicted in Table 2.

The values of the children of group I do not statistically differ from those of the normal controls, either in integrated GH secretion or the maximal peaks attained in the arginine tests. However, the results of group II showed a statistically highly significant ($p < 0.001$) diminution of the integrated GH secretion (by 59%) as well as of the highest peaks reached (by 51%) compared to our normal

Table 1 Sleep-associated GH-Secretion

	P_1	P_2	$P_{3/4}$
Σ GH in 5½ hr	4100 ± 1320	5467 ± 1888	9704 ± 1711
max. peak attained	37 ± 15	49 ± 23	66 ± 27

values. With regard to only the arginine tests (which showed a rather wide variation), no differences were found.

The only exception was the girl with the XO/XX mosaic and spontaneous puberty. Her integrated GH secretion amounted to 4800 ng, which is a normal value for P_2.

CONCLUSIONS

Prior to the normal time of puberty patients with UTS exhibit a normal spontaneous secretion of GH.

Patients older than 9 years of age have a diminished spontaneous GH secretion. Their secretion shows not only no increase with advancing age, but becomes significantly lower than in the prepubertal period. Apparently from the age of 10 years on, sexual hormones are necessary not only to achieve a pubertal growth spurt but even to maintain sufficient GH secretion.

One UTS patient with a XO/XX mosaic and spontaneous puberty exhibited a normal spontaneous GH output.

Table 2 Turner Syndrome—Spontaneous vs. Stimulated GH Secretion

		N	P_1
Σ	TS I	6	3087 ± 863
	TS II	32	1669 ± 880
	contr.	30	4100 ± 1320
max. peaks	TS I	7	28 ± 6
	TS II	32	18 ± 11
	contr.	30	37 ± 15
Arg. test	TS I	5	23 ± 19
	TS II	25	21 ± 13
	contr.	13	19 ± 8

20

Growth Hormone Secretion and Somatomed in C/IGF I Levels in Turner Syndrome and in Patients with Idiopathic Growth Hormone Deficiency

Michael B. Ranke, Werner F. Blum, and Jürgen R. Bierich

*Children's Hospital, University of Tübingen,
Tübingen, Federal Republic of Germany*

Clinical growth hormone deficiency (GHD) is suspected on the basis of its auxological features, including short stature, low height velocity, relative obesity, and retardation of bone age. By "classical" criteria the diagnosis is established if maximal serum GH levels to two standard provocation tests stay below certain limits (e.g., 10 ng/ml). It is assumed that measurements of spontaneously secreted GH can define a state of true GHD by more physiological means. In accepting the endocrine model of somatomedin action, GHD should be reflected by low circulating somatomedin levels. If GHD plays a role in the pathogenesis of the growth disorder in Turner syndrome, growth hormone secretion—at least under the conditions of spontaneous secretion—and subsequently somatomedin levels should, likewise, be subnormal.

In order to investigate whether there are indications for true GHD in Turner Syndrome (TS), we have measured GH levels during 5.5 hours of deep sleep (1) and basal somatomedin (SmC/IGF I (RIA)) levels (2,3) in groups of patients with these disorders.

Maximal GH levels observed during deep sleep in 29 cases with TS and in 25 cases with idiopathic GHD compared to normal prepubertal and pubertal ranges are depicted in Figure 1. In both groups there is a downward trend with bone age progression. During pubertal age most values in both groups are below normal, except for two cases of TS with puberty. There is a tendency of levels in GHD to be lower than in TS. However, there is some overlap between the groups during pubertal age.

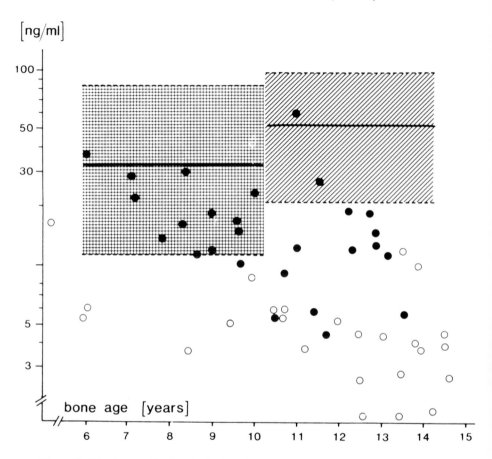

Figure 1 Maximum GH levels during deep sleep in GHD (○) and Turner's syndrome (●) compared to prepubertal and pubertal normal levels (hatched areas).

Figure 2 illustrates SmC/IGF I levels in 30 patients with TS and 43 patients with idiopathic GHD compared to the normal ranges (mean ± 2 SD) for bone age. Except for cases with bone ages below 5 years, when an overlap with the normal range is also known for GHD, levels between the two groups of patients separate distinctively. In the older cases (BA > 10 years) classified as GHD based on stimulation test but with normal SmC/IGF I levels, the diagnosis should be reconsidered.

If one plots SmC/IGF I levels in relation to height assuming that circulating levels may, in part, be a reflection of body size (overflow of SmC/IGF I syn-

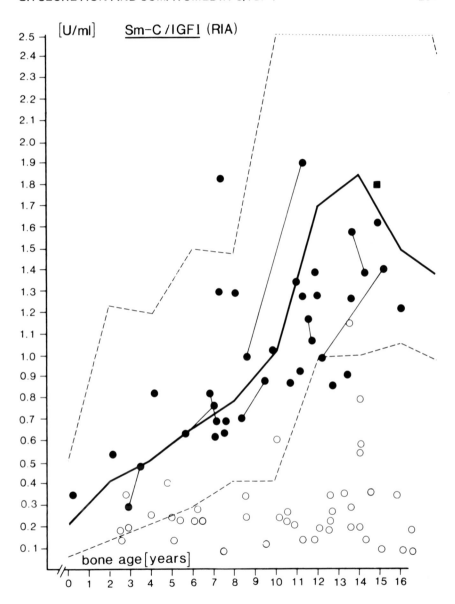

Figure 2 Basal SmC/IGF I serum levels in GHD (○) and Turner's syndrome (●) compared to bone age-related normal ranges.

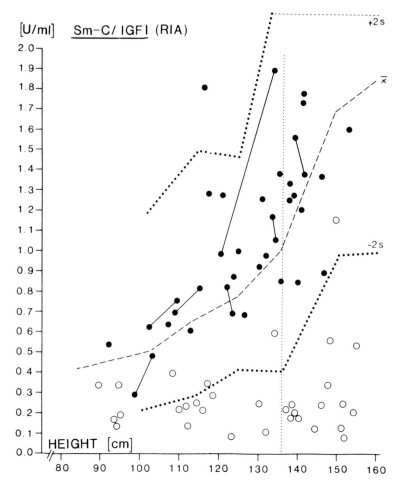

Figure 3 Basal SmC/IGF I serum levels in GHD (○) and Turner's syndrome (●) compared to height-related normal ranges.

thesized at various tissues of the body into the circulation) (Fig. 3), levels of both groups of patients show an even more distinct separation. While levels in TS tend to stay within the high to normal range, levels in GHD tend to be sub-normal.

CONCLUSIONS

1. SmC/IGF I levels in TS and true (by "classical" definitions) GHD differ considerably. In relation to growth hormone secretion and to height, SmC/IGF I levels in TS appear to be too high.

2. Measurements of spontaneously secreted GH may not allow a definite diagnosis of "true" GHD.
3. The findings in TS (high/normal SmC/IGF I with low/normal GH) may be the result of positive influences on SmC/IGF I generation other than GH secretion (related to development of obesity in TS (nutrition/insulin)).

REFERENCES

1. Bierich JR. Minderwuchs. Monatschr Kinderheilk (1983); 131:180–193.
2. Ranke MB, Gruhler M, Rosskamp R, Brügmann G, Attanasio A, Blum WF, Bierich JR. Testing with growth hormone-releasing factor (GRF(1-29)NH2) and somatomedin C measurements for the evaluation of growth hormone deficiency. Eur J Pediatr (1986); 145:485–492.
3. Ranke MB, Blum WF, Haug F, Rosendahl W, Attanasio A, Enders H, Gupta D, Bierich JR. Growth hormone, somatomedin levels and growth regulation in Turner's syndrome. Acta Endocrinologica (Copenh) 1987; 116: 305–313.

DISCUSSION

DR. MILO ZACHMAN: We have been interested for a number of years in studying nitrogen balance using the stable isotope ^{15}N and the response to growth hormone, testosterone, and estrogens. The advantage of this stable isotope, compared to classic nitrogen retention studies, is that you do not need a constant protein intake and the test can be made much shorter.

The test procedure was like this. First, a basal test was carried out, then two injections of human growth hormone were given and the second test was carried out on the third day. This is an older slide which shows 2.6 units of pituitary growth hormone, but we were now interested to see how patients with Turner syndrome would respond to recombinant growth hormone and we gave 3 U/m2. As you know, in classic tests and in our previous studies, patients with true growth hormone deficiency respond with a much more marked nitrogen retention than patients with normal growth hormone secretion.

This is just briefly the test procedure. The patients were given ^{15}N-enriched ammonium chloride, and this was divided into three doses, and a 24-hour urine

Dr. Milo Zachman is at Children's Hospital, University of Zürich, Zürich, Switzerland. Dr. Robert M. Blizzard is at the University of Virginia at Charlottesville, Charlottesville, Virginia. Dr. Sandra L. Blethen is at Schneider Children's Hospital, New Hyde Park, New York. Dr. Gilbert August is at Children's Hospital, Washington, D.C. Dr. Gertrude Costin is at Children's Hospital of Los Angeles, Los Angeles, California.

was collected. We now use only 0.05 g/kg of 99% labeled ammonium chloride, which makes the cost of these tests a bit lower.

The laboratory procedure was first total nitrogen estimation and then an estimation of the percentage of ^{15}N content, considering also the atmospheric ^{15}N content of 0.4%. And then this percentage was estimated either by mass spectrometry or by a special analyzer and from the total nitrogen and the percentage of ^{15}N, the excretion was calculated, and finally the balance from the ingestion and the excretion.

Now, if we look at the data with recombinant growth hormone as to how much ^{15}N is excreted in urine, you can see that patients with proven growth hormone deficiency excrete 11.1 mg/kg, patients with Turner syndrome a little less. That is clear because the patients with growth hormone deficiency have a more negative nitrogen balance.

More interesting are the data of the *balance* in mg/kg. You can see that in the growth hormone-deficient patients the basal balance is considerably lower than in the patients with Turner syndrome. However, when growth hormone is given, the balance in the growth hormone-deficient patients becomes considerably more positive by about 50% of the basal balance, whereas in the patient with Turner syndrome, there is only a slight positive balance change, much less than in the growth hormone-deficient patients.

If you express this in percentage and take the basal balance as 100%, you can see even better that the positive balance change in the growth hormone-deficient patients is much larger than that in the Turner syndrome patients.

I did not include normal values from normal children because these are from previous studies and they were done with pituitary growth hormone. However, I can say that the response of the Turner syndrome patients is exactly the same like in previous studies with normal subjects.

The conclusion from this would be that also metabolically, Turner syndrome patients do not have growth hormone deficiency, and they respond to growth hormone in the same way as normal subjects; I would therefore think that if one wants to treat patients with the syndrome with growth hormone, not the regular replacement doses, but probably considerably higher doses will have to be used. Thank you.

DR. ROBERT BLIZZARD: Could I know the age of your patients?

DR. ZACHMAN: They were all prepubertal and they all had a bone age below 10 years.

DR. SANDRA L. BLETHEN: Circulating GH immunoreactivity is heterogeneous and the peptide known as 22k GH with its 191 a.a. is not the only form present. My colleague, Dr. Chasalow, and I have been interested in studying this microheterogeneity. In order to accommodate the sample volumes available from small children, we have developed sensitive RIAs using different site-specific monoclonal antibodies. These assays are capable of detecting as little as 0.05 ng of GH. While they give equivalent results with authentic pituitary GH, they do not react equally with other GH forms. Pituitary GH provided by the NHPP was used as the standard. Another pituitary GH preparation, Crescormon, showed similar cross-reactivity. In contrast, the 20,000 dalton form of GH did not bind to Ab352 while showing decreased but equal binding to AB 033 and 665.

Samples from 17 normal individuals showed nearly equivalent reactivity with the three Ab. We were able to assay sample from nine girls with Turner syndrome. Five girls had ratios which were outside of the range observed in the controls. These girls were older than the four with normal ratios and there was a statistically significant correlation between serum FSH and [352]/033 ratio. The discrepancy appears to result from a decrease in 033 immunoreactivity.

The Ab used in this study were provided by Dr. E. D. Sevier of Hybritech. Ab 352 and 033 are similar in specificity to the Ab used in the Tandem RIA. Thus, our observation is consistent with Dr. Albertsson-Wikland's findings. They offer the suggestion that ovarian failure in Turner syndrome affects not only the total pituitary output of GH but the type of hormone produced as well.

DR. BLIZZARD: I think you can all see that this is a fascinating topic that probably could take an hour or two, but unfortunately time does not permit us to do that. There are two other people who have asked to make comments pertaining to the data that has been presented so far. Dr. Costin and Dr. August have comments.

DR. GILBERT AUGUST: Gordon Cutler and his group have presented important data on 24-hr secretory rates in normal and in short-statured children. It is also very important, though, to remember that Drs. Bessie Spiliotus, Barry Bercu, Wellington Hung, and I described a highly selected patient population. Not only were these patients short statured, but they also had abnormally low somatomedin-C levels. Except for normal growth hormone responses to standard stimulation tests, they would have fit NHPP criteria for growth hormone deficiency.

We originally thought that we were dealing with, what was then termed bioinactive growth hormone, because these children did have normal responses to pharmacologic stimuli. It was not until we saw a patient who was one of twins that we realized what may be the reason for these children's poor growth rates and short stature. This twin grew identically as her normal twin until she was knocked out in an ice skating accident. Afterwards her growth velocity decreased and she failed to grow as well as her twin. She, however, responded normally to two of three growth hormone stimulation tests.

It was then that we theorized we may be dealing with a group of patients who resembled the monkeys who had received CNS radiation and were under study in this laboratory. Their main defect in growth hormone secretion was a decreased 24-hr secretory rate of growth hormone secretion.

I believe that there is a subgroup of children with a neurosecretory dysfunction in growth hormone secretion who may, if followed long enough, eventually respond as classic growth hormone-deficient children. I do not believe that we should try to extrapolate the data to explain why short-statured children with normal growth rates are short.

DR. GERTRUDE COSTIN: I would like to comment that our results really concur with those of Dr. Cutler and Rose and Dr. Albertsson-Wikland, in that indeed we found a big overlap between the so-called normal growing children, the hypopituitary children, and the Turner's children. Out of 42 normally growing children, 7 to 18 years of age, we have found that the mean growth hormone concentration at 24 hr ranged between 1.5 to 6.7 ng/ml, with a mean of 3 in the prepubertal group and a mean of 4.4 in the pubertal groups, again, with significant overlap with hypopit patients.

In 18 Turner's patients the 24-hr GH concentration ranged from 1.6 to 4.9, again overlapping with normal and hypopituitary children. What was interesting was when we separated the Turner's less than 10 years of age and over 10 years, we found that the younger children had normal growth hormone concentrations, and therefore were not growth hormone-deficient. The older ones greater than 10 years of age had a lower level, which was significantly less than in normals, suggesting again that probably the sex steroids during puberty have an important effect on the 24-hr growth hormone concentration, and confirms what we found, that normal pubertal children secreted significantly greater amounts than prepubertal children.

We need some stimulation tests in Turner patients, again questioning, are they growth hormone-deficient or not. It was interesting that although the 24-hr growth hormone concentrations overlapped with normals, the stimulated level in 7 of 15 children tested with one stimulus were less than 10 ng/ml; half of those or a little less, 40%, had a level less than 7 ng/ml. Of those, 7 patients, half of them had a second stimulation test, and it was also less than 7 ng/ml.

I do not know really what it means. Are they deficient or are they not? Maybe they have some problem in responding to stimulation tests or maybe it is again the fact that they did not have gonadal steroids present. Those patients with very low responses had also 24-hr levels that were low and were in the pubertal age group 10 to 12.

In respect to somatomedin C levels and to Dr. Ranke's remarks, we found that this was normal as a group in the prepubertal and, as a matter of fact, a little higher than normal in the pubertal age group in which it was 1.3 as a mean.

Remember, those patients were never treated and had no gonadal steroids and no effect of puberty. So I think that this was a little higher than what you would expect for a prepubertal state child.

In conclusion, I am as confused as many of you or maybe I am the only one confused, as to whether patients with Turner's are really deficient or maybe their lower GH responses are due to some obesity relative to their height.

21

Growth Plate Biology and the Turner Syndrome

William A. Horton

University of Texas Medical School at Houston
Houston, Texas

INTRODUCTION

The cause(s) of growth deficiency in the Turner syndrome is (are) poorly understood. Although there is evidence for insufficient stimulation of skeletal growth, i.e., low normal to frankly low levels of both growth hormone and insulinlike growth factor 1 (IGF-1) for age (1-4), there is also evidence for a defective response of the growing skeleton. Indeed, Stanescu and colleagues have reported morphologic and histochemical abnormalities of the skeletal growth plate in the Turner syndrome (5). This structure is responsible for linear growth of the skeleton from early in embryonic development through the end of normal puberty. Historically, skeletal development and growth has been poorly understood, making identification or even speculation of possible defects in the Turner syndrome difficult. However, recent advances in this area have made this goal possible. It therefore seems prudent to first review the biology of skeletal formation and growth and then to examine how this process might be disturbed in the Turner syndrome.

NORMAL SKELETAL DEVELOPMENT AND GROWTH

Vertebrate limb development, which has been defined primarily in the chick, begins with the outgrowth of limb buds comprised of mesenchymal tissue covered by a layer of ectoderm. Skeletal primordia form as condensations of the mesenchymal cells (6). Shortly afterwards, the mesenchymal cells differentiate into chondrocytes. This is associated with the synthesis and secretion of typical cartilage matrix containing type II collagen, cartilage proteoglycan, link protein, and the dispersement of the cells within this matrix (7-10). Chondrocytes in the center of the bones-to-be subsequently differentiate into another type of chondrocyte, the hypertrophic chondrocyte, which is much larger than a typical chondrocyte. This cell has a short life span and modifies the cartilage matrix by the secretion of type X collagen, fibronectin, cessation of synthesis of type II collagen and perhaps proteoglycan, and expression of alkaline phosphatase activity (11-17). (To avoid confusion the chondrocytes producing the macromolecules considered typical of cartilage have been called stage I chondrocytes, whereas hypertrophic chondrocytes have been called stage II chondrocytes.) The modifications that accompany the differentiation from stage I to stage II chondrocytes predispose the hypertrophic cartilage to invasion and degradation by vascular tissues. Osteoblasts, which accompany this invasion, deposit bone matrix in place of the degraded cartilage. The vascular invasion and subsequent

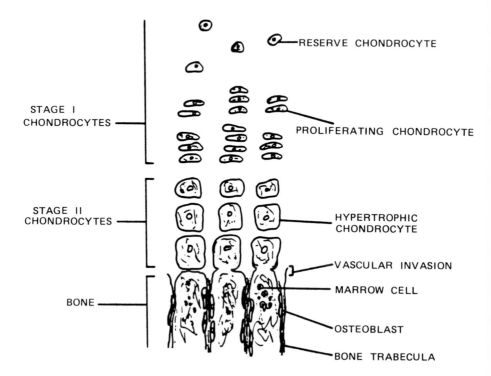

Figure 1 Growth plate.

formation of bone appear to be secondary phenomena dependent upon the modification of the cartilage matrix by the hypertrophic chondrocytes (18-20).

A front is thus created in which cartilage is modified, degraded, and replaced by bone. It spreads rapidly. As it approaches the ends of the bones, another phenomenon occurs: the proliferation of stage I chondrocytes that lie next to the front. The process becomes organized into distinct "zones" of proliferating stage I chondrocytes, cells differentiating from stage I to stage II (hypertrophy), vascular invasion and osteoblastic deposition of bone matrix, i.e., the growth plate (Fig. 1) (18-20). This arrangement allows the growth plate to function as a unit in which chondrocyte proliferation and differentiation match the rate of cartilage degradation and new bone formation.

At the cellular level, linear bone growth is therefore dependent upon three phenomena. First, stage I chondrocytes must proliferate to provide a constant source of cells for subsequent differentiation. Second, stage I chondrocytes must differentiate into stage II chondrocytes. Third, both chondrocyte phenotypes must be properly expressed.

REGULATION OF BONE GROWTH

Bone growth can be viewed as the product of a developmental pathway involving chondrocyte proliferation and differentiation. There are several locations in the scheme where control might be exerted that would influence the rate of new bone formation. One is the proliferation of stage I chondrocytes. Changes in the rate would alter availability of chondrocytes for differentiation. Another has to do with the rate of differentiation from stage I to stage II chondrocytes. Variations in the phenotypes expressed might also be expected to influence the pathway. For example, it has been suggested that the degree to which the hypertrophic chondrocytes enlarge affects the rate at which hypertrophic cartilage is degraded (20). This is variable and seems to depend on the influx of sodium and water into the hypertrophic cells.

Many hormones and growth factors are known or suspected to influence bone growth through this scheme, but precisely how this happens is not clear in most instances. IGF-1, which is strongly affected by growth hormone, stimulates chondrocyte proliferation and production of cartilage matrix (21). The effects of IGF-1 on differentiation are not known, nor is it clear if the active growth factor is circulating IGF-1 that diffuses through the growth plate cartilage or locally produced IGF-1 (22). There is evidence that IGF-1 is generated by proliferating chondrocytes (23). A number of other polypeptide growth factors have recently been isolated from cartilage and bone that may influence growth plate function (Table 1) (24-30). Some of these factors, i.e., IGF-1, IL-1, seem to stimulate proliferation of chondrocytes and expression of the stage I chondrocyte phenotype, while others, such as TGF-β, induce the differentiation of

Table 1 Possible Local Regulators of Skeletal Growth

Factor	Alternate name	Source	Effect(s) on chondrocytes
IGF-1	Somatomedin C	Plasma, chondrocytes	Mitogenic, matrix production
IGF-2		Plasma	Mitogenic, matrix production
IL-1		Macrophages chondrocytes	Mitogenic, matrix production and degradation
CDF		Chondrocytes	Mitogenic, matrix production
CDGF		Chondrocytes	Mitogenic
TFF-B$_1$[a]	CIF-A	Bone, platelets	Cartilage induction
TGF-B$_2$[a]	CIF-B	Bone, platelets	Cartilage induction
PDGF		Platelets	?

Abbreviations: IGF = insulin-like growth factor, BDGF = bone derived growth factor, CDGF = cartilage derived growth factor, CDF = cartilage derived factor, IL = interleuken, BMP = bone morphometric protein, TGF = transforming growth factor, CIF = cartilage inductive factor, PDGF = platelet derived growth factor.

[a] Although distinct, TGF-B$_1$ and B$_2$ are very similar and often referred to simply as TGF-B.

Source: Refs. 24-30.

mesenchymal cells to chondrocytes. Little attention has been given to the effects of the growth factors on the differentiation of stage I chondrocytes to stage II chondrocytes or on the expression of the latter phenotype. Moreover, there are other growth factors, such as platelet-derived growth factor and other peptides produced by bone marrow cells, that are present in the vicinity of the growth plate but have never been tested for effects on chondrocyte behavior. It seems likely, however, that these growth factors regulate and coordinate the chondro-osseous developmental pathway and thereby influence linear bone growth at the local level.

POSSIBLE DEFECTS IN TURNER SYNDROME

How can this new knowledge of growth plate biology be employed to better understand growth deficiency in the Turner syndrome? Probably the most important way is the identification of candidate genes. In other words, genes that reside on the X chromosome and that encode proteins that participate in the chondro-osseous developmental pathway are likely to be responsible for or at least contribute to the growth deficiency when they are missing. Examples would include genes for the polypeptide growth factors, their receptors, and other proteins that affect the action of these factors, intracellular proteins that control the expression of the chondrocyte phenotypes and the differentiation process itself, and even genes expressed as part of the phenotypes. Many of these genes have been mapped, especially those encoding the growth factors and their receptors (Table 2), but none to date have been assigned to the X chromosome (31). Nevertheless, as gene loci continue to be mapped and the developmental scheme becomes better characterized, both of which are currently progressing at a very rapid pace, the identification of the specific candidate genes should become a reality.

Another approach would be to investigate the behavior of chondrocytes in vitro from patients with the Turner syndrome. Methods have very recently been developed in which human chondrocytes (stage I) that have been dedifferentiated in monolayer culture can be grown in agarose suspension culture (32,33). This promotes proliferation as well as the sequential reexpression of the stage I and stage II chondrocyte phenotypes, which would theoretically permit abnormalities in the developmental pathway to be identified (11,16,33).

SUMMARY

Linear bone growth is the product of an extremely complex process that involves the coordinated proliferation and differentiation of growth plate chondrocytes. It appears to be regulated by both circulating hormones and locally generated growth factors. One or more disturbances of this process likely con-

Table 2 Chromosomal Location of Selected Genes Involved in Chondro-osseus Developmental Pathway

	Gene product	Location
Stage I chondrocyte phenotype	Type II collagen	12q13.1 - q13.3
	Proteoglycan core protein	?
	Proteoglycan link protein	?
Stage II chondrocyte phenotype	Type X collagen	?
	Fibronectin	2q32.3 - qter
	Alkaline phosphatase	1
Growth factors	IGF-1	12q22 - q24.1
	IGF-2	11p15.5
	IL-1	2q13 - q21
	CDF	?
	CDGF	?
	TGF-α	2p13
	TGF-β	19q13.1 - q13.3
	PDGF α chain	7pter
	β chain	22q12.3 - q13.1
Growth factor receptors	IGF-1	15q25 - q26
	IGF-2	?
	IL-1	?
	CDF	?
	CDGF	?
	TGF-	?
	TGF-β	?
	PDGF	5q25 - q32

Abbreviations: IGF = insulin-like growth factor, CDF = cartilage derived factor, CDGF = cartilage derived growth factor, IL = interleuken, TGF = transforming growth factor, PDGF = plate-derived growth factor.
Source: Ref. 31.

tributes to the growth deficiency in the Turner syndrome. Candidate gene studies and in vitro investigation of chondrocytes from patients with the syndrome are promising approaches to identifying these disturbances.

REFERENCES

1. Rosenfeld RG, Dollar LA, Hintz RL, Conover C. Normal somatomedin-C/insulin-like growth factor I binding and action in cultured human fibroblasts from Turner syndrome. Acta Endocrinol 1983; 104:502–509.
2. Martinez A, Heinrich JJ, Domene H, Escobar ME, Jasper H, Montuori E, Bergada G. Growth in Turner's syndrome: Long term treatment with low dose ethinyl estradiol. J Clin Endocrinol Metab 1987; 65:253–257.

3. Ross JL, Long LM, Loriaux DL, Cutler GB Jr. Growth hormone secretory dynamics in Turner syndrome. J Pediatr 1985; 106:202-206.
4. Guidoux S, Bozzola M, Larizza D, Schimpff RM. Serum thymidine activity and somatomedin-C levels in children and adolescents with Turner's syndrome: Effect of chronic estrogen and progestogen replacement therapy. Horm Res 1986; 24:256-262.
5. Stanescu V, Pitis M, Ionescu V, Bona C. Histochemical and histoenzymological studies on the growing cartilage in the Turner's syndrome. Acta Histochem 1965; 20:309-330.
6. Solursh M. Cell and matrix interactions during limb chondrogenesis in vitro. In The Role of Extracellular Matrix in Development. Alan R Liss, New York, 1984; pp. 277-303.
7. Dessau W, von der Mark H, von der Mark K, Fisher S. Changes in the patterns of collagens and fibronectin during limb-bud chondrogenesis. Embryol Exp Morphol 1980; 57:51-60.
8. Silver MH, Foidart J-M, Pratt RM. Distribution of fibronectin and collagen during mouse limb and palate development. Differentiation 1981; 18: 141-149.
9. Searls RL. An autoradiographic study of the uptake of S-35 sulfate during differentiation of limb bud cartilage. Develop Biol 1965; 11:155-168.
10. Linsenmayer TF, Toole BP, Trelstad RL. Temporal and spatial transitions in collagen types during embryonic chick limb bud development. Develop Biol 1973; 35:232-239.
11. Castagnola P, Moro G, Descalzi-Cancedda F, Cancedda R. Type X collagen synthesis during in vitro development of chick embryo tibial chondrocytes. J Cell Biol 1986; 102:2310-2317.
12. von der Mark K. Immunological studies on collagen type transition in chondrogenesis. Curr Top Develop Biol 1980; 14:199-226.
13. Dessau W, Sasse J, Timpl R, Jilek F, von der Mark K. Synthesis and extracellular deposition of fibronectin in chondrocyte cultures. J Cell Biol 1978; 79:342-355.
14. Schmid TM, Linsenmayer TF. Developmental acquisition of type X collagen in the embryonic chick tibiotarsus. Develop Biol 1985; 107:373-381.
15. Habachi H, Conrad HE, Gloser JH. Coordinate regulation of collagen and alkaline phosphatase levels in chick embryo chondrocytes. J Biol Chem 1985; 260:13029-13034.
16. Solursh M, Jensen KL, Reiter RS, Schmid TM, Linsenmayer TF. Environmental regulation of type X collagen production by cultures of limb mesenchyme, mesectoderm, and sternal chondrocytes. Develop Biol 1986; 117:90-101.
17. Kosher R, Kulyk W, and Gay S. Collagen gene expression during limb cartilage differentiation. J Cell Biol 1986; 102:1151-1156.
18. Brighton CT. Structure and function of the growth plate. Clin Orthop 1978; 130:22-32.
19. Horton WA, Machado M. Alterations in the extracellular matrix during endochondral ossification in man. J Orthop Res 1988; 6:793-803.

20. Hunziker EB. Growth plate structure and function. Pathol Immunopathol Res 1988; 7:9–13.
21. Phillips LS, Vassilopoulou-Sellin R. Somatomedin. N Engl J Med 1980; 302:371–380.
22. D'Ercole AJ, Applewhite GT, Underwood LE. Evidence that somatomedin is synthesized by multiple tissues in the fetus. Dev Biol 1980; 75:315–328.
23. Nilsson A, Isgaard J, Lindahl A, Dahlstrom A, Skottner A, Isaksson O. Regulation by growth hormone of number of chondrocytes containing IGF-I in rat growth plate. Science 1986; 233:571–574.
24. Castor W. Regulation of connective tissue metabolism. In *Arthritis and Allied Conditions*. DJ McCarty ed. Lea & Febriger, Philadelphia, 1985; pp. 242–256.
25. Centrella M, Canalis E. Local regulators of skeletal growth: A perspective. Endocr Rev 1985; 6:544–551.
26. Seyedin S, Thomas T, Thompson A, Rosen D, Piez K. Purification and characterization of two cartilage-inducing factors from bovine demineralized bone. Proc Natl Acad Sci 1985; 82:2267–2271.
27. Hauschka P, Mavrakos A, Iafrati M, Doleman S, Klagsbrun M. Growth factors in bone matrix. J Biol Chem 1986; 261:12665–12674.
28. Seyedin SM, Thompson AY, Bentz H, Rosen DM, McPherson JM, Conti A, Siegel NR, Galluppi GR, Piez KA. J Biol Chem 1986; 261:5693–5695.
29. Seyedin S, Segarini P, Rosen D, Thompson A, Bentz H, Graycar J. Cartilage-inducing factor-B is a unique protein structurally and functionally related to transforming growth factor-B. J Biol Chem 1987; 262:1946–1949.
30. Ollivierre F, Gublert U, Towle C, Laurencin C, Greadwell B. Expression of IL-1 genes in human and bovine chondrocytes: A mechanism for autocrine control of cartilage matrix degradation. Biochem Biophys Res Comm 1986; 141:904–911.
31. McKusick VA. The human gene map. Proc Hum Gene Mapping Workshop. Updated August 15, 1987.
32. Delbruck A, Dresow B, Gurr E, Reale E, Schroder H. In vitro culture of human chondrocytes from adult subjects. Conn Tissue Res 1986; 15:155–172.
33. Horton WA, Aulthouse AL, Machado MA, Griffey ES, Campbell D. In vitro studies of chondrocyte differentiation in the human chondrodysplasias. Proc Greenwood Genet Center 1988; 7:166.

22

The Potential Role(s) of Bone-Derived Growth Factors as Determinants of Local Bone Formation

David J. Baylink, Thomas A. Linkhart, and John R. Farley

Loma Linda University School of Medicine and Jerry L. Pettis Memorial Veterans' Hospital, Loma Linda, California

Subburaman Mohan

Loma Linda University School of Medicine, Loma Linda, California

Susan G. Linkhart and Robert J. Fitzsimmons

Jerry L. Pettis Memorial Veterans' Hospital, Loma Linda, California

EVIDENCE FOR LOCAL REGULATION OF COMPENSATORY BONE FORMATION PROCESSES— ASSOCIATIONS WITH RELEASE OF BONE-DERIVED GROWTH FACTOR

Skeletal tissues constitute the single largest storehouse of growth factors in the body [1,2]. Our goal in this discussion is to critically evaluate the potential role(s) of these growth factors as determinants of local bone formation within the conceptual framework of bone volume regulation. Although bone is a regenerative organ, the volume of bone is not constant. Bone volume is regulated in response to two aspects of skeletal function: the necessity for structural support and the systemic requirement for mineral homeostasis. Bone volume is decreased (by increasing bone resorption) to adapt to a decreased mechanical load [3] and/or to gain access to the endosteal skeletal reservoir of Ca and Po_4 [4]; conversely, bone volume is increased (by increasing bone formation) to adapt to an increased mechanical load [5] and/or to replace the endosteal bone that had been lost to previous resorption [4]. Recent studies indicate that the skeletal responses to each of these two aspects of bone volume regulation—mechanical loading and mineral homeostasis—may depend on the local activities of bone-derived growth factors for increasing bone formation.

With regard to the effects of mechanical loading on bone, we know that intermittent loading causes increased bone formation and a site-specific increase in bone volume (5) and that the pattern of new bone formation can be predicted from the localized load distribution (6). Furthermore, since this response is mediated by an increase in the rate of bone formation, the mechanism must require localized increases in the number and/or activity of osteoblasts; since both of those activities are characteristic of bone-derived growth factors (see discussion of activity, below), it has been suggested that local release of growth factors—in response to mechanical loading—may provide the mechanism for increasing bone formation (7). This concept is supported by two recent observations: Conditioned culture medium from mouse bone organ cultures contained increased amounts of bone-derived growth factor activity after the bones were subjected to intermittent mechanical loading (7), and conditioned culture medium from chicken bone organ cultures contained increased amounts of bone-derived growth factor activity after the bones had been exposed to an osteogenic electrical field (8,9) (Table 1). Thus, we can hypothesize that bone-derived growth factors may be mediating local increases in the rate of bone formation in response to mechanical loading.

With regard to the role of endosteal bone in mineral homeostasis, previous studies have established that during Ca (or PO_4) deficiency, endosteal bone

Table 1 Effects of Electric Field (EF) Exposure on Indices of Bone Formation and Release of Growth Factor Activity from Skeletal Tissues in Vitro

Tissue[a]	Parameter measured[b]	Length of incubation[c]	Net effect[d]
Calvarial cells	Cell proliferation	18 hr (30 min)	+45%, $p < 0.01$
Calvarial cells	Total DNA	72 hr (30 min/day)	+180%, $p < 0.01$
Calvarial cells	Mitogen activity in CM	72 hr (30 min/day)	+200%, $p < 0.01$
Tibiae	Bone formation	72 hr (30 min/day)	+83%, $p < 0.001$
Tibiae	Mitogen activity in CM	72 hr (30 min/day)	+135%, $p < 0.001$

[a]Skeletal tissues were prepared from embryonic chicks, calvarial cells tested in replicate (n=6) monolayer cultures and tibiae (n=6-10) in organ cultures.
[b]Calvarial cell proliferation assessed by ^{3}[H]-thymidine incorporation into DNA; tibial bone formation assessed by ^{3}[H]-proline incorporation into matrix collagen; mitogen activity in conditioned medium (CM) assessed by the effect on ^{3}[H]-thymidine incorporation in otherwise untreated calvarial cell cultures.
[c]Length of *in vitro* incubation, length of EF exposure in parentheses.
[d]Effect of electric field exposure (capacitively coupled, 10 Hz, sinusoidal-estimated field strength in the culture medium: 10^{-5} V/m) is shown as the percentage change, compared to untreated controls.
(Note: recent studies indicate that EF exposure may mimic the effects of mechanical loading by inducing electric potentials in bone that resemble the stress-generated potentials which are induced by mechanical loading.)
Data from references 8 and 9, with permission of the publishers and authors.

volume is decreased (due to increased bone resorption) as mineral reserves are mobilized to maintain serum Ca (or PO_4) (4). When the normal diet is restored, endosteal resorption is dramatically decreased, and the rate of bone formation is increased, allowing for replacement of the bone that was lost to resorption (i.e., the mineral reserve). This process has been described as coupled bone formation, meaning bone formation which is localized to sites of previous resorption, proportional to the extent of previous resorption, and mediated by an increase in osteoblast number (see reviews in References 4, 10, 11)—all suggestive of a local mechanism. Subsequent studies, demonstrating that a coupled increase in the rate of bone formation, in an organ culture system, was associated with increased amounts of growth factor activity in the conditioned culture medium, not only supported the concept of a local mechanism, but also suggested a possible role for bone-derived growth factors in the process (12,13). More recent studies (12) have further revealed: (a) that the amount of bone-derived growth factor activity released from chicken tibia (i.e., in an organ culture model) was proportional to the extent of bone resorption (14) (Fig. 1); (b) that similar

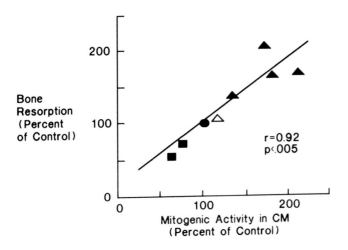

Figure 1 The amount of bone-derived growth factor activity (i.e., mitogen activity, measured by incorporation of ^{3}[H]-thymidine into DNA) in conditioned medium (CM) from tibial organ cultures is proportional to the amount of bone resorption (measured by release of ^{45}Ca from prelabeled embryonic chicken tibiae). Data are shown as percent of untreated controls and represent mean values for groups of 10 tibiae, after treatment with the following effectors: none (i.e., untreated controls), ○; PTH (tested at doses of 1, 3, 10, and 100 pmol/liter), ▲; Cl_2MDP (tested at doses of 10 and 30 μmol/liter), ■; and PTH (10 pmol/liter) plus Cl_2MDP (30 μmol/liter), △. (Data from Ref. 14, with permission of the publishers.)

growth factor activities could also be identified in extracts of bone (15) and in bone cell-conditioned tissue culture medium; and (c) that the amount of bone cell-derived growth factor activity released from osteoblast-line cells in monolayer culture was proportional to the extent of osteoblastic differentiation, whereas the response to bone-derived (or bone cell–derived) growth factors was inversely proportional to differentiation (14) (Figs. 2 and 3). Together, these observations are consistent with the premise that endosteal bone formation might be coupled to resorption, in a local, site-specific manner, by bone-derived growth factor(s), which are released in proportion to the rate (and/or extent) of bone resorption. Our data are also consistent with a mechanistic model (14) in which bone-derived growth factor(s) is produced by osteoblasts and deposited in bone for eventual release by bone resorption, at which time it can act locally to increase osteoblast number (by stimulating the proliferation of osteoprogenitor cells) and, thereby, allow for compensatory, local bone formation.

Thus, we can hypothesize that compensatory bone formation—in response to mechanical loading and for maintenance (replacement) of the endosteal mineral reservoir—may be regulated locally and may depend on the activity of bone-

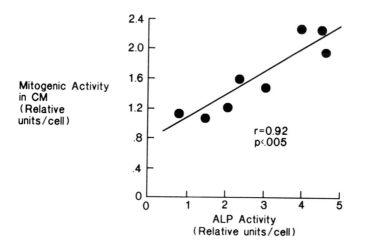

Figure 2 Production of mitogen activity by calvarial cells is proportional to alkaline phosphatase (ALP) activity per cell. Embryonic chicken calvarial cells, prepared from periosteal tissue and from periosteum-free bone, were cultured separately and in graded combination (6 replicate cultures for each combination of cells). Twenty-four-hour conditioned media (CMs) were collected from the wells and used to measure mitogen activity ([3][H]-thymidine incorporation into DNA in otherwise untreated calvarial cell cultures). Data are shown as mean values. (Reproduced from Ref. 14, with permission of the publishers.)

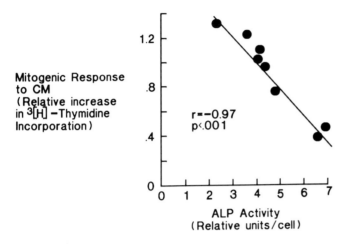

Figure 3 Calvarial cell–derived mitogens stimulate calvarial cell proliferation in inverse proportion to alkaline phosphatase (ALP) activity per cell. Calvarial cells, prepared from periosteal tissue and from periosteum-free bone, were cultured separately and in graded combinations. After overnight plating, the culture media were changed (to remove endogenous growth factors), and aliquots of concentrated, dialyzed calvarial cell conditioned medium (CM) were added to replicate cultures ($n = 6$) for measurement of mitogen activity (i.e., $^3[H]$-thymidine incorporation into DNA). (Reproduced from Ref. 14, with permission of the publishers.)

derived growth factors. If this is true, it follows that we will not understand the local mechanism(s) of bone volume regulation until we have identified these bone-derived growth factors and determined their activities and origins.

IDENTIFICATION OF BONE-DERIVED GROWTH FACTORS

Analysis of the conditioned medium from the studies that showed evidence of coupled bone formation in an organ (chick bone) culture system (see discussion above) led to the identification of a bone-derived growth factor (13), which could also be identified in extracts of chicken bone matrix (15). This activity was characterized as a large molecular weight protein (65-80 kd), and subsequent studies indicated that similar activities could also be identified in extracts of bone from other species (see review in Ref. 11) and in conditioned medium from monolayer cultures of chicken (14) and human (16) bone cells. Additional studies have further revealed that the activities (see discussion below) that had

been associated with this protein could, in fact, be ascribed to a component peptide, and treatment with dissociative agents has since led to purification of the
peptide—which has been described as skeletal growth factor—from bovine and
from human bone (17,18). (The 11 kd peptide has been estimated (18) to comprise 0.00024% of the weight of the organic matrix of human bone). During the
course of these purifications additional bone-derived growth factor activities
were also observed, which did not co-purify with skeletal growth factor (18);
and more recent studies have led to the quantitative identification of a number
of these activities (including insulin-like growth factor I, platelet-derived growth
factor, transforming growth factor-beta, and epidermal growth factor, in addition to skeletal growth factor) in dissociative extracts of human bone matrix
(see Table 2 and Reference 2).

Multiple growth factor activities have also been identified in dissociative extracts of bovine bone matrix (1), based on the criterion of binding to heparin-
sepharose (i.e., gradient elution with NaCl indicated five or six independent activities). Tentative classification indicated the presence of a platelet-derived
growth factor-like activity, anionic and cationic fibroblast growth factor-like ac-

Table 2 Quantitative Identification of Growth Factor Activities in Extracts of
Human Bone Matrix

	Concentration in bone extract[b]	
Growth factor identified[a]	ng/μg G-EDTA protein	μg/g Bone powder
Skeletal Growth Factor (SGF)	1.05	1.26
Transforming Growth Factor-beta (TGF-b)	0.38	0.46
Insulin-like Growth Factor 1 (IGF-1)	0.07	0.085
Platelet-derived Growth Factor (PDGF)	0.055	0.067
Fibroblast Growth Factor (FGF)	Detectable	—
Epidermal Growth Factor (EGF)	Not Detectable	—

[a]Growth factors identified as follows: SGF by radio-receptor assay (RRA), measuring
^{125}[I]-SGF binding to chick calvarial cells (purified SGF as standard); TGF-b by EGF-
dependent NRK cell colony formation in soft agar (purified human TGF-b as standard);
IGF-1 by radio-immuno assay (RIA), using rabbit polyclonal antiserum (NIH) and human
synthetic IGF-1; PDGF was estimated as the difference in mitogen activity in aliquots of
the G-EDTA extract, before and after treatment with PDGF-inhibitory antibodies; FGF by
RIA; EGF by RRA, measuring ^{125}[I]-EGF binding to NRK cells.
[b]Matrix proteins were extracted from human bone powder during demineralization (in
dialysis tubing) in a solution of 10% EDTA plus 4 M Guanidine-HCl and protease inhibitors.
The extracts were desalted before measurements of growth factor activities. (Note: the
amount of TGF-b in the extract may have been underestimated, since we did not subject
the extract to acidic incubation.)
Reproduced from reference 2, with permission of the authors.

tivities, a cartilage growth factor–like activity, and an EGF or IGF-1–like activity (1). Other, less comprehensive analyses have identified the following additional activities in bone: a bone morphogenetic protein (19); a bone matrix-derived chemotactic factor (20); two bone-derived transforming growth factor-beta–like activities (21); and a cartilage-derived growth factor, which appears to be identical to transforming growth factor-beta (22). In vitro studies also indicate that a transforming growth factor-beta activity and another bone-derived growth factor (which is not identical to skeletal growth factor) are released from fetal rat calvariae and may also be present in bone (23,24). Although the latter activity (i.e., the rat calvarial bone-derived growth factor) has been recently identified as β_2-microglobulin (25), this finding has not been confirmed. (Studies in our laboratory indicate that β_2-microglobulin is not active as a bone cell mitogen in vitro, although it can be detected as a contaminant in bone-derived growth factor preparations.)

Thus, it is apparent that skeletal tissues contain a number of growth factors, many of which are known to be produced by osteoblasts—including skeletal growth factor (16), platelet-derived growth factor (26), insulin-like growth factor I (27), and transforming growth factor-beta (28)—and any of which could be released for local regulation of the bone formation process. We should note, however, that our model of compensatory bone formation (14) does not require that the active factor(s) be released from the matrix of bone—only that the osteogenic activity be locally released in proportion to the rate (or the extent) of bone resorption. Therefore, a bone-derived growth factor(s) could be indirectly released from bone matrix or directly released from osteoclasts or macrophages, or from osteoblasts. Since we have previously shown that conditioned medium from cultured osteoclasts (prepared from rat and chicken long bones) did not contain osteogenic growth factors (13), and since macrophages, which can produce growth factors (29), are not known to be required for compensatory bone formation, our data favor the alternatives of osteoblasts and/or bone matrix as the source of growth factor activity. To date, however, only skeletal growth factor, which was identified only as a large molecular weight mitogen (14), and a transforming growth factor-beta, which was identified by anchorage-independent growth of NRK cells (30), have been shown to present in bone-conditioned medium in amounts that were consistent with the rate of bone resorption, and the source of those activities has not yet been determined.

CHARACTERIZATIONS OF BONE-DERIVED
GROWTH FACTOR ACTIVITIES

The rate of bone formation can be defined as the product of osteoblast number (i.e., the number of bone-forming cells) and osteoblast activity (i.e., the amount of bone matrix synthesized per cell per unit time), and all of the bone-derived growth factors that we have considered in this discussion have been shown to increase one or both of these parameters in vitro. For example, skeletal growth factor was first identified, in conditioned culture medium, by its ability to increase embryonic bone formation (12), and subsequent studies (13) indicated that it did so by increasing osteoblast number (osteoblast-line cell proliferation was assessed by the incorporation of ^{3}[H]-thymidine into DNA). More recent studies have confirmed that the purified, small molecular weight form of skeletal growth factor is a potent bone cell mitogen, increasing osteoblast-line cell proliferation at concentrations as low as 0.1 ng/ml, with half-maximal activity at ~1 ng/ml (18) (Fig. 4). The purified skeletal growth factor also had direct effects on osteoblast activity, increasing collagen production per cell in the clonal osteoblast cell line MC3T3-E1 (31) (Fig. 5). This effect on osteoblast activity was significant at 10 ng/ml (half-maximal at ~100 ng/ml) and associated with a corresponding decrease in the rate of MC3T3-E1 cell proliferation (i.e.,

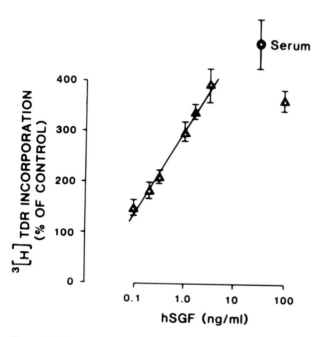

Figure 4 Dose-response curve showing the effect of purified human skeletal growth factor (hSGF) on embryonic chicken calvarial cell proliferation (i.e., ^{3}[H]-thymidine incorporation into DNA). Data are shown as percent of control (mean ± SD, n = 6 wells per dose). (Reproduced from Ref. 18, with permission of the publishers.)

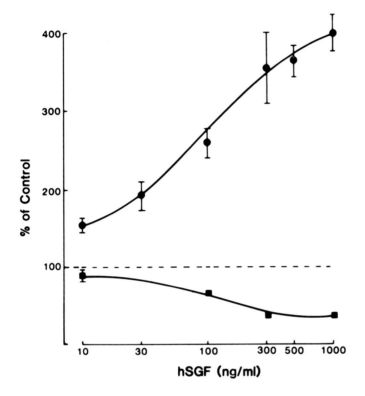

Figure 5 Dose-response curves showing the effects of purified human skeletal growth factor (hSGF) on MC-3T3-E1 cell cultures. [3] [H]-Thymidine incorporation into DNA (■) was measured as an index of effects on cell proliferation, and [3] [H]-proline incorporation into TCA-tannic acid–insoluble material (●) was measured as an index of effects on protein synthesis. Separate studies (i.e., measurements of collagenase-digestible protein and [3] [H]-hydroxyproline incorporation) have confirmed that the effects on [3] [H]-proline incorporation are indicative of the effects on collagen production. Data are shown as percent of untreated controls (mean ± SD). (Reproduced from Ref. 31, with permission of the publishers.)

[3] [H]-thymidine incorporation into DNA). Since we had previously shown that the extent of osteoblastic differentiation in chicken calvarial cell cultures was (a) directly correlated with the rate of growth factor production, and (b) inversely correlated with the proliferative response to exogenous bone-derived growth factors (14) (Figs. 2 and 3), these observations suggested that skeletal growth factor could affect both osteoblast number and osteoblast activity by increasing the proliferation rate of undifferentiated osteoblast progenitors (i.e., a paracrine

effect) while increasing collagen production in more differentiated osteoblasts (i.e., an autocrine effect).

With regard to the in vitro activities of other bone-derived growth factors, insulin-like growth factor I, fibroblast growth factor, epidermal growth factor, and platelet-derived growth factor have all been shown to increase (chicken) osteoblast-line cell proliferation (32). Insulin-like growth factor I has also been shown to increase cell proliferation and (total) collagen production in fetal rat calvariae (33). Epidermal growth factor also stimulated cell proliferation in fetal rat calvaria, but inhibited collagen synthesis (34). The effects of transforming growth factor-beta on osteoblast-line cell proliferation and collagen production are less well defined. Transforming growth factor-beta has been described as a bi-functional effector of bone cell proliferation—being stimulatory or inhibitory, depending upon incubation conditions (35), and recent studies indicate that it can increase (rat) osteoblast-like cell proliferation (36); increase alkaline phosphatase activity in (rat and human) osteosarcoma cells (37); and decrease alkaline phosphatase activity in (mouse) MC3T3-E1 cells, without increasing cell proliferation (38).

Thus, each of the bone-derived growth factors identified in this report have been shown to increase osteoblast-line cell proliferation and/or collagen production, and each is, therefore, capable of acting locally in bone to increase bone formation.

SUMMARY AND CONCLUSIONS

The data summarized in this report are consistent with the premise that compensatory bone formation (in response to mechanical loading and for maintenance of the endosteal bone mineral reservoir) may be mediated locally by release of bone-derived growth factors; however, significant questions remain unresolved. Skeletal tissues contain large quantities of growth factors which are known to act in vitro to increase osteoblast number (by increasing osteoblast-line cell proliferation) and/or osteoblast activity (i.e., collagen synthesis per cell), but it is not known whether any of these bone-derived growth factors have similar activities in vivo. Growth factors are released from bone in vitro in response to intermittent loading (i.e., intermittent compressive force) and in response to bone resorption, but such release has not been shown in vivo. Furthermore, the growth factors which are released from bone in vitro have not yet been specifically identified, nor is it known whether those activities are released from bone cells or bone matrix. And finally, although our hypothesis (that bone formation may be regulated, locally, by release of bone-derived growth factors) is supported by in vitro and animal studies, the evidence, to date, is circumstantial—no bone-derived growth factor has yet been shown to be required for compensatory bone formation, either in vitro or in vivo.

ACKNOWLEDGMENTS

The authors are indebted to George Evans, Chris Hans, Richard Langer, Tracy Moreno, Daniel Russo, Nanine Tarbaux, and Richard Widstrom for technical assistance, and to the secretarial staff of the Mineral Metabolism Unit and the Medical Media staff of the J. L. Pettis Memorial Veterans' Hospital for assistance in the preparation of this manuscript. This research was supported by the NIH, the Veterans' Administration, and the Department of Medicine of Loma Linda University.

REFERENCES

1. Hauschka PV, Mavrokow AE, Iafrati MD, Doleman SE, Klagsbrun M. Growth factors in bone matrix. J Biol Chem 1986; 261:12665-12674.
2. Mohan S, Linkhart TA, Jennings JC, Baylink DJ. Identification and quantification of four distinct growth factors stored in human bone matrix. J Bone Mineral Res (Suppl) 1987; 2:Abstract 44.
3. Uhthoff HK, Jaworski ZFG. Bone loss in response to long term immobilization. J Bone Joint Surg (Br) 1978; 60:420-429.
4. Baylink DJ, Liu CC. The regulation of endosteal bone volume. J Perdontol 1979; 50:43-49.
5. Rubin CT, Lanyon LE. Osteoregulatory nature of mechanical stimuli: function as a determinant for adaptive remodeling in bone. J Orthopaedic Res 1987; 5:300-310.
6. Carter DR, Orr TE, Fyhrie DP, Whalen RT, Schurman DJ. Mechanical stress and skeletal morphogenesis, maintenance, and degeneration. Transactions of the Orthopaedic Res Soc 1987; (Abstract Issue):462.
7. Klein-Nulend J, Veldhuijzen JP, de Jong M, Netelenbos JC, Burger EB. Mechanical stimulation increases the production of bone cell stimulating factors in fetal calvaria in vitro. J Bone Min Res 1987; 2(Supplement 1): Abstract 48.
8. Fitzsimmons RJ, Farley J, Adey WR, Baylink DJ. Embryonic bone matrix formation is increased after exposure to a low-amplitude capacitively coupled electric field, in vitro. Biochim Biophys Acta 1986; 882:51-56.
9. Fitzsimmons R, Farley J, Adey R, Baylink DJ. Electric fields directly increase bone cell proliferation and bone formation in vitro. J Cell Biol 1984; 99:422A.
10. Ivey JL, Baylink. Postmenopausal osteoporosis: proposed roles of defective coupling and estrogen deficiency. Metab Bone Dis Relat Res 1981; 3:3-7.
11. Linkhart TA, Mohan S, Jennings JC, Farley JR, Baylink DJ. Skeletal growth factor. Hormonal Proteins and Peptides 1984; XII:279-297.
12. Howard GA, Bottemiller BL, Turner RT, Rader JI, Baylink DJ. Parathyroid hormone stimulates bone formation and resorption in organ cultures: evidence for a coupling mechanism. Proc Natl Acad Sci USA 1981; 78: 3204-3208.

13. Drivdahl RH, Puzas JE, Howard GA, Baylink DJ. Regulation of DNA synthesis in chick calvarial cells by factors from bone organ culture. Proc Soc Exp Biol Med 1981; 168:143-150.
14. Farley JR, Tarbaux NT, Murphy LA, Masuda T, Baylink DJ. In vitro evidence that bone formation may be coupled to resorption by release of mitogen(s) from resorbing bone. Metabolism 1987; 36:314-321.
15. Drivdahl RH, Howard GA, Baylink DJ. Extracts of bone contain a potent regulator of bone formation. Biochem Biophys Acta 1982; 714:26-33.
16. Wergedal JE, Mohan S, Baylink DJ. Human skeletal growth factor is produced by human osteoblast-like cells in culture. Biochim Biophys Acta 1986; 889:163-170.
17. Jennings JC, Baylink DJ. Bovine skeletal growth factor exists in small and large molecular weight forms. In The Chemistry and Biology of Mineralized Tissues, WT Butler, (ed) 1985; EBSCO Media:48-53.
18. Mohan S, Jennings JC, Linkhart TL, Baylink DJ. Isolation and purification of a low molecular weight skeletal growth factor from human bones. Biochim Biophys Acta 1986; 884:234-242.
19. Urist MR, DeLange RJ, Finnerman GAM. Bone cell differentiation and growth factors. Science 1983; 220:680-686.
20. Somerman M, Hewitt AT, Varner HH, Schiffmann E, Termine J, Reddi AH. Identification of a bone matrix-derived chemotactic factor. Calcif Tissue Int 1983; 35:481-485.
21. Jennings J, Linkhart T, Mohan S, Lundy M, Baylink D. Isolation of two b-transforming growth factors from bovine bone. J Bone Mineral Res 1986; 1:(Supplement 1) Abstract 301.
22. Seyedin S, Thompson AY, Bentz H, Rosen DM, McPherson JM, Conti A, Siegel NR, Gallupi JR, Piez KA. Cartilage inducing factor-A; apparent identity to transforming growth factor-beta. J Biol Chem 1986; 261:5693-5698.
23. Canalis E, Peck WA, Raisz LG. Stimulation of DNA and collagen synthesis by autologous growth factor in cultured fetal rat calvaria. Science 1980; 210:1021-1023.
24. Centrella M, Canalis E. Isolation of EGF-dependent transforming growth factor (TGF-b-like) activity from culture medium conditioned by fetal rat calvaria. J Bone Mineral Res 1987; 2:29-36.
25. Canalis E, McCarthy T, Centrella M. Identity of bone-derived growth factor with beta$_2$ microglobulin. J Bone Mineral Res 1987; 2:(Supplement 1) Abstract 248.
26. Valentin-Opran A, Delgado R, Valente T, Mundy GR, Graves DT. Autocrine production of platelet-derived growth factor-like peptides by cultured normal human bone cells. J Bone Mineral Res 1987; 2:(Supplement 1) Abstract 254.
27. Valentin-Opran A, Delmas PD, Chavassieux PM, Chenu C, Saez S, Meunier PJ. 1,25-Dihydroxyvitamin D$_3$ stimulates the somatomedin C secretion by human bone cells in vitro. J Bone Mineral Res 1986; 1:(Supplement 1) Abstract 139.

28. Young MF, Robey PG, Reddi AH, Roberts AB, Sporn MB, Termine JD. TGF-beta expression in fetal bovine bone forming cells. J Bone Mineral Res 1986;1:(Supplement 1) Abstract 155.

29. Rifas L, Shen V, Mitchell K, Peck WA. Macrophage derived growth factors for osteoblast-like cells and chondroblasts. PNAS USA 1984; 81:4558–4562.

30. Pfeilschifter J, Mundy GR. Modulation of type-beta transforming growth factor activity in bone cultures by osteotropic hormones. Proc Natl Acad Sci USA 1987; 84:2024–2028.

31. Linkhart S, Mohan S, Linkhart TA, Kumegawa M, Baylink DJ. Human skeletal growth factor stimulates collagen synthesis and inhibits proliferation in a clonal osteoblast cell line (MC3T3-E1). J Cell Physiol 1986; 128: 307–312.

32. Linkhart TA, Jennings JC, Wakley GK, Baylink DJ. Characterization of mitogenic activities extracted from bovine bone matrix. Bone 1986; 7: 479–487.

33. Canalis E. Effect of insulin-line growth factor I on DNA and protein synthesis in cultured rat calvaria. J Clin Invest 1980;66:709–719.

34. Canalis E, Raisz LG. Effect of epidermal growth factor on bone formation in vitro. Endocrinology 1979;104:862–869.

35. Centrella M, McCarthy T, Canalis E. Transforming growth factor-beta is a bifunctional regulator of osteoblast replication. J Bone Mineral Res 1986; 1:(Supplement 1) Abstract 156.

36. Chen TL, Mallory JB, Chang SL. Effects of transforming growth factor and its interaction with bFGF and EGF in rat osteoblast-like cells. J Bone Mineral Res 1987; 2:(Supplement 1) Abstract 256.

37. Noda M, Rodan GA. Transforming growth factor beta regulation of alkaline phosphatase expression in rat and human osteosarcoma cells. J Bone Mineral Res 1987; 2:(Supplement 1) Abstract 255.

38. Ibbotson KJ, Oroutt CM, Kumegawa M, D'Souza SM. Inhibition of differentiated function in mouse MC3T3-E1 osteoblast-like cells by transforming growth factor beta. J Bone Mineral Res 1987; 2:(Supplement 1) Abstract 132.

DISCUSSION

DR. JUD VAN WYCK: Bill Horton implied, I think, that palisading of the chondrocytes and maturation of the chondrocytes is a primary effect and that the penetration of blood vessels is secondary. I think that in looking for factors involving local control of bone growth and the growth plate in particular, that the role of angiogenic factors cannot be minimized, and we have an expanding list of angiogenic factors, tumor necrosis factor, the fibroblast growth factors and so on, and the possibility that they are released by interleukins may play a very important role. This is particularly pertinent to the question of the skeletal lesion in Turner syndrome, because we all know that they already have some vascular problems. It is conceivable, at least to me, that a vascular lesion could be ultimately responsible, and we may be looking for something more specifically related to chondrogenesis when we really should look at something related to the vascular penetration and the lining up of the palisades.

DR. DAVID BAYLINK: Yes, that is an interesting idea. I think, physically, it is the change in the cartilage. Cartilage has factors which resist most of those angiogenic factors, but I think that the diffusion of those factors into the cells so that they modify the matrix so that it can be invaded may well be a problem. We are saying the same sort of thing in different sorts of ways. Clearly the in growth of blood vessels into the epiphyseal cartilage, which provides a source of growth factors for the cells that are at the upper end of the growth plate, is obviously very important. But again, that may involve modification of the cartilage matrix which is mediated by the chondrocytes, but perhaps stimulated by those angiogenic factors that diffuse to those cells.

Dr. Judson Van Wyk is at the University of North Carolina at Chapel Hill, Chapel Hill, North Carolina. Dr. David Baylink is at the Loma Linda University School of Medicine and the Jerry L. Pettis Memorial Veterans' Hospital, Loma Linda, California.

23

Skeletal Abnormalities in the Turner Syndrome

Matthew B. Lubin

Cedars-Sinai Medical Center, Los Angeles, California

Helen E. Gruber and David L. Rimoin

*Cedars-Sinai Medical Center and the University of California
at Los Angeles School of Medicine, Los Angeles, California*

Ralph S. Lachman

*Harbor/University of California at Los Angeles Medical Center
Torrance, California*

In addition to the short stature of the Turner syndrome, a number of characteristic skeletal anomalies have been reported. There is a question as to whether the diminished stature in these patients is due to intrinsic abnormalities of bone and cartilage or due to a more generalized growth factor or receptor defect. The onset of the growth retardation is prenatal and continues throughout the growing years. All studies reviewed have revealed intrauterine growth retardation, with mean term birth weights about one standard deviation below normal (1-3). In childhood, growth delay continues with Turner syndrome girls growing slower than controls. Lacking the pubertal growth spurt, these patients continue their growth at a declining rate until fusion of the epiphyses occurs early in the third decade of life. Final heights for women with the Turner syndrome are approximately 3.5 standard deviations below the average normal female adult height, regardless of the particular sex chromosome composition, the development of spontaneous menses, or hormone treatment. Although delayed, the sequence of epiphyseal fusion in all cases of the Turner syndrome is normal, except for the premature fusion of the affected metacarpals.

The correlation coefficient for birth length and final adult height in the general population is about 0.3 (4). In the Turner syndrome the correlation coefficients for birth weight and length and adult weight and height are 0.96 and

0.92, respectively (3). The correlation coefficient for mid-parental height and final adult height in the Turner syndrome was found to be 0.84 (2), and standard deviation scores of first and final heights are almost equal (5). These observations suggest that the variation in height of Turner syndrome patients is primarily the result of familial genetic background.

In addition to the short stature, there are a number of characteristic skeletal abnormalities. Several authors have reported on anthropometric measurements in the Turner syndrome. A number of them have described a sitting height to subischial height ratio greater than that seen in normal females (6-8). Thus, some investigators have considered disproportionately short legs as the primary cause for their short stature. Other body proportions thought to be abnormal are longer arms and greater breadth across the shoulders and chest (6-8). However, in relation to height, Varrela et al. (9) found that sitting height, arm length, and leg length are almost equal to normal. Hughes et al. (10) compared the standard deviation scores for sitting height and subischial leg length in Turner syndrome patients and showed how these were similarly decreased. When he considered sitting height to subischial leg length ratios in the same patients, however, he agreed with other investigators that the legs of the Turner syndrome patients appear to be disproportionately short. It is difficult to say how much of the disproportion is due to the delay in epiphyseal fusion.

Osteoporosis affecting the axial and the appendicular skeleton is very common in these patients. However, fractures due to bone thinning and biconcave vertebrae appear to be uncommon (11,12). There is disagreement on whether or not the osteoporosis of the Turner syndrome is due to decreased bone formation and/or increased bone resorption. Several studies including a retrospective review of radiographs, quantification of cortical area in long bones, and microradiographic analysis suggest a progressive form of osteoporosis (11,13,14). A full discussion of the osteoporosis in Turner syndrome by Rubin is given in Chapter 24.

Numerous reports have appeared in the literature describing anomalies of the skeletal system in the Turner syndrome, which are quite variable. The skull has been the focus of several studies (15-17). In general, the skull is smaller than normal with a tendency towards brachycephaly, though Varrela (9) found measurements very close to normal. Thinning of the parietal bones, consistent with their osteoporosis, has been reported (11). The cranial base angle (nasion to the sella to the anterior of the foramen magnum) is more obtuse, while the cranial base is shorter, especially because of a short clivus. The first cervical vertebra is slender and has a short sagittal diameter. The length of the mandible is decreased and it is more retrognathic in relation to the cranial base. Casts of the alveolar arches of the mandible and maxilla revealed a wider and shorter mandibular arch and a narrow maxillary arch of normal length (15,16). Radiographic studies, however, found a shorter maxillary base in Turner patients and a shorter pharyngeal depth (pterygomaxillary-basion distance) (17).

Several abnormalities of the spine have been noted in the Turner syndrome. Scheuermann's disease (osteochondrosis of the vertebrae) has been described (11,18). The irregular epiphyseal growth rings which may occur in the vertebrae, however, do not cause significant kyphosis or pain as in Scheuermann's disease (18). Schmorl's nodes (herniation of part of the intervertebral disc into the vertebral body due to a defect in the cartilagenous plate of the vertebral body or the underlying bone) are commonly found (11).

The chest may have a minor degree of pectus excavatum (18). Premature fusion of the ossification centers in the sternum is relatively common. The lateral clavicles and posterior ribs are thin. Ikeda et al. (8) noted an increased biachromial breadth.

The long bones are often narrow and the deformities in the upper limb may produce mesomelia. Indeed, we have observed one patient whose Madelung's deformity was severe enough to lead to a diagnosis of dyschondrosteosis (Fig. 1). Abnormalities of the upper extremity include the increased carrying angle (cubitus valgus), which is not associated with obvious bony malformation. Defective growth and early fusion of the medial half of the distal radial growth plate, when accompanied by shortening of the ulna, allows proximal migration of the carpal bones resulting in Madelung's deformity (18). The carpal angle, defined by the intersection of lines drawn tangentially to the scaphoid and lunate, and the triquetrum and lunate, is frequently decreased, from a normal of $131.5°$ to as low as $108°$ (11). Carpal bone fusion occurs in about 0.1% of the normal Caucasian population but is more common in the Turner syndrome. A coarse reticular pattern in the carpal bones is a commonly identifiable feature (19). Shortening of the fourth metacarpal and, less frequently, the fifth and third due to premature fusion of the epiphyses is a characteristic feature (Fig. 2). Short fourth metacarpals can also be seen in type E brachydactyly, pseudohypoparathyroidism, pseudopseudohypoparathyroidism, and the basal cell nevus syndrome. Occasionally the distal phalanges have a "drumstick" appearance (11).

Abnormalities in the lower segment of the skeleton include a more male configuration to the pelvic inlet. The bitrochanteric breadth is decreased (9). The knee has characteristic anomalies (11,18). There may be an accessory ossification center for the proximal tibial epiphysis. The medial portion of the proximal tibial metaphysis is enlarged and projects medially and inferiorly along with the associated epiphysis (Fig. 3). Exostoses of the medial tibial condyle frequently occur. These changes are age-dependent. The medial condyle of the distal femur appears to become larger because of the depression of the medial tibial condyle. In the foot, fusion of the tarsal bones and fusion of the distal interphalangeal joints occur. The fourth metatarsal may be short, and pes cavus is common (11).

We have studied costochondral and iliac crest growth plates from three patients with 45,XO Turner syndrome. The growth plates were qualitatively normal, but the height of the proliferative and hypertrophic cell columns were

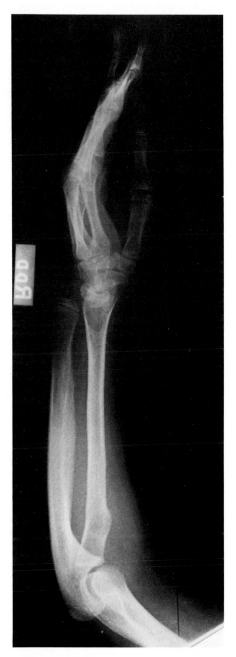

Figure 1 Radiograph of arm and hand of 14-year-old female with 45,XO Turner syndrome and severe Madelung's deformity.

somewhat decreased for age. The bone trabeculae appeared normal. Resting cartilage was somewhat unusual with more intense toluidine blue staining around the chondrocytes. Areas of cartilage degeneration with calcification could be seen in several of the cases (Fig. 4). Thus, in our experience, premature degeneration of resting cartilage appears to be the only unusual morphologic characteristic of the Turner syndrome. Stanescu et al. (20) have reported changes in the growth plate of patients with Turner syndrome. The clustering of chondrocytic columns which they report, however, is similar to what we frequently see in normal individuals, and the growth plate in at least one of our cases had long regular columns.

Thus, Turner syndrome is associated with generalized short stature and characteristic bony anomalies. The skeletal defects, however, do not appear to be sufficiently severe, or generalized, to account for their short stature. If the short stature is not due to the specific skeletal anomalies, could it be due to a more generalized skeletal dysplasia? This is highly unlikely in view of the proportionate appearance to the bones with equal reduction in length and width, and the fact that all organs in these patients are as reduced in size as are the bones. Thus, the growth retardation in Turner syndrome appears to be a generalized growth retardation process affecting all tissues and organs of the body; the growth plate is not the place to look for a specific defect. Indeed, the short stature of Turner syndrome may well be due, in large part, to the nonspecific growth retardation that is characteristic of all aneuploid states, except those associated with extra Y chromosomes. Certainly patients with trisomy 21 and survivors with trisomy 18 and deletion 5p- have marked growth retardation. The cause of their short stature is unknown but is associated with prenatal onset and postnatal continuation of significant proportionate growth retardation, as seen in the Turner syndrome. This would imply that there may not be any specific growth-related genes on the X chromosome. The ovarian dysgenesis, with its lack of estrogen stimulation prepubertally and lack of a pubertal growth spurt–associated lack of the normal hgH and IGF1 surge during puberty, results in a further decrease in final adult height. In addition, the lymphatic and vascular anomalies in utero may well contribute to the specific skeletal anomalies and growth retardation. Thus, it is likely that the growth retardation in Turner syndrome is of multifactoral causation involving the nonspecific growth retardation of aneuploidy, the ovarian dysgenesis and lack of gonadal steroid stimulation of childhood and pubertal growth, the lack of a gonadal steroid-induced hgH and somatomedin spurt during puberty, and a variety of lymphatic and vascular malformations in utero that may also contribute to the bony malformations.

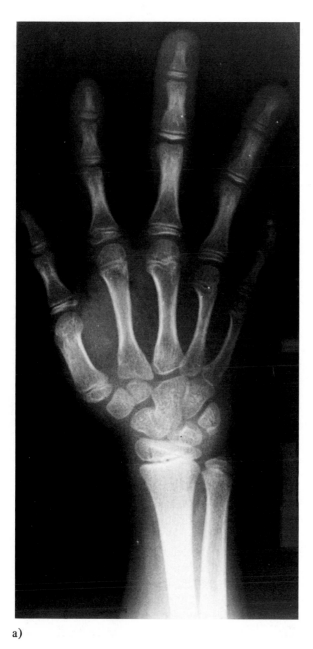

a)

Figure 2 Radiograph of hand of (a) 8-year-old and (b) 14-year-old Turner patients. Note short fourth and fifth metacarpals with premature fusion of their epiphyses in the 14-year-old.

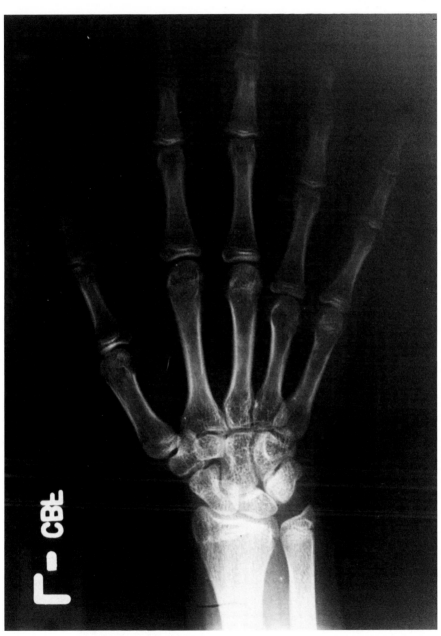

b)

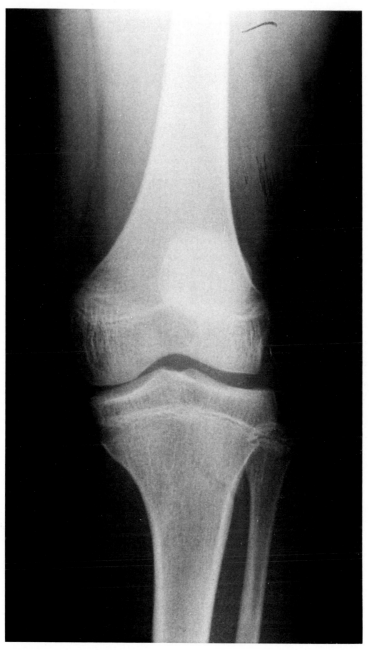

Figure 3 Radiograph of knee in 14-year-old 45,XO Turner patient. Note inferior projection of medial condyle of femur.

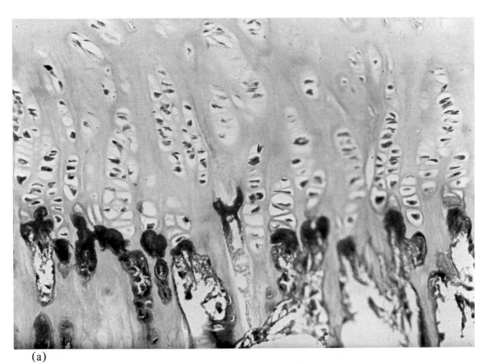

(a)

Figure 4 Chondroosseous histomorphology in Turner syndrome. (a) Costochondral junction growth plate from 11-year-old; (b) resting costochondral
cartilage from 14-year-old with focal areas of degenerating calcifying matrix; and
(c) costochondral resting cartilage from 19-year-old with large calcified area extending around the chondrocytes.

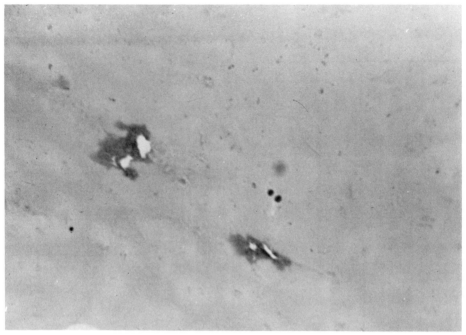

(b)

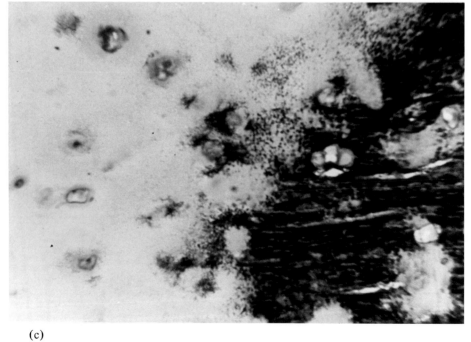

(c)

Figure 4 (Continued)

ACKNOWLEDGMENTS

We wish to thank Sue Lane, Mary Ann Priore, and Loyda Nolasco for their help in preparing this manuscript. This project was supported in part by a USPHS NIH Program Project Grant (HD22657).

REFERENCES

1. Ranke MB, Pflüger H, Rosendahl W, Stubbe P, Enders H, Bierich JR, Majewski F. Turner syndrome: spontaneous growth in 150 cases and review of the literature. Eur J Pediatr 1983; 141:81-83.
2. Brook CGD, Mürset G, Zachmann M, Prader A. Growth in children with 45,XO Turner syndrome. Arch Dis in Child 1974; 49:789-795.
3. Park E, Bailey JD, Cowell CA. Growth and maturation of patients with Turner's syndrome. Pediatr Res 1983; 17:1-7.
4. Tanner J. Growth as a target-seeking function. In Falkner F and Tanner JM, eds. Human Growth, a Comprehensive Treatise. Vol. 1. 2d ed. New York: Plenum Press, 1986; 173.
5. Lyon AJ, Preece MA, Grant DB. Growth curve for girls with Turner syndrome. Arch Dis in Child 1985; 60:932-935.
6. Neufeld ND, Lippe BM, Kaplan SA. Disproportionate growth of the lower extremities. A major determinant of short stature in Turner's syndrome. Am J Dis Child 1978 March; 132:296-298.
7. Miller R, Ross WD, Rapp A, Roede M. Sex chromosome aneuploidy and anthropometry: a new proportionality assessment using the phantom stratagem. Am J Med Gen 1980; 5:125-135.
8. Ikeda Y, Higurashi M, Egi S, Ohzeki N, Hoshina H. An anthropometric study of girls with the Ullrich-Turner syndrome. Am J Med Gen 1982; 12:271-280.
9. Varrela J, Vinkka H, Alvesalo L. The phenotype of 45,X females: an anthropometric quantification. Ann Hum Biol 1984; 11(1):53-66.
10. Hughes PCR, Ribeiro J, Hughes IA. Body proportions in Turner's syndrome. Arch Dis in Child 1986; 61:506-517.
11. Preger L, Steinbach HL, Moskowitz P, Scully AL, Goldberg MB. Roentgenographic abnormalities in phenotypic females with gonadal dysgenesis. A comparison of chromatin positive and chromatin negative patients. AJR 1968 Dec; 104(4):899-910.
12. Smith MA, Wilson J, Price WH. Bone demineralization in patients with Turner's syndrome. J Med Gen 1982; 19:100-103.
13. Garn SG, Poznanski AK, Nagy JM. Bone measurement in the differential diagnosis of osteopenia and osteoporosis. Radiology 1971 Sept; 100:500-518.
14. Brown DM, Jowsey J, Bradford DS. Osteoporosis in ovarian dysgenesis. J of Ped 1974 June; 84(6):816-820.
15. Laine T, Alvesalo L, Lammi S. Palatal dimensions in 45,X—females. J of Crainiofac Gen and Dev Bio 1985; 5:239-246.

16. Laine T, Alvesalo L. Size of the alveolar arch of the mandible in relation to that of the maxilla in 45,X females. J Dent Res 1986 Dec; 12:1432–1434.
17. Jensen BL. Craniofacial morphology in Turner syndrome. J of Crainiofac Gen and Dev Bio 1985; 5:327–340.
18. Beals RK. Orthopedic aspects of the XO (Turner's) syndrome. Clin Ortho and Rel Research 1973 Nov–Dec; 97:19–30.
19. Bercu BB, Kramer SS, Bode HH. A useful radiologic sign for the diagnosis of Turner's syndrome. Pediatrics 1976 Nov; 58(5):737–739.
20. Stanescu V, Pitis M, Ionescu V, Bona C. Histochemical and cytoenzymological studies on growing cartilage in Turner's syndrome. Acta Histochem. (Jena), 1965; 20:309–330.

DISCUSSION

DR. RAPHAEL RAPPAPORT: I just wanted to discuss a few slides on Turner's syndrome that I borrowed from Dr. Stanescu, who is a pathologist in our hospital. There have been very little data in the literature, and this very elegant and stimulating talk from Dr. Rimoin urged me to show you some of these slides, as the interpretation of Dr. Stanescu goes perhaps in a different line. These are cartilage biopsies performed in normal children (Figures 5, 7, and 9) and from children with Turner syndrome (Figures 6, 8, and 10) as part of a previously published study (Stanescu et al, Acta Endocrinologica Kbh 9, 659–688, 1972). Fragments of upper tibial growth cartilage were obtained from 5 patients with Turner's syndrome and were compared with fragments of the same cartilage with the same location obtained from 10 children of comparable age with apparent normal growth (orthopedic intervention after accidents or death due to traffic accidents). The organization of the upper tibial growth cartilage showed evident differences between the two groups. In children with apparent normal growth the columns were well organized with a well developed proliferating and hypertrophic zones. Individual columns or groups of 2 to 3 columns were separated by narrow and long septa. The primary trabeculae were thin and regularly arranged. The growth zone in patients with Turner's syndrome was narrower. The cell arrangement was different, in oval shaped or triangular groups with both proliferative and hypertrophic zones reduced. The primary trabeculae were thicker and irregularly arranged. Even the appearance of an obliquely cut normal cartilage can be easily distinguished from the arrangement of cells seen in

Dr. Raphael Rappaport is at Hospital des Enfants-Malades, Paris, France. Dr. David Rimoin is at the Cedars-Sinai Medical Center, Los Angeles, California. Dr. William Horton is at the University of Texas Medical School at Houston, Houston, Texas.

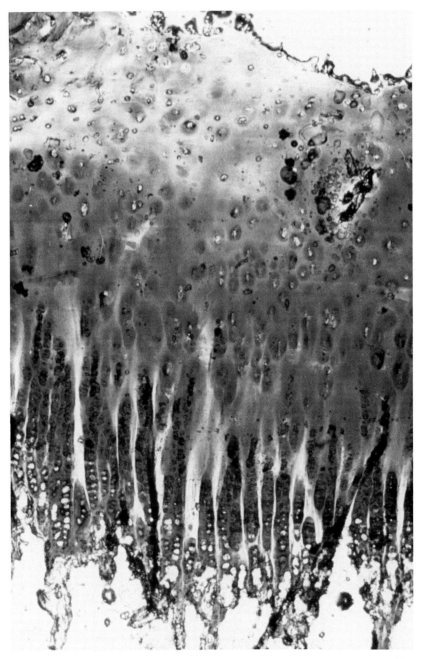

Figure 5 Upper tibial cartilage. Normal child (died after a traffic accident), aged 9 yrs. Fresh frozen section, Azur A pH 2, obj 4. Long, regularly disposed columns.

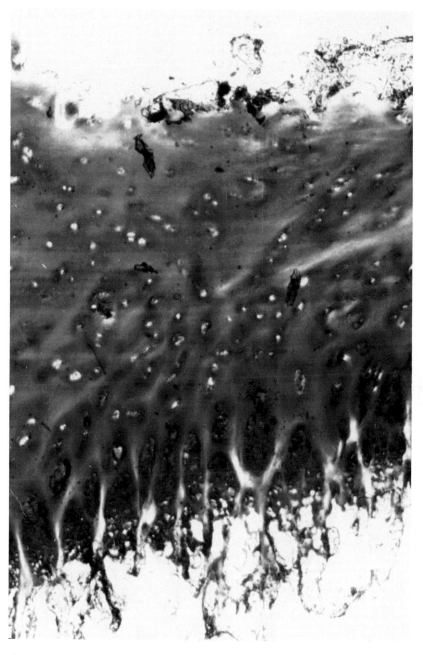

Figure 6 Upper tibial cartilage. Turner's syndrome XO, untreated, aged 10.5 yrs. Fresh frozen section. Azur A pH 2, obj 4. Narrow proliferative and hypertrophic areas. Ovoid arrangement of cells of the growth zone.

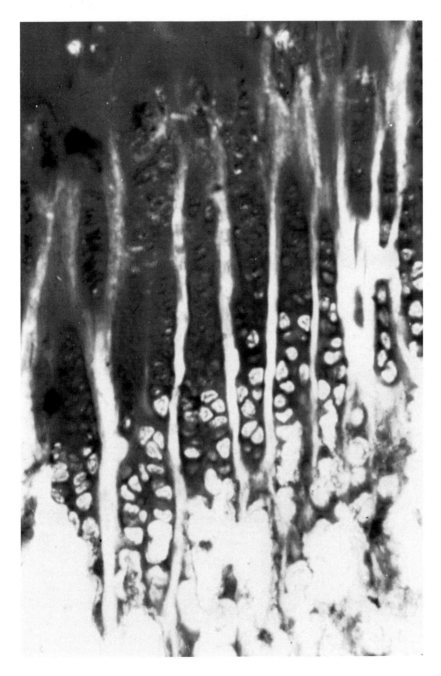

Figure 7 Upper tibial cartilage. Normal child aged 9 yrs. Fresh frozen section, Azur A pH 2, obj 10. The columns of the growth zone are long with well developed proliferative and hypertrophic areas.

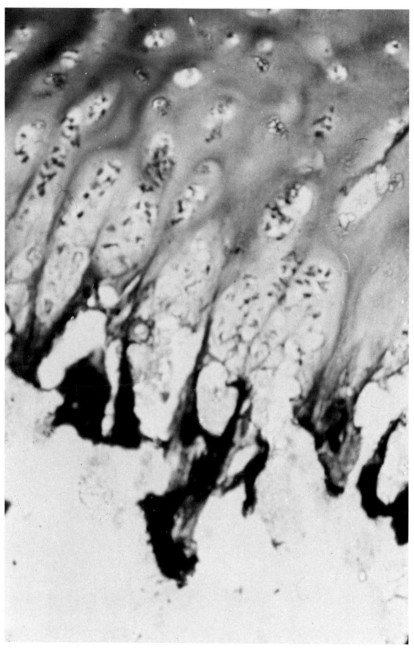

Figure 8 Upper tibial cartilage. Turner's syndrome XO, untreated, aged 10.5. Fresh frozen section, Mallory staining, obj 10. Narrow hypertrophic area and still narrower proliferative area. The cells are grouped in ovoid formations separated by septa.

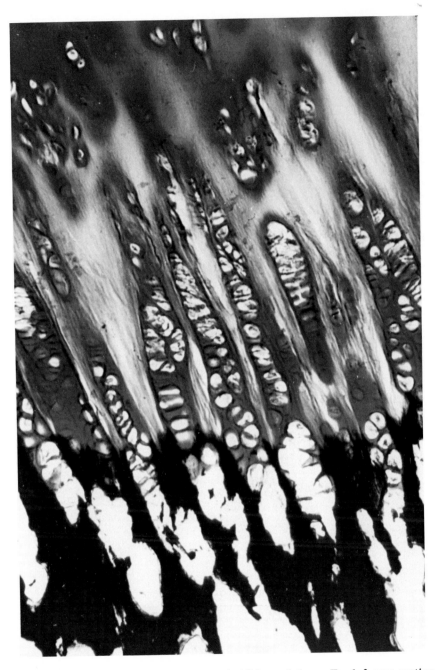

Figure 9 Upper tibial cartilage. Normal child, aged 6 yrs. Fresh frozen section, Von Kossa staining, neutral red counter staining, obj 10. Regular thin columns, regularly arranged thin primary trabeculae.

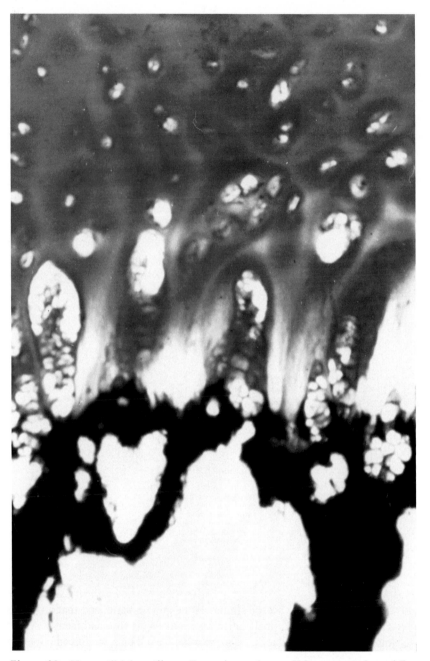

Figure 10 Upper tibial cartilage. Turner's syndrome XO, untreated, aged 7 yrs. Fresh frozen section, Von Kossa staining, neutral red counterstaining, obj 10. Short ovoid groups of cells separated by wide septa, thick and irregular primary trabeculae.

the cartilage of patients with Turner's syndrome. In 3 cases of pituitary dwarf-ism (data not shown) the tibial cartilage was narrow, with short but regularly ar-ranged columns separated by rather wide septa, and with thin and short primary trabeculae. The pattern was different from that seen in Turner's syndrome. It is important to mention that in normals the apophyseal iliac crest growth plate is narrower and less well organized and has a more irregular grouping of cells than the upper tibial cartilage. Only cartilages with the same location can be properly compared. In addition, in several syndromes with growth disturbances, altera-tions were found in the tibial or fibular growth plates, whereas the apophyseal growth cartilage of the iliac crest presented little or no changes compared with the normal (Dr. Stanescu).

In conclusions, I would propose that in spite of a proportional and diffuse shortening of bone length, a primary abnormality in the cartilage function cannot be ruled out. This defect in growth may be due to a specific lesion rela-tive to Turner's syndrome that deserves further investigation by modern election microscopy and histochemical studies if cartilage becomes available.

DR. DAVID RIMOIN: I think that we see this type of clustering normally, and in the three patients of Turner's syndrome that I showed you, two of them had some clustering, while one of them had perfectly long straight columns. In quan-titative analysis of the cells and the columns, they were perfectly normal or slightly decreased, so I think this is a variable finding that we find in normal individuals. And again, if you were to say that this was causing the growth re-tardation in Turner's syndrome, you would have to say that something really abnormal was going on in periosteal bone formation, or else you would end up with a short, wide bone, because they are proportionally decreased in length and in width, and the width is caused by membranous ossification, the length is caused by endochondral ossification.

DR. RAPPAPORT: I have reported the comments made by Dr. Stanescu who is a well known pathologist in the field of cartilage abnormalities. I would add that the mechanism of bone growth in Turner syndrome is still open for studies.

DR. WILLIAM HORTON: I completely agree with Dave in that I think these are probably normal, and one of the main reasons I say that is a few years ago we decided to do histomorphometric studies of the growth plate, and that forced us to look at an awful lot of normal controls from different sites and from different ages. And even within one specimen so we would avoid bias, we forced ourselves to look at preselected points. And what we discovered was that the normal growth plate is considerably more variable than we ever appreciated, and these sorts of clustering and lack of cells can typically be seen. In fact, we have done a large study on growth hormone-deficient children who were biopsied before and after treatment, and we could not even discover a difference there. Again, we saw areas that looked just like this in some of them, but it did not change when we treated them. The other comment I want to make is that I think that we are putting too much emphasis on what we call this thing, whether you try to shove it into a skeletal dysplasia, an endocrinopathy, a variant of normal or something like that. It seems to me that we used to be able to distinguish skeletal dysplasias from normal variants, from endocrinopathies and so on, but as we began to understand the biology of the growth plate these distinctions are clearly beginning to merge, and there is a lot of overlap, and I think we need to think of all this as a unit in which something is not quite right, but we do not know quite what it is, and there are probably a whole bunch of things that are not quite right, since we are missing an awful lot of genes in this instance.

24

Osteoporosis in Turner Syndrome

Karen R. Rubin

University of Connecticut Health Center
Farmington, Connecticut

INTRODUCTION

The frequent observation of radiographic "osteopenia" (1) together with the reports of low bone mineral content (BMC) in Turner syndrome (TS) individuals have led many investigators to consider osteoporosis an additional feature in this disorder, despite the lack of reports of symptomatic fractures. It remains controversial whether or not the skeletal demineralization represents an intrinsic bone defect due to the missing X chromosomal material, is related to an abnormal hormonal milieu, or is due to a combination of both. Understanding the cellular and endocrine basis for these bone-related findings in this well-defined subpopulation of females will play an important part in deciphering the heterogeneous nature of osteoporosis in the general population. Following a brief overview of osteoporosis at large and of what constitutes our present understanding of the normal patterns of bone accretion and loss, the relevant findings in TS will be presented. Lastly, the potential clinical significance of these findings and tentative conclusions about the etiology of osteopenia in TS will be discussed.

CURRENT CONCEPTS IN OSTEOPOROSIS

Osteoporosis can be defined as an absolute decrease in the amount of bone and a loss of bone strength, leading to an increase in fractures after minimal trauma, particularly of the vertebral bodies, proximal femur, and distal radius. Osteoporosis is often a silent disease with the decreased bone mass and strength existing for some time prior to the onset of fractures. However, because of the multiplicity of factors which are thought to contribute to the development of osteoporosis, we are unable to accurately predict the development of clinically significant osteoporosis before it reaches an irreversible stage with fractures.

The risk of fracture can be estimated indirectly by measuring bone mineral content or bone density. In the absence of significant trauma, fractures do not occur until bone density falls below a value which is termed the "fracture threshold." With decreases in bone density below this theoretical fracture threshold, the incidence of hip fractures and the prevalence of vertebral fractures increase (2,3).

The correlation between bone mass and strength forms the basis for the use of measurements of bone density in the diagnosis of osteoporosis. However, these measurements appear to be an imperfect predictor of the propensity to fracture. The geometric structure of the trabecular skeleton may be weakened to a greater or lesser extent than might be expected from an absolute measurement of BMC or bone density. In the nonosteoporotic individual, trabecular bone is comprised of numerous plates distributed in a fairly uniform manner. In the osteoporotic, one sees a reduction in the number of plates and a conversion of plates to rodlike structures (4). Excessive thinning of these rods can result in microfractures. Such qualitative structural changes might occur more readily in older bone as compared to nonaged bone. It is the loss of structural elements and/or the accumulation of microfractures that is thought to result in increased bone fragility and subsequent fractures.

Bone density during the later decades is determined by the amount of bone made during the active bone-forming years of childhood, adolescence, and young adulthood and its subsequent rate of loss. Although most efforts in the field of osteoporosis prevention have been aimed at slowing down the rate of bone loss with aging, a number of important findings suggest that suboptimal accumulation of bone mass by young adulthood or the inadequate development of "peak bone mass" predisposes an individual to fractures later in life when age-related bone loss occurs. For example, black men and women have a greater bone mass at all ages, which is associated with a lower fracture rate at all ages (5). Because women have a lower peak bone mass than men and an accelerated rate of postmenopausal loss, they are more susceptible to fractures with age than men (6). Women with mild osteogenesis imperfecta who have less peak bone mass experience an increased fracture rate after the menopause (7). These observations serve to emphasize the role of "peak bone mass" in the development of adult osteoporosis. Whether or not the young woman with TS who enters adult life with deficient "peak bone mass" is at greater risk for symptomatic osteoporosis with aging remains unclear.

Our present understanding of the rates and patterns of bone accretion in the cortical and trabecular skeleton during the active bone-forming years of childhood and adolescence is limited. The work of Garn, based upon micrometric measurements at mid-shaft of the second metacarpal, made a major contribution to our understanding of cortical bone accretion during childhood. Throughout childhood cortical bone is formed at the subperiosteal surface and resorbed at the endosteal surface, with an excess of periosteal appositional growth resulting in net bone accretion. At puberty, presumably due to the rise in sex steroid levels, there is continued formation of new bone on the outer surface and a shift from endosteal bone resorption to formation, a phase which is reported to be abnormal in TS. This pattern of bone accretion continues into early adulthood, where after a relatively short period of stability, age-related bone loss begins. On the basis of his data, Garn concluded that approximately 50% of maximum cortical mass is obtained during childhood, 45% is added during the adolescent years, and the remaining 5% is added beyond the age of 18 (8). The only widely available bone density data in children utilizing the newer noninvasive method of bone densitometry are the standards of Mazess and Cameron, which normalize single photon bone mineral measurements at the distal radius for sex, age, height, weight, and bone width (9). Ideally, longitudinal bone density data to assess the rates and patterns of bone accretion in normal children and adolescents at both cortical and trabecular sites are needed to better enable us to evaluate children with known or potential abnormalities in osteogenesis.

Over their lifetimes women lose approximately 35% of their cortical bone and 50% of their trabecular bone (10,11). Cortical bone is present to the greatest extent in the shaft of the long bones, whereas trabecular bone predominates in the vertebrae, the flat bones of the skull, pelvis, and shoulder girdle, and in the ends of the long bones. Trabecular bone is a metabolically more active tissue than cortical bone with a higher turnover rate and therefore more responsive to changes in mineral homeostasis, endogenous hormonal changes, or to any therapeutic intervention, than cortical bone.

A combination of anatomic and densitometric data reveals a biphasic pattern of bone loss for both cortical and trabecular bone that occurs in both sexes and a transient accelerated phase that occurs in women in their early postmenopausal years. Although some of the data is controversial and incomplete, certain trends are apparent. In both sexes the onset of trabecular bone loss occurs at least a decade earlier than the onset of cortical bone loss. In females, the extent of premenopausal trabecular bone loss is much greater than the extent of cortical bone loss, and the accelerated postmenopausal phase of trabecular bone loss may have a faster initial rate than for cortical bone but an overall shorter duration (2).

The skeleton is a dynamic tissue undergoing continuous remodeling throughout life at discrete foci called bone remodeling units (12). Each remodeling cycle begins with the appearance of osteoclasts along an inactive bone surface, and over an approximate 2-week time period, the osteoclasts form resorption bays or lacuna in cortical bone or on the trabecular surface. The osteoclasts are then replaced by osteoblasts, which fill in the resorption bays over a 3- to 4-month period, thereby creating a new structural unit of bone. The rate of bone turnover or the frequency of activation of these new bone-forming units is regulated by a variety of circulating hormones and a number of locally produced factors. Low bone mass may result from impaired bone formation, accelerated resorption, or a combination of both.

OSTEOPOROSIS IN TS

Skeletal demineralization has been detected in approximately 60–80% of subjects with TS by a variety of methods. The degree of demineralization does not appear to be related to cytogenetic findings. Radiographic "osteopenia" or skeletal demineralization is commonly observed in Turner subjects during both the pre- and postpubertal years. Changes in the spine are reported to worsen with age and include a prominence of the vertebral stress trabeculae and a decreased number of the thinner horizontal trabeculae, resulting in a coarse trabecular pattern (1). Similarly, a coarse trabecular pattern of the carpal bones, seen on conventional hand-wrist films, has been reported in TS (13). Garn was the first to use radiogrammetry as a quantitative method to assess the amount of cortical bone in a study of 17 subjects with TS 15–65 years of age. The results indicated a failure to shift to endosteal bone growth during the adolescent years, leading to osteopenia mostly due to deficiency of bone growth at the endosteal surface (8).

Barr measured metacarpal cortical thickness, metacarpal diameter, and medullary width in 184 hand films from 67 Turner subjects aged 4 months to 25 years utilizing radiogrammetry (14). The results suggested that in children less than 11 years of age, periosteal appositional growth was deficient. However, in those patients greater than 11 years of age, the results indicated a lack of the pubertal shift from endosteal resorption to formation and thereby supported the results of Garn.

The method of single beam photon absorptiometry (SBPA) with ^{125}I as the source of photon has been used to quantitate BMC in TS. This method is widely accepted due to the fact that the single photon measurements have been shown to be highly correlated with total body calcium as measured by neutron activation. The method involves minimal radiation exposure (2–5 mr), is highly accurate (1–3% error), and has a reproducibility of 1–3% (15). As can be seen in Table 1, there have been at least four cross-sectional studies in Turner patients measuring bone BMC in g/cm at the radius, one-third of the length from its distal end, and one cross-sectional study measuring BMC at the os calcis (16–20). The

Table 1 Summary of Studies to Access BMC Utilizing SBPA

Skeletal site	n	Age range (yr)	Mean % of normal	Ref.
Radius	8	9–19	71%	16
Os calcis	6	17–28	72%	20
Radius	11	18–57	73%	17
Radius	17	9–23	75%	18
Radius	23	8–18	78%	19

measurement at the radius represents a skeletal site with a predominance of cortical bone. The os calcis is a site which is comprised mostly of trabecular bone. These five studies utilizing the single photon method report a BMC between 71 and 78% of normal, with a cumulative age range between 8 and 57 years of age.

The major limitation of the single photon method is that it cannot measure the spine where the largest changes in trabecular bone mass occur during growth and with aging. This drawback has been circumvented by dual beam photon absorptiometry (DBPA), which can assess the bone density of vertebra and correct for underlying and overlying soft tissue. The radiation exposure, and accuracy, are similar to that for SBPA, and the reproducibility in experienced hands is approximately 2-5%. DBPA measures the entire lumbar vertebrae for L2-L4, which is about 70% trabecular bone. Although quantitative CT scan can measure exclusively the center of the vertebral body, which is entirely trabecular, the radiation exposure (500-1000 mr) is too high to utilize for serial measurements in asymptomatic healthy subjects.

At present, only preliminary data utilizing DBPA in Turner subjects are available. These include observations of low lumbar bone density in a group of adult women with TS, mostly between 20 and 40 years of age (J. Siebert, unpublished observations). Preliminary data obtained at our institution (K. R. Rubin and E. S. Dalkowski, unpublished observations) suggests that this deficiency in lumbar bone mass first develops during the pubertal years and is not present during early childhood. As can be seen in Figure 1, the mean lumbar bone density in TS is not statistically different from age-matched controls until age 14 and beyond. Then the mean lumbar bone density in the Turner group is significantly lower than that of age-matched controls ($p < 0.001$) with a 16% decrease in bone density. Long-term serial single and dual beam measurements are needed to determine what the ultimate deficiencies in the cortical and trabecular skeleton are in TS. The patients enter adulthood, and age-related bone loss begins.

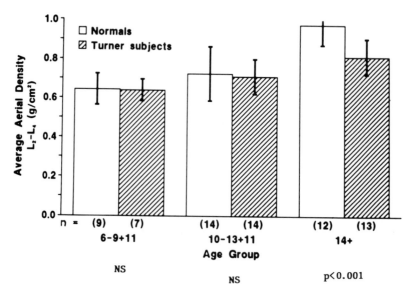

Figure 1 Comparison of mean lumbar bone density by age group in normal vs. Turner subjects.

CLINICAL MANIFESTATIONS OF OSTEOPOROSIS IN TURNER SYNDROME

Although the association between idiopathic scoliosis and osteoporosis is well established, the cause of the association remains unknown. Epidemiologically, both conditions primarily affect white females and spare blacks. Over the past decade, there has been an increased understanding of the biochemical basis of several inherited single-gene disorders associated with osteogenesis imperfecta in which mild to severe scoliosis is present. Scoliosis and osteoporosis have also been observed to occur together in a number of distinct chromosomal disorders. For example, the presence of low bone mass in Prader-Willi Syndrome (PWS) has recently been reported (21), a syndrome in which there is also an increased incidence of scoliosis and kyphosis. Similarly, in TS, an increased incidence of scoliosis occurs together with osteopenia.

We utilized the safe and accurate method of digital radiography of the spine to assess spinal curvature in patients from our young TS population. Twelve (41%) of 29 patients evaluated had scoliosis. However, the scoliosis was felt to be compensatory to a pelvic tilt in seven of these subjects with the remaining five or 17% diagnosed as having idiopathic scoliosis. Although most of the curves are mild, a small number of patients develop severe scoliosis requiring bracing or surgery.

There is a paucity of information on the development of kyphosis in TS, and it has not been determined whether the kyphosis which does occur in TS is largely a musculoskeletal or positional phenomenon, secondary to Scheuermann's disease (irregularities of epiphyseal rings), or secondary to osteoporotic changes with age. A longitudinal clinical, radiographic, and bone densitometric study of a large Turner population into their later adult years is needed to document the prevalence of vertebral abnormalities (anterior wedging, Schmorl's nodes, loss of anterior and/or posterior height, compressions) and to determine whether or not they have clinical consequences such as the development of kyphosis, loss of height, episodes of back pain, and compression fractures. It would also be important to determine whether or not these vertebral abnormalities and their progression, if any, are related to changes in bone density.

The vertebral crush fracture syndrome, which is associated with the greatest degree of physical deformity and causes the most psychological and physical pain, and Colles fractures, both of which are associated with decreased trabecular bone mass and strength, have not been reported to occur widely in TS. It is possible that some degree of underreporting has occurred since most academic centers caring for adult Turner have few patients who have reached the fifth decade or beyond. In addition, a significant percentage of compression fractures are essentially asymptomatic. Therefore, before it is definitely concluded that there is no increased incidence of vertebral crush fractures in TS, an older population of Turner individuals should be followed and screened with spinal X-rays. Furthermore, long-term follow-up care of older Turner patients into their seventh and eighth decades would be necessary to determine whether or not there is an increased hip fracture rate in TS.

BONE BIOPSY DATA IN TURNER SYNDROME

Noninvasive methods to assess bone mass describe the tissue on a gross level and do not define the state of bone remodeling. To provide such information, invasive methods requiring transcortical iliac crest bone biopsy are needed. The first invasive study of bone morphology in Turner syndrome was reported by Brown and co-workers on eight girls aged 9 to 19 years (16). The authors reported an increased percentage of bone surfaces undergoing resorption in six of the eight subjects. Brown utilized the method of quantitative microradiography on iliac crest bone biopsy material. The major limitation of this method is that it infers where the actual bone-forming osteoblasts and bone-resorbing osteoclasts are, and the results are not compared to a stained section where the actual cells can be seen on the bone surfaces.

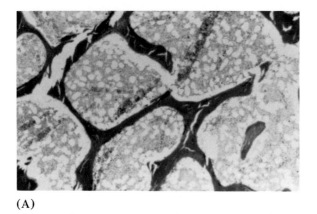

(A)

(B)

Figure 2 (A) Low-power micrograph of inner trabeculae of biopsy section from 13-year-old girl with mild juvenile osteoporosis: 19% trabecular bone volume. (B) Low-power micrograph of inner trabecular of biopsy section from 14-year-old girl with Turner syndrome: 12% trabecular bone volume.

At our center, transcortical iliac crest bone biopsies were obtained on two un-treated Turner patients aged 12 and 14 years, and the biopsy sections were analyzed by the newer method of quantitative histomorphometry (K. R. Rubin, M. Gunness-Hey, N. D. Adams, unpublished observation). The most striking findings from these two biopsies was the low percentage of trabecular bone volume and the lack of active bone-forming surfaces. There was no evidence of a mineralization defect. Figures 2A and 2B compare a low-power light micrograph of the inner trabeculae of a biopsy section from a 13-year-old girl with a mild form of juvenile osteoporosis to a section from a 14-year-old patient with TS. The comparison illustrates the markedly reduced trabecular bone volume present in the Turner patient with 12% trabecular bone volume, as compared to 19% in the juvenile osteoporosis patient, and 28% for a normal child. The percentage of total active surfaces taking up the double tetracycline label in the TS patient is 6.9%, which is less than half of the value of 15.6% in the juvenile osteoporotic, and half of the expected adult value of 14%. Where there was bone formation, it occurred at a normal rate. The results of these static and dynamic variables indicate a low turnover state and suggest a problem with osteoblast renewal and differentiation.

ENDOCRINE STATUS AND ITS POTENTIAL ROLE IN THE PATHOGENESIS OF OSTEOPENIA

It is likely that a fundamental bone defect exists in TS despite the lack of data to demonstrate an underlying genetic abnormality. A number of hormonal factors have been identified which may contribute to the osteopenia in TS and/or exacerbate the presumed bone defect (see Table 2).

Calcium-Regulating Hormones

The calcium-regulating hormones are essential for the body's mineral homeostasis and, in serving this function, exert major effects on bone. Brown and coworkers studied various biochemical markers of bone turnover in eight Turner's patients between 9 and 19 years of age (16). The authors reported normal serum levels of calcium, phosphorus, immunoreactive parathyroid hormone (PTH), and

Table 2 Summary of Endocrine Status and Its Potential Role in the Osteopenia of TS

Endocrine factor(s)	Evidence for significant role in osteopenia
1. Calcium-regulating hormones (PTH, calcitriol, calcitonin)	No
2. Growth-regulating hormones	
GH, IGF-1	Yes
Thyroid hormones	No
Cortisol	No
Insulin	No
3. Sex steroids	
Estrogen	Yes
Progestin	Maybe
Androgen	No
4. Obesity	Maybe

normal amounts of 24-hr urinary hydroxyproline. The only abnormal finding was an elevated serum alkaline phosphatase in five of the eight subjects. However, we have not been able to confirm the elevated alkaline phosphatase levels in 11 untreated Turner patients between age 8 and 13 years (T. Carpenter and K. R. Rubin, unpublished observations). Parathyroid function and vitamin D metabolism are presently being studied in this same patient group both prior to and during growth hormone therapy. Decreased basal levels of calcitonin (CT), an inhibitor of bone resorption, were reported in one study of 11 untreated Turner subjects aged 14 to 43 years (22). Even if a CT deficiency were confirmed in additional studies, it is unlikely that this hormone plays a role in the pathogenesis of osteopenia in TS, since neither deficiency of CT in athyreotic patients or CT excess in patients with medullary thyroid carcinoma affects bone mass (23). Overall, the present evidence including the bone biopsy data does not suggest an important role for any of the calcium-regulating hormones in determining the osteopenia in TS.

Growth-Regulating Hormones

Skeletal growth and maturation and achievement of "peak bone mass" by young adulthood depends on the integrated action of a number of systemic growth-regulating hormones including thyroid hormone, growth hormone, glucocorticoids, and insulin. Growth hormone (GH), a powerful determinant of bone mass, is thought to act indirectly through the production of insulin-like growth factor 1 (IGF-1) or somatomedin-C. IGF-1, one of the best characterized somatomedins, stimulates DNA, collagen, and noncollagen protein synthesis in cultured bone (24). Evidence has accumulated that IGF-1 production is not limited to the liver, but is produced locally in numerous tissues, including bone, where it presumably mediates the effect of GH on bone formation (25). An additional but important effect of GH on bone may be an indirect anabolic effect by increasing muscle mass. Skeletal stresses from muscle contractions stimulate osteoblastic function, and it has been shown that muscle mass and bone mass are directly related (5).

Abnormalities in the GH-IGF-1 axis in TS have been documented by a number of investigators. Ross and co-workers performed 24-hr physiological GH testing on 30 Turner patients aged 2 to 20 years (26). GH secretion patterns from the younger Turner girls between 2 and 8 years were indistinguishable from age-matched normal girls, in contrast to the older subjects aged 9 to 20, who showed significantly decreased mean 24-hr GH levels, peak amplitude, and peak frequency, as compared to age-matched controls.

Cuttler and associates (27) evaluated IGF-1 levels in 36 untreated Turner girls age 4 to 16 years. As compared with levels in 153 age-matched normal girls, the author reported that IGF-1 levels were significantly decreased in Turner girls aged 11 to 16 years. Eight of these older Turner patients, when administered low dose estrogen, showed a significant rise in their IGF-1 levels. Most pediatric endocrinologists have concluded from these and similar studies that the gradually increasing levels of gonadal sex steroids augment endogenous GH secretion, causing the elevation in IGH-1 that occurs during normal puberty. The relative deficiency in both GH and IGF-1 that occurs in the pubertal-aged Turner individual may contribute not only to their short adult stature but to their adult osteopenia or insufficient peak bone mass.

Thyroid hormones increase bone turnover but with a relatively greater increase in resorption than formation so that thyroid hormone excess can lead to decreased bone mass. The incidence of Hashimoto's thyroiditis with overt hypothyroidism is increased in TS. A less than average degree of skeletal demineralization has been observed in several of our untreated hypothyroid Turner patients and may represent a protective effect of their low thyroid status. However, it should be noted that treatment of Turner patients with exogenous thyroid hormone in excessive doses could induce bone loss and thereby contribute to the baseline osteopenia.

Endogenous glucocorticoid secretion has not been reported to be abnormal in Turner syndrome and therefore is presumed not to contribute to the osteopenia. Although an increased incidence of insulin resistance has been reported in TS with the potential to develop non-insulin dependent diabetes, insulin status is probably not an important contributing factor to the osteopenia since diabetes in general is not associated with an increased risk for osteoporosis (38).

Sex Steroids

Estrogen deficiency is a major determinant in the development of postmenopausal osteoporosis. The major effect of estrogen withdrawal is an increase in bone resorption with a smaller increase in bone formation, resulting in net bone loss. Endogenous progestins may also have additional bone-enhancing effects (29). The mechanism of estrogen action remains uncertain. No consistent changes in the serum levels of the calcium-regulating hormones occur as a result of estrogen withdrawal. Two recent studies have demonstrated that cultured bone cells can have estrogen receptors (30,31). It is possible that estrogen may act indirectly via one or more of the local mediators of bone metabolism, i.e., prostaglandins, IGF-1, etc.

The vast majority of girls with TS have bilateral streak gonads, experience no spontaneous feminization, and are estrogen-deficient during both their pre- and postpubertal years. It is possible that chronically low levels of estrogen secretion in the normal prepubertal girl may contribute to the normal bone growth during early childhood. The lack of rising estrogen levels in the pubertal-aged Turner subject may be largely responsible for failure to the shift to endosteal appositional bone growth and perhaps a diminished "accelerated" phase of trabecular bone formation. Therefore, estrogen deficiency in the Turner individual may play a significant role in the development of osteopenia.

The skeletal demineralization present in TS, however, is not analogous to postmenopausal osteoporosis or cases of surgical menopause, which are usually characterized by a phase of accelerated bone loss. These conditions represent states of estrogen withdrawal, in contrast to the untreated Turner patient who experiences lifelong estrogen deficiency with no true withdrawal effect. The bone density and bone biopsy studies to date show no evidence of a phase of accelerated bone loss during the adolescent and young to mid-adult years, but rather suggests a slow phase of suboptimal bone accretion which persists into young adulthood. Interrupted and/or abbreviated courses of estrogen therapy may have deleterious effects on trabecular bone by producing an estrogen withdrawal state with accelerated bone loss like that seen in postmenopausal osteoporosis.

Androgens are believed to play an important role in the development of osteoporosis in men but may also enhance bone accretion in females as well. Adrenarche is presumed to be normal in TS despite clinical observations of incomplete and/or delayed adrenarche in some Turner individuals. Measurement of dehydroepiandrosterone sulfate (DHEA-S), an androgen synthesized exclusively in the adrenal gland, revealed normal levels based on pubic hair stage in a group of 11 of our untreated Turner patients aged 8 to 13 years (T. Carpenter and K. R. Rubin, unpublished observations). It is probably safe to conclude that androgen deficiency in TS does not contribute significantly to the observed osteopenia. However, serum levels of additional androgens need to be measured.

Results of large epidemiological studies have shown obesity to be protective against the development of osteoporosis (32,33). The mechanism of this protective effect is unknown but may be related to increased peripheral fatty conversion of androgenic precursors to estrone, in addition to a generalized increase in skeletal loading. The development of mild to moderate obesity is common in TS. It usually becomes apparent during the pubertal-aged years and may be exacerbated by hormone therapy. Whether or not significant obesity in TS exerts an independent beneficial effect on bone mass has not been explored.

EFFECTS OF HORMONE TREATMENT ON BONE MINERAL CONTENT IN TURNER'S SYNDROME

To date there have been several studies investigating the short-term effects of hormonal therapy on BMC in TS subjects (see Table 3). One of three cross-sectional studies which examined the effect of estrogen treatment on radial BMC shows opposite results. Smith et al., who studied 11 Turner subjects aged 18 to 50 years, saw no effect of discontinous and relative short-term use of estrogen

Table 3 Summary of Studies to Assess Effects of Hormones on BMC

1. Cross-Sectional Studies

Skeletal site	Hormone Rx	Total n	Age range	Results
Radius	Estrogen	11	18–50	No effect
Radius	Estrogen	17	9.7–23	+ effect
Radius	Estrogen, anavor, 6H, alone or combination	34	8–19	No effect

2. Longitudinal Studies

Skeletal site	Hormone Rx	Mean Rx duration (months)	Total n	Age range	Results
Radius	Ox plus 6H	12	4	9.6–11.25	+ effect
Lumbar spine	Halotestin plus pre-marin	9	12	14–19	+ effect

treatment on radial BMC (17). The authors concluded that this negative result may be due to the finding that any gain in BMC is lost once estrogen is discontinued. A cross-sectional analysis of single photon measurements of the distal radius in 23 of our untreated and 11 of our treated patients aged 8-14 years showed no significant effect of hormone therapy (K. R. Rubin and E. S. Dalkowski, unpublished observations). We also attributed the negative results to the relative short-term of treatment. Shore et al. studied a group of 17 Turner girls aged 9.7 to 23 years and showed that the older, estrogen-treated girls had less skeletal demineralization than the younger, untreated subjects (18).

A short-term longitudinal study to assess the effect of human growth hormone (GH) plus oxandrolone (Ox), a weak synthetic androgen, on radial BMC was carried out at our center on four girls with TS aged 9.6 to 11.25 years at the start of the study (K. R. Rubin and D. Carey, unpublished observations). BMC was measured twice during the 6-month lead-in period and at 6-month intervals during the one-year treatment period. Their initial percentage of expected bone mineral (%EBM) ranged from 60.7 to 78.2% for chronological age, which is below the 3rd percentile for the normal population. The expected bone mineral (EBM) for the single photon method is derived from measurements which normalize for sex, age, height, weight, and bone width. Eighty percent or less of EBM is below the 3rd percentile for the normal population. The effect of combination hormone therapy was assessed by the change in the %EBM, which normalizes for the other important variables which can affect the bone mineral

Table 4 Radial BMC Pre- and Post–Combination Hormone Therapy, % Expected Bone Mineral (%EBM)

Patient	Baseline	Oxandrolone plus hGH
S.N.	60.7	62.3
J.H.	69.9	74.5
D.W.	78.2	84.4
J.J.	76.5	79.7
	mean %EBM 71.4	mean %EBM 74.5

mean %D in EBM = +3.1%

measurement. As can be seen in Table 4, the mean change in %EBM at the end of the one-year treatment period was 3.1%. Although the number of patients studied was small and they showed some degree of biological variability, these preliminary data suggest that combination hormone treatment, which is presently being used in TS to enhance short-term growth rate and potentially ultimate height, may also be beneficial in enhancing bone deposition in this population. Unfortunately, the small gain in BMC on therapy was not maintained in the posttreatment period.

Several nonprotocol patients followed in our TS program being treated with various hormonal regimens (estrogen, estrogen plus oxandrolone, etc.) have had two or more serial bone density measurements over a 2- to 3-year period which suggest, for the most part, a beneficial effect on bone density independent of the effect of increased age, height, and weight.

Line et al. reported results of a longitudinal study designed to assess the effects of combination hormone treatment with oral premarin 0.15 mg plus oral halotestin 0.1 mg daily on lumbar bone density utilizing DBPA for L2 through L4. Twelve Turner subjects between 14 and 19 years of age were studied on treatment for a mean of 9 months. The results reported in abstract (34) suggest a positive effect of combination sex steroid therapy on lumbar bone density in these young Turner patients. Collectively, these studies indicate the need for long-term intervention studies with various hormonal regimens to resolve the issue of whether or not such treatment can be effective in ultimately enhancing bone mass and, in some cases, preventing symptomatic osteoporosis.

SUMMARY

The characteristic "osteopenic" appearance to the bone, together with the results of some of the invasive and noninvasive studies discussed suggests a state of impaired bone formation in TS. The diminished bone deposition may be due to an intrinsic bone defect related to the absent X chromosomal material. The development of hormonal abnormalities which become apparent during the pubertal-aged years may exacerbate the underlying bone defect. These hormonal factors may ultimately have a greater impact at trabecular sites.

The nature of this postulated bone defect is not known. The osteoblasts may have an inability to produce normal matrix or may produce a matrix hyporesponsive to one or more of the numerous systemic and/or local regulators of bone turnover. The increased mortality in TS from dissection of the aorta (35) suggests the presence of a connective tissue defect in the blood vessels, a defect which may involve bone matrix as well. Collagen studies have not yet been reported on skin or bone material from Turner patients. Lysyl oxidase, an X-linked enzyme essential for cross-link formation in collagen and elastin, is a candidate connective tissue gene in need of evaluation in TS (36).

It has been well established that there is a low fracture incidence during childhood, adolescence, and through the fourth adult decade in TS. It is possible that the "idiopathic scoliosis" in TS represents a potentially important clinical manifestion of the observed osteopenia.

Whether or not the osteopenia in TS progresses to clinically significant osteoporosis with aging has not been adequately determined. Although most physicians involved in the care of adult Turner patients at academic centers have not been impressed with the presence of significant symptomatology, only a small percentage of their patient populations have reached to or beyond the fifth decade of life. It is premature to conclude with certainty that the osteopenia of TS represents a nonprogressive bone defect of little or no clinical consequence. Long-term surveillance of a large Turner population into their later adult years with the current methodologies are needed before any definitive conclusions are reached.

At the present time, it is prudent to recommend early institution of a bone-enhancing regimen in most Turner patients. The components of such a program should include assuring adequate daily calcium intake, encouraging frequent weight-bearing exercise, and the institution of continuous hormonal therapy aimed at enhancing linear height prior to epiphyseal fusion and at enhancing bone deposition, both pre- and postpubertally. Even if the longitudinal studies ultimately show no significant progression of the so-called "preclinical" stage of osteopenia in TS, it would be important to identify the factors which, in the presence of low bone density, are protective against the development of clinically significant osteoporosis.

REFERENCES

1. Preger L, Steinbach HL, Moskowitz P, Scully AL, Goldberg MB. Roentgenographic abnormalities in phenotypic females with gonadal dysgenesis. AJR 1968;106:899–910.

2. Riggs BL, Melton LJ III. Involutional osteoporosis. N Engl J Med 1986; 314:1676–1686.
3. Melton LJ III, Riggs BL. Epidemiology of age-related fractures. In Avioli LVC, ed. The Osteoporotic Syndrome. New York: Grune & Stratton, 1983; 45–72.
4. Dempster DW, Shane E, Horbert W, Lindsay R. A simple method for correlative light and scanning electron microscopy of human iliac crest bone biopsies: qualitative observations in normal and osteoporotic subjects. J Bone Min Res 1986; 1:15–21.
5. Cohn SH, Abesamis C, Yasumura S, Aloia JF, Zanzi F, Ellis KJ. Comparative skeletal mass and radial bone mineral content in black and white women. Metabolism 1977; 26:171–178.
6. Raisz LG. Osteoporosis. J Am Geri Soc 1982; 30:127–138.
7. Paterson CR, McAllion S, Stellman JL. Osteogenesis imperfecta after the menopause. N Engl J Med 1984; 310:1694–1696.
8. Fransancho AR, Garn SM, Ascoli W. Subperiosteal and endosteal bone apposition during adolescence. Human Biol 1970; 42:639–662.
9. Mazess RB, Cameron JR. Bone mineral content in normal U.S. whites. In "International Conference on Bone Mineral Measurements." R. Mazess RB, ed. U.S. Department of Health, Education and Welfare Publ. (NIH)-75-683, Washington, 1974; 228–237.
10. Mazess RB. On aging bone loss. Clin Orthop 1982; 165:239–252.
11. Riggs BL, Wahner HW, Dunn WL, Mazess RB, Offord KP, Melton LJ III. Differential changes in bone mineral density of the appendicular and axial skeleton with aging: relationship to spinal osteoporosis. J Clin Invest 1981; 67:328–335.
12. Parfitt AM. Quantum concept of bone remodeling and turnover: implications for the pathogenesis of osteoporosis. Calcif Tissue Int 1979; 28:1–5.
13. Bercu BB, Kramer SS, Bode HH. A useful radiologic sign for the diagnosis of Turner's syndrome. Pediatrics 1976; 58:737–739.
14. Barr DGO. Bone deficiency in Turner's syndrome measured by metacarpal dimensions. Arch Dis Child 1974; 49:821–822.
15. Mazess RB. Non-invasive measurement of bone. In Osteoporosis II, Barzel WS, ed. New York: Grune and Stratton, 1979; 5–26.
16. Brown, DM, Jowsey J, Bradford DS. Osteoporosis in ovarian dysgenesis. J Pediatr 1974; 84:816–820.
17. Smith MA, Wilson J, Price WH. Bone demineralization in patients with Turner's syndrome. J Med Genet 1982; 19:100–103.
18. Shore RM, Chesney RW, Mazess RB, Rose PG, Bargman GJ. Skeletal demineralization in Turner's syndrome. Calcif Tissue Int 1982; 34:519–522.
19. Rubin KR. Unpublished observations.
20. Risch WD, Banzer DH, Moltz L, Schneider U, Rudloff R. Bone mineral content in patients with gonadal dysfunction. AJR 1976; 126:1302.
21. Cassidy SF, Rubin KG, Mukaida C. Osteoporosis in Prader-Willi syndrome. Amer J Human Genet 1985; 37:Abstract A49.
22. Zseli J, Boszze P, Szalay F, Szucs J, Horvath C, Kollin E, Szathmari M,

Loszlo J, Hollo F. Calcitonin secretion in streak gonad syndrome (Turner's syndrome). Calcif Tiss Int 1986; 39:297–299.

23. Hurly DL, Tiegs RD, Wahner HW, Heath H III. Axial and appendicular bone mineral density in patients with long-term deficiency or excess of calcitonin. N Engl J Med 1987; 317:537–541.

24. Canalis E. Effect of insulin-like growth factor I on DNA and protein synthesis in cultured rat calvaria. J Clin Invest 1980; 66:709–719.

25. Schlechter NL, Russel SM, Spencer EM, Nicoll CS. Evidence suggesting that the direct growth-promoting effect of growth hormone on cartilage in vivo is mediated by local production of somatomedin. Proc Nal Acad Sci USA 1986; 83:7932–7934.

26. Ross JL, Long LM, Loriaux DL, Cutler Jr GB. Growth hormone secretory dynamics in Turner syndrome. J Pediatr 1985; 106:202–206.

27. Cuttler L, Vliet GV, Conte FA, Kaplan SL, Grumbach MM. Somatomedin-C levels in children and adolescents with gonadal dysgenesis: differences from age-matched normal females and effect of chronic estrogen replacement therapy. J Clin Endocrinol Metab 1985; 60:1087–1092.

28. Heath H III, Melton LJ III, Chu CP. Diabetes mellitus and risk of skeletal fracture. N Engl J Med 1980; 303:567–570.

29. Christiansen C, Riis BJ, Nilas L, Rodbro P, Deftos L. Uncoupling of bone formation and resorption by combined oestrogen and progestagen therapy in postmenopausal osteoporosis. Lancet 1985; II:800–801.

30. Eriksen EF, Berg NJ, Graham ML, Mann KG, Spelsbert TC, Riggs BL. Evidence of estrogen receptors in human bone cells. J Bone Min Res 1987; 2(S1):Abstract 238.

31. Komm BS, Sheetz L, Baker M, Gallegos A, O'Malley BW, Haussler MR. Bone related cells in culture express putative estrogen receptor mRNA and [125]I-17B-estradiol binding. J Bone Min Res 1987; 2:Abstract 237.

32. Daniell HW. Osteoporosis of the slender smoker-vertebral compression fractures and loss of metacarpal cortex in relation to postmenopausal cigarette smoking and lack of obesity. Arch Intern Med 1976; 136:298–304.

33. Dalen N, Hallberg D, Lamke B. Bone mass in obese subjects. Acta Med Scand 1975; 197:353–355.

34. Lin TH, Kirkland RT, LeBlanc AD, Evans H, Hausinger SA, Kirkland JL. Changes in bone density induced by sex steroid hormones in children with Turner syndrome. J Bone Min Res 1986; 1:117.

35. Price WH, Clayton JF, Collyer S, DeMay R, Wilson J. Mortality ratios, life expectancy, and causes of death in patients with Turner's syndrome. J Epid Comm Health 1986; 40:97–102.

36. Rowe DW, McGoodwin EB, Martin GR, Grahn D. Decreased lysyl oxidase activity in the aneurysm-prone mottled mouse. J Biol Chem 1976; 252:939–942.

25

Effects of Hormonal Therapy on Bone Mineral Density in Turner Syndrome

Rebecca Trent Kirkland, Tsu-Hui Lin, Adrian D. LeBlanc
and John L. Kirkland

Baylor College of Medicine, Houston, Texas

Harlan J. Evans

Krug International, Houston, Texas

Children with Turner syndrome (TS) frequently have asymptomatic osteopenia by radiologic diagnosis. Growth hormone (GH) has been considered as a therapeutic or preventive measure for osteoporosis. GH also has been demonstrated to be effective in improving growth velocity in children with TS. Sex steroid hormone has been demonstrated to be important in maintaining bone density in postmenopausal women. This study was designed to determine the changes in bone density associated with GH and to compare these with the changes observed previously with sex steroid hormone therapy. The bone density changes were assessed by dual photon absorptiometry (DPA) (1) with a program modified for children. The area studied was L2-L4. Bone density was measured every 6 to 9 months. Thirty children with TS (45,X in 15, mosaicism in 15), age 10.7 ± 0.4 (5-15 years) had bone density measured before any hormonal therapy was initiated. Twelve of them had bone density measured again 6 months later. The change of bone density in 6 months served as "control." Nine of these 12 girls were treated with growth hormone (Protropin, 0.125 mg/kg/dose, subcutaneously, three times weekly) for 6 months; six of them were treated for 12 months. Another 13 girls with TS were treated with Premarin 0.15 mg and Halotestin 1-2 mg daily for 11.8 ± 2 months (4-29 months). Our study results indicated (a) bone density in children with TS is significantly lower than normal children (0.655 ± 0.020 versus 0.860 ± 0.030 gm/cm^2, $p < 0.001$, $n = 30$); (b) in girls with TS, the changes in bone density during the control period are not significantly different from the changes in 6 months (0.005 ± 0.023 for control period versus 0.012 ± 0.020 gm/cm^2/yr for GH treatment, n = 9) or 12 months (0.003 ± 0.036 for the control period versus 0.054 ± 0.021 gm/cm^2/yr for GH treatment, n = 6) of GH treatment. However, the changes during the second 6 months (0.096 ± 0.019 gm/cm^2/yr) are significantly greater than the first 6 months (0.007 ± 0.031 gm/cm^2/yr, p = 0.013, by paired t-test, n = 6) of GH therapy. This suggests that with longer duration of therapy, GH may have beneficial effects on bone density in girls with TS; (c) in girls with TS, treatment with sex steroid hormone significantly increases the change of bone density (0.063 ± 0.008 gm/cm^2/yr, n = 13) in comparison to the age comparable controls with TS (-0.007 ± 0.023 gm/cm^2/yr, n = 8 by unpaired t-test, $p < 0.005$).

INTRODUCTION

Skeletal demineralization or asymptomatic osteopenia has been reported to exist in children with Turner syndrome (TS). The reported abnormalities have been

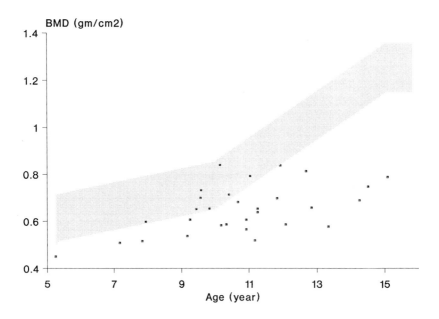

Figure 1 Vertebral bone density in normal children (shaded area) and in 30 children with Turner syndrome before any hormone therapy was initiated. Normal DPA data in children. (Courtesy of Johnston and Miller, University of Indiana.)

determined by radiographic assessment of bone and by single beam photon absorptiometry. We have confirmed this observation by dual beam photon absorptiometry (DPA), as demonstrated in Figure 1. The etiology of the demineralization is unknown. Both estrogen deficiency and intrinsic defects of bone formation inherent in the chromosomal abnormality have been proposed as responsible factors. In 1982 we began to test the hypothesis that treatment with conjugated estrogen (Premarin) and anabolic steroid (Halotestin) might improve the bone density in Turner syndrome. Subsequently, we reported that Premarin and Halotestin improved the bone density in TS (2). In addition, recent reports have documented that children with TS may have various forms of growth hormone deficiency. We hypothesized that diminished growth hormone also may contribute to the etiology of the observed demineralization. The following relates our study of bone density by DPA of the vertebral bone in several girls after 6 months to one year of treatment with growth hormone administration. This report compares these bone density changes with those of the girls with TS who received sex steroid hormone therapy.

PATIENTS, METHODS, AND MATERIALS

Table 1 indicates the bone density data on 30 girls with Turner syndrome (45,X in 15 and mosaicism in the remaining girls) who had measurement of bone density at least one time prior to administration of any hormonal therapy. Five girls had only one single measurement of bone density and did not have any measurements following hormone therapy. Twelve girls (1-12) had bone density measured 6 months later (Fig. 2). The change of bone density in 6 months was the control. Nine of these 12 (1-8,10) received growth hormone (Protropin, 0.125 mg/kg/dose, subcutaneously, three times weekly) for 6 months to one year (Fig. 3, Table 2). Thirteen (a-m) received Premarin 0.15 mg and Halotestin 1-2 mg daily for 11.8 ± 2 months (4-29 months) (Fig. 4, Table 3). Heights were assessed by stadiometer techniques at each visit.

Table 1 Bone Density (gm/cm^2) in 30 Children with Turner Syndrome Compared to Age-Matched Normal Children Prior to Any Hormone Treatment

	Age	BMD	Mean for age	5th Percentile for age
Mean	10.73	0.655	0.860	0.760
SE	0.39	0.020	0.030	0.030

The bone density was significantly reduced by 24% ($p < 0.001$).
Source: Ref. 3.

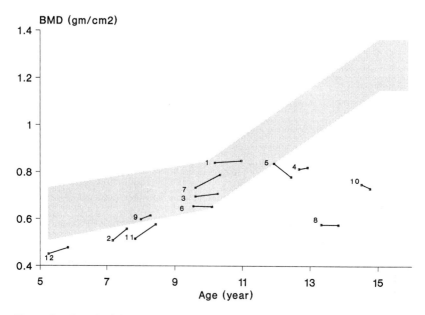

Figure 2 Vertebral bone density in normal children (shaded area) and in those children with Turner syndrome during control period. Normal DPA data in children. (Courtesy of Johnston and Miller, University of Indiana.)

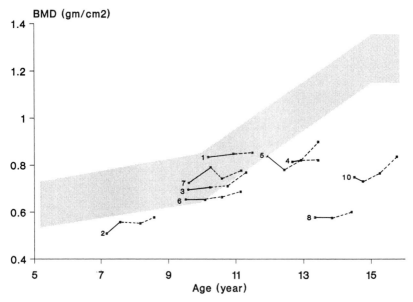

Figure 3 Correlation of changes in bone density in girls with Turner syndrome before (solid line) and during (dotted line) GH treatment. There is a highly significant ($p = 0.006$) negative linear correlation ($r = 0.939$) between pretreatment and 12 months of GH treatment.

Table 2 Bone Density Changes (gm/cm² /year) Observed During Pretreatment and GH Treatment Periods

	Before GH	0-6 Months of GH	6-12 Months of GH
Mean	.0199*	.0120	.0962**
SE	.0196	.0203	.0191
n	12	9	6

*$p > 0.05$ when compared with 0-6 months or 6-12 months of GH treatment (paired t).
**$p < 0.02$ when compared with 0-6 months of GH treatment (paired t).

The bone density assessments were measured by dual photon absorptiometry (DPA). Bone density of L2-L4 was measured every 6 to 9 months with a program modified for children. The reproducibility, precision, and standardization of the data from this laboratory has been reported (1). The DPA normal data for children was courtesy of Johnston and Miller at the University of Indiana (3).

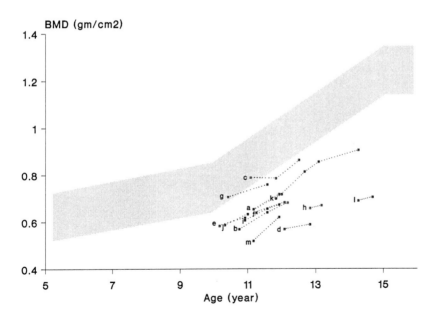

Figure 4 Vertebral bone density in normal children (shaded area) and 13 (a–m) girls with Turner syndrome during Premarin (0.15 mg qd) and Halotestin (1–2 mg qd) therapy (dotted line). Normal DPA data in children. (Courtesy of Johnston and Miller, University of Indiana.)

Table 3 Bone Density Changes for Patients Observed During Premarin and Halotestin Treatment Period Compared to Age-Comparable Controls with Turner Syndrome and GH Treatment

	Control	Premarin + Halotestin 4–29 months	Growth hormone 6–12 months
Mean	−.007	.0632*	.0962**
SE	.023	.0078	.0191
n	8	13	6

*$p < 0.005$ compared to control.
**$p > 0.05$ compared to Premarin and Halotestin treatment.

RESULTS

The bone density by DPA in the 30 children with Turner syndrome when compared to age-matched normal children (3) prior to any hormonal treatment was significantly reduced by 24% (0.655 ± 0.020 versus 0.860 ± 0.030 gm/cm^2, $p < 0.001$) (Table 1). In girls with TS treated with GH, the changes in bone density during the control period were not significantly different from the changes in 6 months (0.005 ± 0.023 for control period versus 0.012 ± 0.020 gm/cm^2/yr for GH treatment, $n = 9$) or 12 months (0.003 ± 0.036 for the control period versus 0.054 ± 0.021 gm/cm^2/yr for GH treatment, $n = 6$) of GH treatment. However, the changes during the second 6 months (0.096 ± 0.019 gm/cm^2/yr) were significantly greater than the first 6 months (0.007 ± 0.031 gm/cm^2/yr, $p = 0.013$, by paired t-test, $n = 6$) of GH therapy. Treatment with sex steroid hormone significantly increased the change of bone density (0.063 ± 0.008 gm/cm^2/yr, $n = 13$) in comparison to the age-comparable controls with TS (-0.007 ± 0.023 gm/cm^2/yr, $n = 8$ by unpaired t-test, $p < 0.005$). Since growth hormone seemed to have a beneficial effect the second 6 months of treatment,

Table 4 Growth Rates (cm/year) in Response to GH or Sex Steroid Hormone Treatment

	Pretreatment growth rate (cm/yr)	Treatment growth rate (cm/yr)	Change in growth rate (cm/yr)
Growth Hormone			
mean ± SE	2.86 ± 1.63	6.64 ± 1.37*	3.88 ± 1.51
Premarin + Halotestin			
mean ± SE	3.81 ± .30	6.83 ± .40*	2.75 ± .56

*$p < 0.01$ compared to pretreatment.

the second 6 months of growth hormone was compared with the Premarin- and Halotestin-treated groups. Changes of bone density during sex steroid hormone treatment did not differ significantly from GH treatment during the 6 to 12-month period (Table 3). Treatment with either GH or sex steroid hormone significantly improved growth rates in TS (Table 4) (5).

CONCLUSIONS

Children with Turner syndrome have a significant reduction of bone density in vertebral bone as measured by DPA. As reported previously (4), administration of growth hormone (Protropin, 0.125 mg/kg/dose, t.i.w.) during 6 months, and in this report of a 12-month treatment period does not result in significant changes of bone density. However, there is a significant improvement of changes in bone density during the second 6 months of GH treatment in comparison to the first 6 months of GH treatment. This may imply that longer periods of GH treatment may be necessary in order to observe the beneficial effects of GH on bone density. As noted in our previous report (2) sex steroid hormone treatment for 11 ± 2 months improves bone density compared to a control period of no hormone treatment for 6 months. Studies of the effects of a combination of growth hormone and sex steroids on bone density in Turner syndrome should be conducted.

ACKNOWLEDGMENT

Supported in part by M01-RR-00188 GCRC-NIH.

REFERENCES

1. LeBlanc AD, Evans HJ, Marsh C, Schneider V, Johnson PC, Jhingran SG. Precision of dual photon absorptiometry measurements. J Nucl Med 1986; 27:1362.
2. Lin TH, Kirkland RT, LeBlanc AD, Evans H, Hausinger SA, Kirkland JL. Changes in bone density induced by sex steroid hormones in children with Turner syndrome. American Society for Bone and Mineral Research, June 1985 (Abstract).
3. Conrad Johnston, M.D. and Judy Miller, Ph.D. Departments of Medicine and Nuclear Medicine, University of Indiana, October 1987, in press.
4. Kirkland RT, Lin TH, LeBlanc AD, Evans H, Kirkland JL. Growth hormone and bone density in Turner syndrome. Presented to the International Symposium on Growth Hormone: Basic and Clinical Aspects. Tampa, Florida, June 15, 1987 (Abstract).
5. Kirkland RT, Lin TH, Kirkland JL. Growth hormone studies and therapeutic trials with sex steroid hormones and growth hormones in Turner syndrome. Texas Pediatric Society, 1987.

26

Serum Osteocalcin in Turner Syndrome

Paul Saenger, Morri E. Markowitz, and Frank Gasparini

Montefiore Medical Center/Albert Einstein College of Medicine
Bronx, New York

Caren Gundberg

Yale University School of Medicine, New Haven, Connecticut

Barry M. Sherman

Genentech, Inc., South San Francisco, California

Accurate measurement of skeletal growth and bone metabolism in children with growth disorders is desirable. Alkaline phosphatase is mainly related to bone mineralization and may not be as sensitive an index for appositional bone growth (1). Somatomedin-C is synthesized by a variety of tissues and is thus not specific for bone (2).

We wish to present preliminary data on osteocalcin measurements in children with Turner syndrome. The question of osteocalcin measurements in these children in the baseline state is of particular interest, as Dr. Rubin indicates that children with Turner syndrome may have osteopenia.

Osteocalcin is the most abundant noncollagenous protein of the bone matrix (3). It is synthesized in bone by osteoblasts, and its synthesis is stimulated by $1,25\text{-}(OH)_2D_3$ (4). In adults several studies have shown that osteocalcin provides a sensitive and useful marker for bone metabolism in a variety of disease states such as osteoporosis, primary hyperparathyroidism, and renal osteodystrophy (5-9).

It is thought that the circulating pool of osteocalcin represents a small fraction of newly synthesized protein which is not adsorbed to bone but is released directly into the blood. Since osteocalcin is synthesized by osteoblasts, serum levels may, therefore, reflect the amount of osteoblastic activity in the bone.

We have measured osteocalcin according to previously described methods (10) in 15 children participating in the collaborative Turner study sponsored by Genentech, Inc. (11).

In the baseline state osteocalcin levels were slightly below the low normal range. In response to treatment with GH, osteocalcin rises. The rise is only measurable 4 months after initiation of treatment with GH (see Fig. 1). The rise does not correlate with the observed growth velocity. An unexpected drop at 6 months may be due to improper handling of samples as repeated freeze-thaw cycles may falsely lower osteocalcin levels (12). A sluggish rise in osteocalcin levels was also observed by Albertsson-Wikland and co-workers (13) in growth-deficient children treated with growth hormone. The slow rise in osteocalcin seen here is at variance with the rapid rise reported by Castells et al. (14) and Delmas et al. (15), who observed a rise in osteocalcin after treatment of growth hormone–deficient children with growth hormone. Delmas (15) measured osteocalcin only after 6 months of therapy; it remains, therefore, unclear at present how soon osteocalcin rises after growth hormone therapy.

Of further note is that the group of children with Turner syndrome receiving growth hormone *and* oxandrolone showed at 9 and 12 months significantly higher osteocalcin levels than the group receiving gorwth hormone alone. This group showed the highest growth velocity throughout the first year of study (11).

Diurnal rhythms of ionized calcium, phosphate, and PTH have been demonstrated in humans. These changes may, in part, reflect changes in bone cell metabolism (16-19). Since the serum level of osteocalcin is thought to be related to the rate of bone remodeling, similar rhythms may be present in circulating osteocalcin levels.

Gundberg et al. (10) have indeed demonstrated a circadian rhythm in circulating osteocalcin concentrations: nocturnal peaks are observed with a fall during daytime hours. Averaging levels of nine individuals and subjecting the data to median smoothing yields the useful model of circadian osteocalcin levels shown in Figure 2. The twofold fluctuations in osteocalcin concentrations over the 24-hr period stress how important it is to regulate the time of blood collection for this measurement.

There were no consistent correlations between osteocalcin concentration and circulating levels of Ca^{2+} and PO_4.

We have now measured hourly osteocalcin levels from 2000 hours to 0800 hours in five untreated girls with Turner syndrome (ages 8-12, prepubertal) using a slightly different assay for osteocalcin (Incstar Corp., Stillwater, MN). A similar nighttime elevation with lower daytime levels was seen in these meaned 12-hr studies (Fig. 3). Baseline levels are within the normal range as defined for children in our laboratories (nl 8.95 ± 2.5 mean ± SD for prepubertal children, ages 5-12).

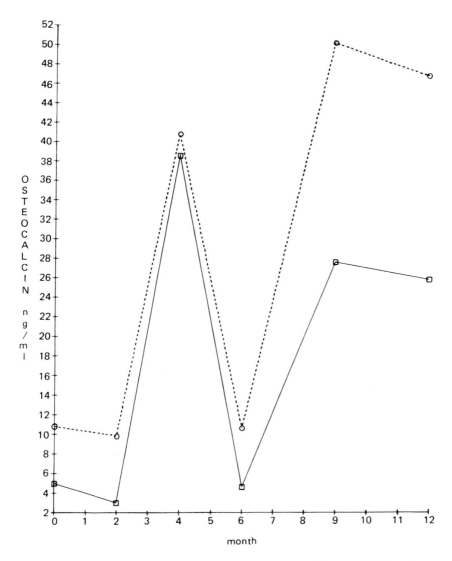

Figure 1 Serum osteocalcin levels at 0, 2, 4, 6, 8, and 12 months in patients with Turner syndrome treated with growth hormone (—□—) and growth hormone and oxandrolone (---○---). (For details of patients and methodology, see Ref. 11.)

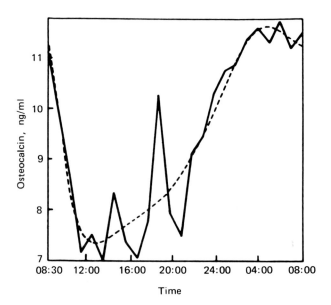

Figure 2 Mean serum osteocalcin levels determined every 60 minutes in six normal 20- to 30-year-old men: ——, Mean values; – – –, the osteocalcin polynomial. The correlation between the mean raw data and the smoothed data was 0.93. The curve is described by the equation: $y = 0.152 \times 10^2 - 0.4336 \times 10^3$ $(x) + 0.9822 \times 10^4$ $(x^2) - 0.1136 \times 10^6$ $(x^3) + 0.7137 \times 10^6$ $(x^4) - 0.2245 \times 10^7$ $(x^5) + 0.2749 \times 10^7$ (x^6). (Reprinted with permission from JCEM 60:736, 1985.)

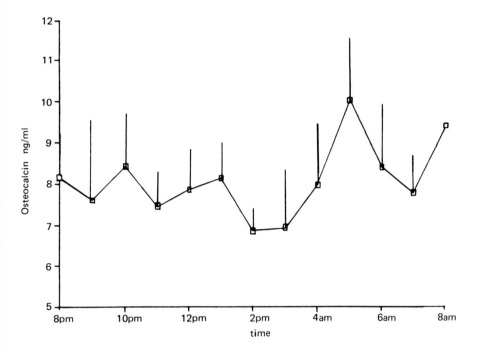

Figure 3 Twelve-hour fluctuations of serum osteocalcin in five untreated patients with Turner syndrome.

SUMMARY

Osteocalcin does not appear to be decreased in children with Turner syndrome. Osteocalcin levels rise with growth hormone treatment, showing no correlation with achieved growth rate. Osteocalcin levels show nocturnal peaks in Turner syndrome, making standardization of sampling criteria necessary.

REFERENCES

1. Krabbe S, Christiansen C, Rodero P, Transbol I. Pubertal growth as reflected by simultaneous change in bone content and serum alkaline phosphatase. Acta Pediatr Scand 1980; 69:49.
2. Underwood LE, Van Wyk JJ. Normal and aberrant growth. In William's Textbook of Endocrinology, Wilson, J.D., Foster, D.W. eds. Philadelphia: W.B. Saunders, 1985; 155.
3. Price PA, Otsuka AS, Poser JW, Kristaponis J, Raman N. Characterization of a γ-carboxyglutamic acid containing protein from bone. Proc Natl Acad Sci USA 1976; 73:1447.

4. Price PA, Baukol SA. 1,25-Dihydroxyvitamin D_1, increases synthesis of the vitamin K dependent bone protein by osteosarcoma cells. J Biol Chem 1980; 255:11660.
5. Price PA, Parthermore JG, Deftos LJ. New biochemical marker for bone metabolism. J Clin Invest 1980; 66:878.
6. Deftos LJ, Parthermore JG, Price PA. Changes in plasma bone GLA-protein during treatment of bone disease. Calcif Tissue Int 1982; 34:121.
7. Delmas PD, Wahner HW, Mann KG, Riggs BL. Assessment of bone turnover in postmenopausal osteoporosis by measurement of serum bone GLA-protein. J Lab Clin Med 1985; 102:470.
8. Slovik DM, Gundberg CM, Neer RM, Lian JB. Clinical evaluation of bone turnover by serum osteocalcin. J Clin Endocrinol Metab 1984; 59:228.
9. Brown JP, Delmas PD, Malaval L, Edouard C, Chapuy MC, Meunier PJ. Serum bone GLA-protein: a specific marker for bone formation in postmenopausal osteoporosis. Lancet 1984; I:1091.
10. Gundberg CM, Markowitz ME, Mizruchi M, Rosen JF. Osteocalcin in human serum: A circadian rhythm. J Clin Endocrinol Metab 1985; 60:736.
11. Rosenfeld RG, Hintz RL, Johanson AJ, Brasel JA, Burstein S, Chernausek SD, Clabots T, Frane J, Gotlin RW, Kuntze J, Lippe BM, Mahoney PC, Moore WV, New MI, Saenger P, Stoner E, Sybert V. Methionyl human growth hormone and oxandrolone in Turner syndrome: Preliminary results of a prospective randomized trial. J Peds 1986; 109:936–943.
12. Gundberg CM, Wilson PS, Gallop PM, Parfitt AM. Determination of osteocalcin in human serum: results with two kits compared with those by a well-characterized assay. Clin Chem 1985; 31/10:1720.
13. Lindstedt G, Wejkum L, Lundberg PA. Increase in serum osteocalcin concentration is a slow indicator of therapeutic effect in children treated for somatropin deficiency. Clin Chem 1986; 32:1589.
14. Castells S, Rebong K, Greig F, Yasumuru S, Smith S. Human growth hormone administration increases plasma osteocalcin concentrations in growth hormone deficiency. Ped Res 1987; 4:245A. (Abstract).
15. Delmas PD, Chatelain P, Malaval L, Bonne G. Serum bone GLA-protein in growth hormone deficient children. J Bone Mineral Res 1986; 1:333.
16. Markowitz M, Rotkin L, Rosen JF. Circadian rhythms of blood minerals in humans. Science 1981; 213:672.
17. Markowitz ME, Rosen JF, Laxmenarayan S. Circadian rhythms of blood minerals during adolescence. Pediatr Res 1984; 18:456.
18. Jubiz W, Canterbury JM, Reiss E, Tyler FH. Circadian rhythm in serum parathyroid hormone concentration in human subjects: correlation with serum calcium, phosphate, albumin and growth hormone levels. J Clin Invest 1972; 51:2040.
19. Robinson MF, Body J, Offord KP, Heath H. Variation of plasma immunoreactive parathyroid hormone and calcitonin in normal and hyperparathyroid men during daylight hours. J Clin Endocrinol Metab 1982; 55:538.

DISCUSSION

DR. FELIX CONTE: I just wanted to discuss some data that was published in 1985 from the University of California, generated by Drs. Leona Cuttler, Guy Van Vliet, Grumbach, Kaplan, and me. Data in girls with Turner syndrome somatomedin-C levels show that the somatomedin-C levels in our laboratory were not significantly different prior to the age of onset of puberty, but thereafter the girls with Turner syndrome did not experience a significant rise in somatomedin-C level, as opposed to the age-matched controls.

We had the opportunity of looking at the isolated effect of estrogen on SM-C. We were treating these girls with doses of ethinylestradiol in the range of 100 to 200 ng/kg/day. As you can see, they had a significant rise in their somatomedin-C level, and then when they were off the ethinylestradiol, the somatomedin-C levels dropped. They then went back up again with later estrogen therapy. We apparently saw a sex steroid–induced change in somatomedin-C levels. The statistical difference between before and ethinylestradiol therapy and on ethinylestradiol is significant. We unfortunately did not measure 24-hr growth hormone secretion in these patients.

DR. ROBERT BLIZZARD: What did you want to conclude?

DR. CONTE: The question is whether this is a permissive effect of growth hormone on somatomedin-C or whether, and this is heretical, estrogen may have a direct effect on somatomedin-C generation given its direct effect, as Corvol and Rappaport have shown, on cartilage, etc. Is it being mediated through growth hormone secretion or is there another effect of sex steroids, or both?

DR. BLIZZARD: Estrogen to hypopituitary patients does not elevate the somatomedin-C determination.

DR. CONTE: That true, Bob, but Friesen has an articel in *Molecular Endocrinology* in July showing that estrogen increases the expression of IGF-I message

---

Dr. Felix Conte is at the University of California at San Francisco. Dr. Robert M. Blizzard is at the University of Virginia at Charlottesville, Charlottesville, Virginia. Dr. Raphael Rappaport is at Hospital des Enfants-Malades, Paris, France. Dr. Judith Hall is at the University of British Columbia, Vancouver, Canada. Dr. Annlis Soderholm is at the Social Service Center, Helsinki, Finland. Dr. William Horton is at the University of Texas Medical School at Houston, Houston, Texas. Dr. Arthur Robinson is at the University of Colorado Health Science Center, and the National Jewish Center, Denver, Colorado. Dr. Leslie Plotnick is at the Johns Hopkins Medical Institutions, Baltimore, Maryland.

in the rat uterus in the hypox animal, even though it didn't affect the circulating levels of IGF-I, so that, at least, provides a possible mechanism for synergism between estrogen and growth hormone that would work, where estrogen is working directly.

DR. BLIZZARD: And the question of dose is also important, because of the biphasic effect of estrogen on somatomedin-C generation. That is the problem with the literature. If you use high doses, you get suppression, whereas low doses may stimulate somatomedin-C production at least at the cellular level, and it is also age dependent.

DR. RAPHAEL RAPPAPORT: In the old textbooks, hypertension was quite a frequent complication of Turner's syndrome, but it has disappeared from the program of this meeting, I just do not know why. So probably it is not any more of a problem in Turner's syndrome, except for coarctation and vascular abnormalities, which have been discussed yesterday. Therefore I went through my files and I want just to show you one slide.

We looked at blood pressure in 33 girls. Most of them were seen at age of 10 years before estrogen therapy and at age of 15 years while treated with ethinyl estradiol (EE). The girls who had elevated blood pressure while receiving 20–25 μg/day EE were switched to transdermal estradiol. Blood pressure returned to normal except in two cases. Three girls had a specific clinical histology: familial history of essential hypertension (▲), immune glomerulopathy (Berger disease) on single kidney (○), kidney hypoplasia (△), and two patients had essential hypertension (◊ and ♦) (Figure 4). In patients without overt kidney disease plasma renin activity was normal. Aortic stenosis was ruled out in all cases.

From these data we can draw some conclusions: 1. Some patients develop an ethinyl estradiol induced hypertension and their condition is improved by changing to transdermal administration of estradiol. 2. Some of our patients were slightly overweight but we could not correlate this finding with the occurence of high blood pressure. 3. We cannot conclude on the basis of that limited study an increased risk of hypertension. The most apparent cause of hypertension was the administration of oral ethinyl estradiol. In one of our patients high BP occured for a dosage as low as 5 μg per day.

DR. BLIZZARD: Does anyone have a comment about the hypertension that we sometimes see?

DR. JUDITH HALL: It is a significant problem in adults with Turner syndrome aside from those who have coarcts or renal problems. A fair number of patients do have problems with hypertension. In our experience, however, it is related to obesity. In fact, women can usually control their hypertension by losing weight. We have not looked specifically at which estrogens they are on, but a

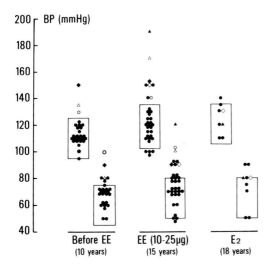

Figure 4 Blood pressure in children with Turner syndrome and effect of estrogen replacement therapy.

very large number of our adult women with Turner syndrome go off their estrogens, because they get disillusioned with taking them.

DR. ANNLIS SODERHOLM: I studied 62 adult patients with Turner syndrome, and of the 62 patients 13 patients had hypertension.

DR. WILLIAM HORTON: Do you know, since genes from the family are important determinants for hypertension, if those people who did develop that had a family history of hypertension?

DR. RAPPAPORT: These paients did not have a history of familial hypertension.

DR. ARTHUR ROBINSON: I think this is very interesting, because in the old days we observed hypertension, and we could never be sure whether they had minor coarcts or some renovascular, relatively minor, anomaly, and we did not have the technology, except very interventionalist. Do you really feel now that you have excluded, by your imaging techniques, those two possibilities?

DR. RAPPAPORT: Yes, we feel so.

DR. LESLIE PLOTNICK: In our adults we have as well, and have excluded familial histories.

Summary of Part III

Robert M. Blizzard

University of Virginia at Charlottesville
Charlottesville, Virginia

The purpose of this session was to consider the alternative causes of the growth retardation that accompanies Turner syndrome.

An evaluation of the data and concepts which were presented permits the participants to conclude that patients with Turner syndrome are not growth hormone-deficient in relation to their state of deficient sexual development, although the parameters of GH production at ages 10-14 in non-steroid-treated patients are low as compared to normal children who have developed sexually. Prior to this meeting there were some who interpreted the relatively low IGF-1 and GH concentrations, which are observed in teenage females with Turner syndrome, as indicative of growth hormone deficiency. This consideration was challenged. Participants agreed that true GH deficiency probably does not exist. This is not to say that treatment with growth hormone might not be beneficial by increasing growth velocity, but if effective, this may be attributable to a pharmacologic and not a physiologic action.

The portion of the program related to chondrogenesis was exceedingly helpful to the participants. The speakers enlightened the audience regarding chondrogenesis—normal and abnormal. The considerations that the growth retardation observed in Turner syndrome was related to abnormalities of skeletal formation were discussed extensively. Dr. Rimoin thought that we should differentiate skeletal dysplasias, which refer to generalized abnormalities of cartilage and/or bone growth and development, from dysostoses, which refer to malformations

337

of individual bones singly or in combination. Dr. Rimoin concluded that the short stature in Turner syndrome is not attributable to a defect in the growth plate. Logical deductions will need pursuit to find abnormalities in the growth plate. He readily admits, however, that he does not understand, and can't explain, the short stature which begins in utero.

The use of photonometry to evaluate decreased bone density was discussed by Dr. Rubin and Dr. Kirkland. The data presented are conclusive only in that decreased bone density occurs, as we all have known for 30 years, but the etiology of the osteomalacia remains obscure. There are still distinct limitations to measuring bone density, but further evaluation by dual beam photonometry and other techniques are desirable.

In summary, the etiology of the short stature associated with Turner syndrome remains unexplained, as is the etiology of the decreased bone density. Most discussants agree that there must be a defect in skeletal formation, but do not know where the defect lies. This session was both informative and exciting. The subjects discussed were clarified even though the pathophysiology remains unexplained and sets the stage for the subsequent section regarding the therapeutic approaches in Turner syndrome.

Part IV

Endocrine Treatment

27

Use of Anabolic Steroids in Turner Syndrome

Nathan J. Blum

The Johns Hopkins University School of Medicine, Baltimore, Maryland

Leslie P. Plotnick

Johns Hopkins Medical Institutions, Baltimore, Maryland

INTRODUCTION

Short stature is one of the predominant phenotypic characteristics of Turner syndrome. It occurs in nearly 100% of patients with a 45,XO karyotype and in approximately 95% of patients with X chromosome deletions or mosaic karyotypes (1,2). In 30% of the cases short stature may be the only phenotypic characteristic of Turner syndrome at the time of diagnosis (2).

The short stature of Turner syndrome results from growth retardation occurring during three phases of life. First, intrauterine growth is retarded with both mean birth weight and length being approximately one standard deviation below that of normal newborns (3). The cause of the intrauterine growth retardation is not known, but Park et al. (2) have demonstrated that in Turner syndrome birth weight correlates with adult height and weight to a much greater degree than in the general population. This suggests that changes in fetal development affect growth potential throughout life in Turner syndrome.

Up to approximately 3 years of age, children with Turner syndrome appear to have a normal growth velocity, but subsequently there is a progressively greater decline in growth velocity than is seen in the general population (3,4). Thus, by the time normal females are entering pubertal growth, their mean height is already 15 cm taller than that of children with Turner syndrome (3). Due to the

---

Current affiliation: The Children's Hospital of Philadelphia, Philadelphia, Pennsylvania

absence of a pubertal growth spurt, the mean height of children with Turner syndrome is four standard deviations below that of normal females during the early to mid-teenage years (3). Finally, due to a prolonged period of slow growth, patients with Turner syndrome reach a mean adult height of approximately 143 cm (4,5), which is two to three standard deviations below that of the general female population. It is this severe growth retardation, especially during adolescence, that has stimulated the search for agents that increase growth in Turner syndrome.

Interest in the use of synthetic derivatives of testosterone in the treatment of short stature came from the observation that while testosterone stimulated growth velocity, it caused both virilization and bone age progression (out of proportion to height age) potentially reducing adult height (6,7). Thus, it was hoped that synthetic derivatives of testosterone, termed anabolic steroids, that stimulated linear growth to a greater degree than bone maturation and had less androgenic side effects could be developed. This led to the synthesis and use of nandrolone phenylpropionate, methandrostenolone (8), fluoxymesterone (9), and oxandrolone (10-12) in the treatment of short stature of multiple etiologies. Initial studies with oxandrolone were especially encouraging as Ray et al. (10) and Danowski et al. (11) failed to demonstrate bone maturation out of proportion to linear growth when patients were treated with this anabolic steroid. However, subsequently it has been found that in younger children (12,13) and at high doses (14) oxandrolone can cause skeletal maturation out of proportion to linear growth. Indeed, the significance of using low doses is emphasized by the recent demonstration that at low doses even testosterone can stimulate linear growth without a disproportionate increase in skeletal maturity (15). Nonetheless, it is the synthetic derivatives of testosterone that have been most extensively used in the treatment of short stature in Turner syndrome.

EFFECT OF ANABOLIC STEROIDS ON GROWTH VELOCITY IN TURNER SYNDROME

While Prader (8) initially reported that patients with Turner syndrome failed to increase their growth velocity in response to methandrostenolone and nandrolone phenylpropionate, subsequent reports have refuted this claim (16,17). Moreover, all studies of oxandrolone and fluoxymesterone in Turner syndrome have demonstrated an increase in mean growth velocity of 2 cm to >4 cm per year in the first year of treatment (Table 1). The criteria that determine the magnitude of this response are not well defined. Multiple investigators have now demonstrated that in Turner syndrome (16,17), as well as other conditions associated with short stature (6,10,13), changes in growth velocity are unaffected by anabolic steroid dose over a wide range of dosages. The minimal dose to maximally stimulate growth velocity in Turner syndrome has not been determined for any anabolic steroid.

Table 1 Effect of Anabolic Steroids on Growth Velocity During the First Year of Treatment

No. of patients	Age (yr)	Treatment period	Dose (mg/kg/day)	Growth (cm/yr)	Velocity (SDS)	ΔGV (cm/yr)	Ref.
26	8.5–18	Pretreatment		3.3			9
		Fluoxy	0.12–0.18	6.6[a]		+3.3	
9	8.8–17.8	Pretreatment		1.9			24
		Oxan	0.07–0.125	6.4		+4.5	
21		Pretreatment		4.1			23
		Oxan	0.25	6.7		+2.6	
25	9.1–17.2	Pretreatment			+0.05[b]		18
		Fluoxy	0.06–0.17		+5.03		
17		Pretreatment		2.6			20
		Oxan	0.07–0.125	6.2		+3.6	
25	10–17	Pretreatment		2.8			22
		Oxan	0.1	5.3		+2.5	
16	11.1–16.3	Pretreatment		2.3			19
		Oxan	0.1	5.5		+3.2	
26[c]		Pretreatment		2.9	−0.3		21
		Oxan	0.1	5.0	+3.0	+2.1	
17	4.7–12.4	Pretreatment		4.1	−0.1		26
		Oxan	0.125	7.9	+3.7	+3.8	

Fluoxy = Fluoxymesterone; Oxan = Oxandrolone.
[a] Treatment period was 7–12 months.
[b] Pretreatment data available on 17 of the 25 patients.
[c] Twenty-six one-year treatment periods for 20 patients.

BLUM AND PLOTNICK

Table 2 Effect of Duration of Treatment on Growth Velocity

No. of patients	Pretreatment GV		GV during 1st yr		GV during 2nd yr			GV during 3rd yr			Ref.
	cm/yr	SDS	cm/yr	SDS	No. of patients	cm/yr	SDS	No. of patients	cm/yr	SDS	
9	1.9		6.4		6	4.2					24
21	4.1		6.7		11	4.3		11	3.5		23
15			3.4		15	2.5		15	2.0		17
25		+0.05[a]		+5.03			+4.09				18
17	2.6		6.2		5	4.7		4	3.3		20
25	2.8		5.3		10	3.9			2.8		22

[a]Pretreatment data available on 17 of the 25 patients.

Pretreatment growth velocity (18) and Turner syndrome karyotype (9,20) have also been shown not to predict the magnitude of the response to anabolic steroids. The effect of age at the onset of treatment is less clear. Joss and Zuppinger (21) found that height velocity correlated negatively with bone age from the ages of 8 to 13 years, and Heidemann et al. (22) found that patients less than 14 years old had a greater increase in height velocity than those over 14. However, other investigators have not found any correlation between chronologic age or bone age and growth velocity (9,18,20).

The only factor that has been found to consistently correlate (negatively) with growth velocity is the duration of treatment. Some have reported that after an initial increase, growth velocity begins to decrease during the first year of treatment (21,23) and mean growth velocity during the second year of treatment is always found to be less than for the first (Table 2). Nonetheless, growth velocity during the second year is usually found to be greater than pretreatment growth velocity (18,20,22). It seems likely that this is a manifestation of the growth-stimulating effect of anabolic steroids, because in untreated patients with Turner syndrome growth velocity tends to decrease from early childhood until growth ceases in the early twenties (3,4,18). While the effect of anabolic steroid dose on growth velocity during the second year of treatment has not been systematically investigated, it is interesting to note that Moore et al. (23), who failed to demonstrate a significant beneficial effect of oxandrolone during the second year of treatment, were using a dose at least twice as high as that used by other investigators. By the third treatment year growth velocity has usually fallen close to or below pretreatment levels (20,22,23).

Thus, it seems well established that anabolic steroids increase growth velocity in Turner syndrome. However, this response is transient, only occurring over approximately the first 2 years of treatment. Moreover, there is no evidence that higher doses of any anabolic steroid have greater effect on growth velocity than lower doses over the dosage range commonly used.

EFFECT OF ANABOLIC STEROIDS ON ADULT HEIGHT IN TURNER SYNDROME

The influence of anabolic steroids on adult height has consistently been one of the most controversial issues involving the use of these medications for the treatment of short stature. While initially this controversy centered on whether anabolic steroids decreased adult height, more recently it has centered on whether they can be used to increase adult height. In general, this question has been addressed using three methods: comparison of changes in height age with changes in bone age ($\Delta HA/\Delta BA$) during treatment, assessment of changes in predicted adult height during treatment, and comparison of actual adult heights in a treatment and control group.

Use of the $\Delta HA/\Delta BA$ ratio is based on the theory that if this value is less than one, then skeletal maturation is progressing at a rate proportionately greater than linear growth and final adult height will be compromised. As one might expect from the prevalence of short stature in Turner syndrome, untreated patients have a $\Delta HA/\Delta BA$ ratio less than one (23,26). In contrast, those treated with anabolic steroids are usually found to have a $\Delta HA/\Delta BA$ ratio closer to or even exceeding one during the treatment interval (Table 3). This type of data has relieved some of the concern about anabolic steroids decreasing adult height.

However, the validity of using height age as a measure of linear growth when comparing patients of a wide variety of ages has been questioned (18). Therefore changes in predicted adult height have been used to assess the effect of anabolic steroids on ultimate height. The Bayley-Pinneau (B-P) (27) adult height prediction (28) and Lenko's (29) index of potential height (IPH) (21) have been shown to be the most accurate methods of predicting adult height in untreated or estrogen-only-treated patients with Turner syndrome. When these methods have been used in determining the change in predicted height during treatment with anabolic steroids, significant variability in individual responses has been seen (18,25). However, in four of five studies the mean height prediction increased (Table 4), and in all of these cases was greater than any increase in predicted height seen in a control group or pretreatment control interval (Table 4). It has been suggested that both in children with Turner syndrome (25) and in children with constitutional delay (13,14), predicted adult height is most likely to decrease in those with bone ages less than 7-10 years. Joss and Zuppinger (21) found that two patients with bone ages less than 7 experienced disproportionately rapid bone age progression during treatment with oxandrolone, but in patients between the chronologic ages of 9 and 17, Lenko et al. (18) found no correlation between change in height prediction and chronologic or bone age.

Table 3 Change in Height Age:Bone Age Ratio

Treatment	Dose mg/kg/d	Mean $\Delta HA/\Delta BA$	Ref.
Oxandrolone	0.075–0.125	1.66[a]	24
Control		0.84	23
Oxandrolone	0.25	0.98	23
Oxandrolone	0.07–0.125	0.82	20
Control		0.80[a]	26
Oxandrolone	0.125	0.98[a]	26

[a]Median value.

Table 4 Change in Predicted Adult Height During Treatment

Treatment	Dose (mg/kg/day)	Duration (yr)	Change in predicted height			Ref.
			B-P (cm.)	IPH (SDS)	Range (SDS)	
Fluoxy	0.1	0.7–3		−0.5	−2.1, + 0.9	25
Pretreatment		1		−0.03[a]		18
Fluoxy	0.06–0.17	1		+0.32[a]	−0.6, +1.3	18
Oxan	0.1	1	+2.6			22
Oxan	0.1	3	+5.5			22
Control		1–2	−0.6			21
Oxan	0.1	1–2	+1.4			21
Control		1	+1.2			26
Oxan	0.125	1	+2.5			26

Fluoxy = Fluoxymesterone; Oxan = Oxandrolone.
[a]Used modified IPH method.

Even in cases where adult height prediction increases, the significance of this finding can be questioned. Some have suggested that after stopping treatment with anabolic steroids, skeletal maturation continues at an accelerated rate while growth velocity returns to pretreatment levels (6,12). If this occurs in patients with Turner syndrome, adult height prediction could fall to pretreatment levels during the posttreatment interval. In a study of 16 boys treated with anabolic steroids, Blethen et al. (30) have demonstrated that despite an increase in predicted adult height at the end of the treatment interval, ultimate height did not differ from pretreatment predicted height. Thus, evidence that an increase in predicted adult height leads to an increase in ultimate stature is lacking.

Therefore, in attempting to answer the question of whether anabolic steroids increase adult height, one must rely on controlled studies of patients reaching adult height. Of the five such studies performed, three have demonstrated an increase in adult height while two have not (Table 5). Unfortunately, no definitive conclusions can be drawn. In the three studies which demonstrate an increase in adult height, historical controls made up at least part of each group, and the mean final adult height ranged from 139.0 cm (21) to 140.6 cm (20). Recent studies suggest that untreated patients have a mean final adult height of approximately 143 cm (4) with no study reporting a mean of less than 142 cm (2,3,5,31). This suggests that a secular trend in adult height may account for some of the difference observed in these studies. However, in most cases the treatment groups did have mean adult heights above 143 cm.

Sybert (32) performed a retrospective review of 27 anabolic steroid–treated and 37 untreated patients and could find no difference in adult height. However,

Table 5 Adult Height in Treated and Untreated Patients

No. of patients	Treatment	Dose (mg/kg/day)	Duration (yr)	Adult ht. (cm)	Ref.
12	Control			143.2	17
15	a	a	3	143.3 $p > 0.1$	17
10	Control			140.3	23
6	Oxan	0.25	2.67[b]	146.4 $p < 0.001$	23
21	Control			140.6	20
7	Oxan	0.07–0.125	1.7–3.8	145.7 $p < 0.025$	20
7	Control			139.0	21
7	Oxan	0.1	1	140.5	21
8	Control			139.8	21
8	Oxan	0.1	2	145.7	21
37	Control			146.9	32
27	Oxan[b]	0.13–0.29	0.8–8.2	147.9 $p > 0.1$	32

Oxan = Oxandrolone.
[a]Patients treated with either methandrostenolone 5 mg/day or nandrolone 25 mg/wk.
[b]One patient received fluoxymesterone.

the control group had a mean height of 146.9 cm, suggesting the possibility that there was a tendency not to treat taller patients. Lev-Ran (17) randomized patients to no therapy or treatment with methandrostenolone or nandrolone phenpropionate and found no difference in adult height. However, none of these patients were treated before age 13, and the growth velocity during the first year of treatment with these steroids was approximately 40% less than in patients treated with oxandrolone or fluoxymesterone.

While it is not possible to reach a conclusive answer to the question of whether anabolic steroids can increase adult height, it would seem that any tendency to increase adult height must be small and probably will remain difficult to demonstrate. In contrast, with the possible exception of children treated before 7–10 years of age, anabolic steroids do not compromise adult height when used in Turner syndrome at low doses.

SIDE EFFECTS OF TREATMENT WITH ANABOLIC STEROIDS

The most common side effects of anabolic steroid treatment in females include deepening of the voice, clitoromegaly, acne (7), hirsutism, weight gain, and edema (9). These side effects are dose-related (9,18,20) and occur relatively infrequently at the doses currently used in the treatment of short stature in Turner syndrome. When Urban et al. (20) treated 20 patients with 0.1 mg/kg/day of oxandrolone, treatment was stopped in only two patients: one developed facial hair and one developed a deep voice and clitoromegaly. Using this same dose Joss and Zuppinger (21) noticed no side effects in the 20 patients they treated. Similar findings have been reported with low doses of fluoxymesterone (18).

Anabolic steroids have also been reported to cause various types of liver damage including: cholestasis, elevation in serum transaminases (7), peliosis hepatis (33), and hepatocellular carcinoma (34). These alterations in liver function are felt to be most common with 17-alpha alkylated steroids (which include oxandrolone and fluoxymesterone) and are reversible when the steroid is stopped or replaced with a steroid that is not alkylated at the 17 position (35).

Despite the fact that we know of no cases of hepatocellular carcinoma developing in patients with Turner syndrome during or after treatment with anabolic steroids, reports of an association between hepatocellular carcinoma and anabolic steroids are of great concern. However, the available data on this association is confusing. Ishak (36) reviewed the literature and found 24 reports of anabolic steroid treatment associated with the development of liver tumors (19 carcinomas; 5 adenomas). In 15 of 19 patients with carcinomas the underlying diagnosis was anemia (usually aplastic or Franconi's). In addition, only two patients had evidence of metastases, and subsequent reports have questioned whether metastases were really present in one of these cases (37). While 18 of the 24 patients reviewed by Ishak (36) had died, most died from their underlying illness. In two cases of androgen-induced carcinoma developing in patients without life-threatening diseases, the tumor regressed after withdrawal of the anabolic steroid (34). Both of these patients were alive more than 10 years after the diagnosis without evidence of tumor on liver scan (37). Furthermore, in one case where the tumor did not regress, the patient died of a myocardial infarction 10 years after the tumor was diagnosed (37).

Therefore, this tumor, although called hepatocellular carcinoma, does not behave like a typical hepatocellular carcinoma, and it is very rare in conditions not associated with anemia. Thus, while we continue to be concerned about both the risk of androgen-induced hepatocellular carcinoma in Turner syndrome and the meaning of the diagnosis, we feel that the current data suggests the risks are small. Nonetheless, our understanding of this condition is still evolving, and we recommend prompt discontinuation of the anabolic steroids once they are no longer effectively stimulating growth velocity.

ANABOLIC STEROIDS VS. HUMAN GROWTH HORMONE

Over the past 2-3 years it has been unequivocally demonstrated that human growth hormone (hGH) can increase growth velocity in Turner syndrome (26, 38). This has raised the question of whether growth hormone, anabolic steroids, or a combination of these is the most beneficial treatment for patients with Turner syndrome.

In a randomized trial of oxandrolone (0.125 mg/kg/d), hGH (0.125 mg/kg 3 times a week), or combination therapy (at these doses), Rosenfeld et al. (26) demonstrated that during the first year of treatment the group receiving oxandrolone increased their growth velocity by 3.8 cm/yr over the pretreatment rate while the group receiving hGH only increased their growth velocity by 2.1 cm/yr. The change in B-P predicted adult height in these two groups was equivalent. In addition, as occurs in patients treated with anabolic steroids (21,23), after the initial increase in growth velocity, those treated with growth hormone experience a decreasing growth velocity during the first year of treatment (38). Thus, while it has not yet been possible to investigate the effect of hGH on adult height, hGH alone appears to offer no advantage over oxandrolone in increasing growth velocity.

However, Rudman et al. (39) have suggested that there may be a synergistic interaction between anabolic steroids and hGH. Indeed, Rosenfeld et al. (26) showed that patients receiving combination therapy had a mean increase in growth velocity of 5.5 cm/yr, suggesting at least an additive effect. Moreover, while growth velocity did decrease during the second year of treatment, it remained greater than four standard deviations above that of untreated patients with Turner syndrome (40). B-P predicted adult height increased by 5.0 cm in this group, but it is not possible to compare this to the oxandrolone-alone group, as they received combination treatment during the second year. Thus, in contrast to hGH alone, combination therapy does appear to be superior to oxandrolong alone in increasing growth velocity, but analysis of effect on adult height must await completion of ongoing studies.

RECOMMENDATIONS FOR TREATMENT

Given our current level of knowledge, the question of whether to routinely treat patients with Turner syndrome for short stature is a legitimate one. It is clear that no treatment regimen has yet been conclusively demonstrated to increase adult height. However, we and others (25,41) feel that even if adult height cannot be increased, there may be significant psychological benefit to increasing growth velocity during childhood and adolescence so that these girls do not lag so far behind their peers. Clearly, this benefit will vary among patients, and thus the decision to treat needs to be made on an individual basis.

In cases where the decision is made to treat, combination therapy will produce the best growth rates. However, the cost of growth hormone is high, and oxandrolone will also increase growth velocity. If combination therapy does not significantly increase adult height, the high cost of the growth hormone might not be acceptable. Decisions on cost/benefit issues await the determination of the ultimate stature of those treated with combination therapy (26,40).

When oxandrolone alone is used, it will effectively stimulate growth velocity for about 2 years. Most investigators have used a dose of 0.1 mg/kg/day, and higher doses do not seem to be more effective. Risk of rapid skeletal maturation seems to be greatest in those less than 10 years old, although we recommend frequent bone-age monitoring (approximately every 6 to 8 months) for all children during treatment. Oxandrolone should be discontinued if bone age progresses significantly more rapidly than height age or when the patient's growth velocity returns to pretreatment levels.

REFERENCES

1. Ferguson-Smith MA. Karyotype-phenotype correlations in gonadal dysgenesis and their bearing on the pathogenesis of malformation. J Med Genet 1965; 2:142-155.
2. Park E, Bailey JD, Cowell CA. Growth and maturation of patients with Turner's syndrome. Pediatr Res 1983; 17:1-7.
3. Ranke MB, Pfluger H, Rosendahl W, Stubbe P, Enders H, Bierich JR, Majewski F. Turner syndrome: spontaneous growth in 150 cases and review of the literature. Eur J Pediatr 1983; 141:81-88.
4. Lyon AJ, Preece MA, Grant DB. Growth curve for girls with Turner syndrome. Arch Dis Child 1985; 60:932-935.
5. Pelz L, Timm D, Eyermann E, Hinkel GK, Kirchner M, Verron G. Body height in Turner's syndrome. Clin Genet 1982; 22:62-66.
6. Sobel EH, Raymond S, Quinn KV, Talbot NB. The use of methyltestosterone to stimulate growth: relative influence on skeletal maturation and linear growth. J Clin Endocr 1956; 16:241-248.
7. Bierich JR. Effects and side effects of anabolic steroids in children. Acta Endocr 1962; 63(suppl):89-103.
8. Prader A. The influence of anabolic steroids on growth. Acta Endocr 1962; 63(suppl):78-88.
9. Johanson AJ, Brasel JA, Blizzard RM. Growth in patients with gonadal dysgenesis receiving fluoxymesterone. J Pediatr 1969; 75:1015-1021.
10. Ray CG, Kirschvink JF, Waxman SH, Kelly VC. Studies on anabolic steroids III. The effect of oxandrolone on height and skeletal maturation in mongoloid children. Am J Dis Child 1965; 110:618-623.
11. Danowski TS, Lee FA, Cohn RE, D'Ambrosia RD, Limaye NR. Oxandrolone therapy of growth retardation. Am J Dis Child 1965; 109:526-532.
12. Zangeneh F, Steiner MM. Oxandrolone therapy in growth retardation of children. Am J Dis Child 1967; 113:234-241.
13. Bettmann HK, Goldmann HS, Abramowicz M, Sobel EH. Oxandrolone treatment of short stature: effect on predicted mature height. J Pediatr 1971; 79:1018-1023.

14. Jackson ST, Rallison ML, Buntin WH, Johnson SB, Flynn RR. Use of oxandrolone for growth stimulation in children. Am J Dis Child 1973; 126:481–484.
15. Rosenfield RL. Low-dose testosterone effect on somatic growth. Pediatrics 1986; 77:853–857.
16. Whitelaw MJ, Thomas SF, Grahaw W, Foster TN, Brock C. Growth response in gonadal dysgenesis to the anabolic steroid norethandrolone. Am J Obst Gyn 1962; 84:501–504.
17. Lev-Ran A. Androgens, estrogens and the ultimate height in XO gonadal dysgenesis. Am J Dis Child 1977; 131:648–649.
18. Lenko HL, Perheentupa J, Soderholm A. Growth in Turner's syndrome: spontaneous and fluoxymesterone stimulated. Acta Paediatr Scand 1979; 277(suppl):57–63.
19. Stahnke N, Willig RP. Effect of oxandrolone on growth in Turner's syndrome. (ESPE, 18th meeting Ulm, 1979) Pediatr Res 1979; 13:1194.
20. Urban MD, Lee PA, Dorst JP, Plotnick LP, Migeon CJ. Oxandrolone therapy in patients with Turner syndrome. J Pediatr 1979; 94:823–827.
21. Joss E, Zuppinger K. Oxandrolone in girls with Turner's syndrome. A pair-matched controlled study up to final height. Acta Paediatr Scand 1984; 73:674–679.
22. Heidemann P, Stubbe P, Beck W. Oxandrolone treatment for growth promotion in Turner's syndrome. (ESPE, 18th meeting Ulm, 1979) Pediatr Res 1979; 13:1194.
23. Moore DC, Tattoni DS, Ruvalcaba RHA, Limbeck GA, Kelly VC. Studies of anabolic steroids VI. Effect of prolonged administration of oxandrolone on growth in children and adolescence with gonadal dysgenesis. J Pediatr 1977; 90:462–466.
24. Rosenbloom Al, Frias JL. Oxandrolone for growth promotion in Turner syndrome. Am J Dis Child 1973; 125:385–387.
25. Perheentupa J, Lenko HL, Nevalainen I, Niittymaki M, Soderholm A, Taipale V. Hormonal treatment of Turner's syndrome. Acta Paediatr Scand 1975; 256(suppl):24–25.
26. Rosenfeld RG, Hintz RL, Johanson AJ, Brasel JA, Burstein S, Chernausek SD, Clabots T, Frane J, Gotlin RW, Kuntze J, Lippe BM, Mahoney PC, Moore WV, New MI, Saenger P, Stoner E, Sybert V. Methionyl human growth hormone and oxandrolone in Turner syndrome: preliminary results of a prospective randomized trial. J Pediatr 1986; 109:936–943.
27. Bayley N, Pinneau SR. Tables for predicting adult height from skeletal age: revised for use with Greulich-Pyle standards. J Pediatr 1952; 40:423–441.
28. Zachmann M, Sobradillo B, Frank M, Frisch H, Prader A. Bayley-Pinneau, Roche-Wainer-Thissen and Tanner height predictions in normal children and in patients with various pathologic conditions. J Pediatr 1978; 93: 749–755.
29. Lenko HL. Prediction in adult height with various methods in Finnish children. Acta Paediatr Scand 1979; 68:85–92.

30. Blethen SL, Gaines S, Weldon V. Comparison of predicted and adult height in short boys: effect of androgen therapy. Pediatr Res 1984; 18:467–469.
31. Snider ME, Solomon IL. Ultimate height in chromosomal gonadal dysgenesis without androgen therapy. Am J Dis Child 1974; 127:673–674.
32. Sybert V. Adult height in Turner syndrome with and without androgen therapy. J Pediatr 1984; 104:365–369.
33. Turani H, Levi J, Zevin D, Kessler E. Hepatic lesions in patients on anabolic androgenic therapy. Israel J Med Sci 1983; 19:322–327.
34. Farrell GC, Uren RF, Perkins KW, Joshua DE, Baird PJ, Kronenberg H. Androgen-induced hepatoma. Lancet 1975; 2:430–432.
35. Lowdell CP, Murray-Lyon IM. Reversal of liver damage due to long term methyltestosterone and safety of non-17-alpha alkylated androgens. Brit Med J 1985; 291:637.
36. Ishak KG. Hepatic neoplasms associated with contraceptive and anabolic steroids. In Lingeman CH. Carcinogenic Hormones. Recent Results Cancer Res 1979; 66:73–128.
37. McCaughan GW, Bilous MJ, Gallagher ND. Long-term survival with tumor regression in androgen induced liver tumors. Cancer 1985; 56:2622–2626.
38. Raiti S, Moore WV, Van Vliet G, Kaplan SL, and the National Hormone and Pituitary Program. Growth-stimulating effects of human growth hormone therapy in patients with Turner syndrome. J Pediatr 1986; 109:944–949.
39. Rudman D, Goldsmith M, Kutner M, Blackston D. Effect of growth hormone and oxandrolone singly and together on growth rate in girls with X chromosome abnormalities. J Pediatr 1980; 96:132–135.
40. Rosenfeld RG, Hintz HL, JOhanson AJ, Sherman B, and the Genentech Collaborative Group. Results from the first 2 years of a clinical trial with recombinant DNA-derived human growth hormone (Somatrem) in Turner's syndrome. Acta Pediatr Scand 1987; 331(suppl):59–66.
41. Lippe BM, Morris A, Kaplan SA. Androgen therapy in Turner syndrome. J Pediatr 1984; 105:503.

28

Oxandrolone Therapy in Turner Syndrome

Patricia A. Crock

Monash University
Melbourne, Australia

George A. Werther and H. Norman B. Wettenhall

Royal Children's Hospital
Melbourne, Australia

The role of androgen therapy in increasing final height in Turner syndrome remains controversial (1,2).

Thirty-five patients with Turner syndrome (XO, 54%; variants, 46%), aged 8.2-16.3 years, were treated with oxandrolone for a mean of 33 months (range 12 months to 6 years) at a mean dosage of 0.136 mg/kg/day (range 0.07-0.26 mg/kg).

Oxandrolone therapy significantly increased height velocity from 3.3 ± 0.1 cm/year (pretreatment) to 5.8 ± 0.3 cm/year at 12 months ($p < 0.001$). There was a significant increase in estimated mature height EMH (Bayley-Pinneau-method) pretreatment from 140.4 ± 1.1 cm to 144.4 ± 1.1 cm. posttreatment ($p < 0.001$).

Final height available in 22 patients at mean age 19.4 ± 0.4 years was 145.5 ± 1.3 cm. In these patients there was no statistical difference between actual final height and EMH posttreatment of 145.2 ± 1.3 cm.

Final height SDS (according to data of Ranke (3)) was 0.22 ± 0.21, which was significantly greater than pretreatment SDS of -0.23 ± 0.3 ($p = 0.001$) (Fig. 1).

Mild facial hirsutism and mild clitoral enlargement were seen in 10 patients.

In conclusion, oxandrolone therapy in Turner syndrome increases height velocity, and the magnitude of this increase is related both to lower chronological age and lower bone age at onset. Oxandrolone therapy increases height prediction and final height, which correlates with mid–parental height.

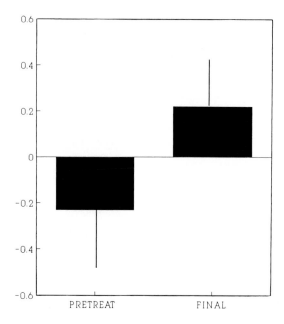

Figure 1 Height SDS ± SE pre-oxandrolone therapy and at age 18 (close to final height). $n = 22; p < 0.001$.

REFERENCES

1. Joss E, Zuppinger K. Oxandrolone in girls with Turner's syndrome: a pair-matched controlled study up to final height. Acta Paediatr Scan 1984; 73: 674–679.
2. Sybert VP. Adult height in Turner syndrome with and without androgen therapy. J Pediatr 1984; 104:365–369.
3. Ranke MB, Pflüger M, Rosendahl W, et al. Turner syndrome: spontaneous growth in 150 cases and review of the literature. Eur J Pediatr 1983; 141: 81–88.

DISCUSSION

DR. JAAKKO PEERHENTUPA: Dr. Heideman has presented his data on the final height of 27 patients at the ESPE meeting. There was a treatment period of between 2 and 6 years, and the mean height of this group was 150 ± 6 cm or so, while the control group had a mean height of 146 cm. I think that is the largest sample of patients that has been presented as yet, and it also indicates that oxandrolone improves final height.

DR. MILO ZACHMAN: I would like to bring up a methodological point about the Bayley-Pinneau height prediction. If two children have the same height and the same bone age, the one with the retarded bone age has a lower height prediction than the one with the normal bone age. It may be that you increase the Bayley-Pinneau height prediction by changing from the retarded percentage values to the normal percentage values, and that is rarely taken into account. A second point I would like to make is about oxandrolone. I do not know why everybody is using oxandrolone, because to my knowledge and to the knowledge of people from Ciba-Geigy, who have spent years in animal and in vitro experiments, there is no evidence that any anabolic steroids can do anything different than testosterone.

DR. CHARLES BROOK: I do not use testosterone because it certainly causes hirsutism and clitoromegaly.

DR. JAMES TANNER: What did Norman Wettenhall do about the induction of puberty in those girls?

DR. GEORGE WERTHER: He delayed the commencement of estrogens as late as he could, in general, and they started between ages 14 and 16 with conventional low dose estrogen, 10 μg/day.

DR. BROOK: So, the final heights may be underestimated. If they used large doses of estrogen at age 14, that would have finished all growth.

Dr. Jaakko Peerhentupa is at the Children's Hospital, Helsinki, Finland. Dr. Milo Zachman is at Children's Hospital, University of Zürich, Zürich, Switzerland. Dr. Charles Brook is at The Middlesex Hospital, London, England. Dr. James Tanner is at the University of Texas Health Center, Houston, Texas. Dr. George Werther is at the Royal Children's Hospital, Melbourne, Victoria, Australia. Dr. Robert Rosenfield is at the University of Chicago, Chicago, Illinois.

DR. TANNER: What Dr. Brook is saying is, if you had not used those doses of estrogen, you would have gotten still further height increase.

DR. ROBERT ROSENFIELD: In defense of testosterone, I think if it is used in very low doses for modest periods of time, it has a seeming anabolic effect on growth without causing undue virilization. I published that in *Pediatrics* a year ago in June. I think it is an important concept because theoretically I would think testosterone might be better than oxandrolone because it is a aromatizable. The issue of whether its effect on potentiating somatomedin-C production through growth hormone secretion, whether that is or is not mediated by estradiol generation in the brain, is a real possibility. Properly designed studies might show that it is better for growth than oxandrolone. I have a question for Dr. Werther. The average duration of anabolic steroid treatment was 2 years, and yet you talk about following people to final height. Can you explain how many patients were followed to final height? Did you treat them for 2 years and then follow them to final height for another 10?

DR. WERTHER: These are not my patients. Dr. Wettenhall treated them for 2 years and followed them to final height. Most of them are in their twenties.

DR. BROOK: That clarifies actually something that confused me slightly. You predicted the final height before treatment. Then you had another predicted height which was a very accurate prediction of final height at the end of treatment, 2 years later—2, 3, 4 years later. Then there was a further gap of 3 or 4 years, during which they were still growing. If you keep on predicting the final height until final height is achieved, your prediction gets wonderfully good. I should say that I would like to underline what Dr. Zachman said, that there are various ways of doing the prediction of adult height. You do not get the same results from all of the various ways of doing it, and you have to watch your step and know really quite well what you are doing.

DR. ROSENFIELD: Let me pursue it since I now begin to understand the design of the study. After you finished your 2 years of androgen treatment and then followed them to final height, what was done then? Were they treated with estrogen or did you, like Dr. Ranke, just let them drift until they finally reached their final height?

DR. WERTHER: No, as I said earlier, they were given estrogen from about age 14, some of them not until about 16.

DR. ZACHMAN: I would like to oppose the idea that there is not a difference between testosterone and oxandrolone. The difference really is that if you give testosterone and get a growth response of the same magnitude that you would get with a dose of oxandrolone, and then stop therapy with testosterone or any of the old steroids, you will most probably get an advancement of bone age after you have stopped the treatment, which you do not get with oxandrolone. And we have just finished some extensive animal experiments on testosterone and various anabolics looking into the anabolic, androgenic, and growth effects. I think there is a tremendous difference between oxandrolone and other anabolic steroids because its structure is also different from the other ones.

DR. BROOK: We also have seen the continuation of skeletal maturation after you have stopped testosterone. There is a built-in delay in the bone age mechanism. I guess that has to be taken into account. It is not against what you say, so long as you have taken it into account.

DR. ZACHMAN: I did not say there was no difference between anabolic steroids. I only wanted to say that people who have been studying androgen receptors for many years have been unable to dissociate the anabolic growth-promoting from the androgenic effect. If Dr. Brook gets hirsutism in his patients with testosterone, it means that he has given disproportionately more testosterone. Of course, there are differences among steroids, but if comparable doses are given, I am convinced that all the anabolic steroids have the same effect.

29

Estrogen Therapy in Turner Syndrome

Judith L. Ross

Hahnemann University
Philadelphia, Pennsylvania

Gordon B. Cutler, Jr.

National Institute of Child Health and Human Development
Bethesda, Maryland

INTRODUCTION

Girls with Turner syndrome are short during childhood, lack a pubertal growth spurt, and are severely short as adults (1–3). This review will address the following aspects of estrogen therapy in Turner syndrome. First, what dose of estrogen is optimal for short-term growth in these patients? Second, does the combination of estrogen and growth hormone offer any advantage in increasing short-term growth in these patients? Finally, how should the long-term effects of estrogen and growth hormone on adult height be evaluated?

RELATIONSHIP BETWEEN ESTROGEN DOSE AND SHORT-TERM GROWTH RATE

Since one of the consequences of the genetic defect in Turner syndrome is hypogonadism, we have sought to correct the estrogen deficiency in a way that would be optimal for adult height. We predicted, however, that a detailed knowledge of the dose-response relationship between estrogen dose and growth rate would be critical for determining the optimal growth-promoting dose of estrogen for the following reasons.

First, the pubertal growth spurt is the earliest sign of puberty in girls (4). Tanner (5) estimated that approximately 20% of the normal pubertal growth spurt is completed before the first appearance of breast budding or pubic hair.

361

This observation suggests that very low levels of estrogen can stimulate growth. The second reason that we predicted that the estrogen dose would be critical in achieving growth stimulation is that even moderate doses of estrogen inhibit growth.

Van den Bosch et al. showed that as little as 50 μg per day of ethinyl estradiol, a dose contained in oral contraceptive pills, decreased the 3-week ulnar growth rate by more than 75% in pubertal girls who were receiving treatment for tall stature (6). Withdrawal of estrogen in a subset of these girls led to a resumption of growth, which indicated that the growth deceleration with estrogen could not be attributed solely to ongoing epiphyseal fusion. Thus, we postulated that estrogen has a biphasic effect on growth, with stimulation at very low concentrations and with inhibition at higher doses.

To evaluate this hypothesis, we studied the effects of estrogen dose on short-term growth rate in 19 patients with Turner syndrome, age 5 to 15 (7). Short-term growth was assessed with the ulnar measuring device, which is a sensitive index of short-term growth that correlates with longer-term height growth (8).

Patients underwent the following protocol: Baseline measurements of ulnar length were made monthly for 2 months. The mean of the two 1-month velocities defined the ulnar growth rate during the pretreatment period. Patients then received oral ethinyl estradiol daily for 1 month. All the measurements were repeated at 1 and 2 months after starting estrogen treatment. The mean of those two ulnar velocities defined the treatment period ulnar growth rate. This treatment period rate included the first month following estrogen treatment because the growth response to estrogen persisted during this month.

Children with bone ages below 10 years received 0, 50, 100, 200, or 400 ng/kg of ethinyl estradiol per day for 28 days. Children with bone ages above 10 years received one of the same doses or 800 ng/kg/day. For a 40-kg patient, this corresponded to 0, 2, 4, 8, 16, or 32 μg of ethinyl estradiol per day. The dosages in each patient were assigned in random sequence and a double-blind fashion.

Increasing doses of ethinyl estradiol had a biphasic effect on ulnar growth rate. The relatively low dose of 100 ng/kg/day (approximately 4 μg/day) of ethinyl estradiol produced the maximal growth response, an 83% increase above the baseline ulnar growth rate. The doses corresponding to approximately 16 and 32 μg of ethinyl estradiol per day actually produced no growth stimulation. By contrast, the vaginal maturation index score (an index of estrogen effect on vaginal mucus) and the serum concentrations of prolactin and testosterone binding globulin did not change at the 100 ng/kg dose.

These observations indicated that estrogen has a biphasic effect on growth, that the optimal ethinyl estradiol dose for growth is about 4 μg/day, and that standard ethinyl estradiol doses in Turner syndrome (10-50 μg/day) are not optimal for ulnar growth and may conceivably impair growth potential.

At this point, we investigated whether the short-term growth seen at 100 ng/kg/day would be sustained over a longer period, whether this low dose of estrogen would stimulate breast development, and whether estrogen would increase the rate of bone maturation or alter predicted adult height (9).

The study design involved the administration of ethinyl estradiol at the dose of 100 ng/kg/day or placebo for 6 months. The sequence of ethinyl estradiol and placebo was selected randomly, and the study was double-blind. After the initial 6 months, there was a period of 2 months without treatment and the subjects were then crossed over to the other treatment group for an additional 6 months.

The ethinyl estradiol-treated group had significantly increased height vleocity compared to the placebo group [5.9 ± 0.5 vs. 3.7 ± 0.2 cm/yr ($p < 0.001$)]. The 69% increase in growth rate was similar to the 83% increase observed with the 1-month estrogen treatment period in the original study that measured ulnar growth rate.

We measured serum somatomedin C at the end of the estrogen and placebo treatment periods to assess the contribution of circulating somatomedin to the growth stimulation by estrogen. The concentration of somatomedin C at the end of the estrogen treatment period did not differ from the concentration at the end of the placebo period (1.01 vs. 1.03 U/ml).

Increased growth rate occurred in 15 of the 16 girls, whereas breast budding occurred in only 6 of the 16 girls during the 6 months of estrogen treatment. Thus, growth was a more sensitive index of estrogen effect than breast development. This is consistent with Tanner's observation of the growth spurt as the earliest sign of puberty in girls (5).

Skeletal maturation, expressed as Δ bone age/Δ chronologic age, did not differ between the 6-month estrogen treatment period and the placebo period (0.92 ± 0.23 vs. 0.96 ± 0.31, $p = $ NS).

Predicted adult height was calculated using the Roche-Wainer-Thissen (RWT) method (10) because the bone ages in some of our patients were too low (< 7 yr) for the Bailey-Pinneau method (11). Over a 6-month treatment period of our study, predicted height decreased significantly during the placebo period (-0.85 ± 0.32 cm, $p < 0.05$) but increased slightly during the estrogen treatment period (0.35 ± 0.38 cm). This yielded a net improvement of 1.20 cm in the predicted height after the estrogen compared to the placebo treatment period ($p < 0.03$).

We concluded that 6 months of treatment with ethinyl estradiol increases growth rate without bone age acceleration and improves predicted adult height in girls with Turner syndrome. The acceleration of growth rate did not appear to be mediated by changes in circulating somatomedin C.

This short-term study could not address the issues of whether the acceleration of growth rate would continue with more prolonged estrogen treatment and whether the improvement in predicted adult height would actually be achieved.

Resolution of these questions will require long-term controlled studies in which final adult height is the end point.

EFFECT OF LOW-DOSE ESTROGEN, GROWTH HORMONE, AND THE COMBINATION ON SHORT-TERM GROWTH RATE

We next investigated whether growth hormone and ethinyl estradiol combined would have an additive effect on growth, such that the combination of the two hormones would stimulate more growth than either alone in girls with Turner syndrome.

The study design involved 2 months of treatment with estrogen at 100 ng/kg/ day and placebo (for growth hormone), growth hormone at 0.15 u/kg subcutaneously three times weekly and placebo (for estrogen), or the combination of estrogen and growth hormone.

Patients had lower leg measurements performed every 2 months with the lower leg measuring device, which is also a sensitive index of short-term growth (12). After a 2-month baseline period, they received one of the three treatments in a randomized, double-blind fashion. After a 2-month washout period they restarted the same sequence.

Lower leg growth rate increased significantly with all three regimens. However, there was no significant difference between growth rate achieved with growth hormone alone and the combination of ethinyl estradiol and growth hormone (Fig. 1).

Somatomedin C levels were measured before and after each treatment period. Somatomedin C concentrations increased significantly with growth hormone

Table 1 Serum Somatomedin C Levels Before and at the Conclusion of Treatment for 2 Months with Ethinyl Estradiol, Growth Hormone, for the Combination in Girls with Turner Syndrome

	Somatomedin C (U/ml) (mean ± SEM)	
Treatment regimen	Baseline	After treatment
Ethinyl estradiol (EE$_2$) 100 ng/kg/day	1.4 ± 0.2	1.4 ± 0.2
Growth hormone (GH 0.15 U/kg tiw	1.3 ± 0.1	1.8 ± 0.1[a]
Combination of GH and EE$_2$	1.5 ± 0.1	2.0 ± 0.2[a]

[a]$p < 0.001$, compared to baseline (two-tailed paired Student t-test).

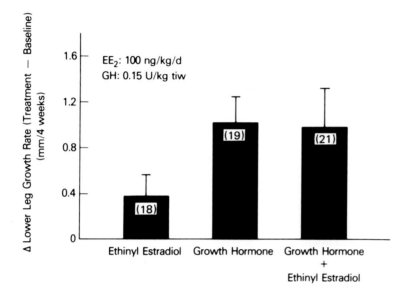

Figure 1 Mean (± SEM) change in lower leg growth rate (treatment–baseline) with ethinyl estradiol, growth hormone, or the combination. The number of patients in each treatment group is indicated.

treatment and the combination of ethinyl estradiol and growth hormone treatment (Table 1). We concluded that addition of low-dose estradiol to an optimal dose of growth hormone did not cause any apparent increase in short-term lower leg growth rate.

EFFECT OF LOW-DOSE ESTROGEN AND OF GROWTH HORMONE ON ADULT HEIGHT

Our studies and those of other investigators have shown a short-term increase in growth rate during treatment with low-dose estrogen and with growth hormone. However, patients, parents, and their physicians are interested primarily in whether these agents can increase the final adult height of girls with Turner syndrome.

To address the question of the effects of therapy on adult height, a long-term, double-blind, placebo-controlled trial has been initiated at Hahnemann University and the National Institute of Child Health and Human Development. The study design involves four treatment groups (Fig. 2): a control group receiving placebo, one receiving early low-dose estrogen, one receiving growth hormone, and one receiving both early low-dose estrogen and growth hormone.

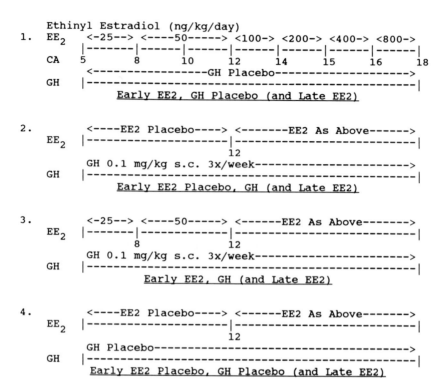

Figure 2 Schematic representation of the protocol for the long-term study of growth in Turner syndrome. Numbers at left correspond to the four treatment groups in the Turner study.

Girls with Turner syndrome are accepted into the study between their fifth and twelfth birthdays. The end point of the study will be adult height (<0.5 cm gain in height over the previous year). From age 12 until they reach adult height, all four groups will receive estrogen according to the same schedule, beginning with the 100 ng/kg/day dosage of ethinyl estradiol that was optimal for the short-term growth rate. Once menstruation begins, cyclic monthly administration of medroxyprogesterone acetate will be started, and the estrogen dose will not be increased beyond that required to achieve regular, normal menses. The ethinyl estradiol dosages from ages 5 to 8 (25 ng/kg/day) and from ages 8 to 12 (50 ng/kg/day) were set below the optimal growth-promoting dosage to avoid breast budding in younger children and to decrease the possibility that a long duration of low-dose estrogen therapy in this age group might cause bone age advancement (which was not observed in the 6-month study of the 100 ng/kg/day dosage).

The estrogen dosages selected for the 5- to 12-year-old girls in this study represent an attempt to approximate the physiological replacement dosage for a normal prepubertal girl. Some of the clinical and laboratory features of girls with Turner syndrome, such as their decreased growth rate, delayed bone ages, and low bone density and somatomedin C levels, may be attributable in part to their presumed deficiency of normal prepubertal estrogen secretion. Major increases in growth rate would not be expected with estrogen at these replacement dosages. Clinically significant gains in adult height, however, may result if small increases in growth rate are sustained over time. Additionally, the administration of small amounts of estrogen during these years might enhance the response to growth hormone, which would be analogous to the interaction of sex steroids and growth hormone during the pubertal growth spurt (5,13).

In summary, both low-dose estrogen and growth hormone can increase the short-term growth rate in girls with Turner syndrome. To determine the effect of therapy on adult height, long-term trials must be undertaken. The design of such trials is complex. Decisions must be made concerning drug dosage, the time and frequency of administration, the age of onset of estrogen treatment and adjustment of the estrogen dosage schedule with age, the number of treatment groups, and the nature of the control group. No one study can address all of these issues, and different investigators are likely to reach different conclusions concerning which issues to address first. Despite these uncertainties, however, we conclude that it is appropriate to begin such long-term controlled trials.

REFERENCES

1. Brooke CGD, Murset G, Zachmann M, Prader A. Growth in children with 45,XO Turner's syndrome. Arch Dis Child 1974; 49:789.
2. Ranke MB, Pfluger H, Rosendahl W, et al. Turner syndrome: Spontaneous growth in 150 cases and review of the literature. Eur J Pediatr 1983; 141:81.
3. Lyon AJ, Preece MA, Grant DB. Growth curve for girls with Turner syndrome. Arch Dis Child 1985; 60:932.
4. Frisch RE, Revelle R. Height and weight of girls and boys at time of initiation of adolescent growth spurt in height and weight and relationship to menarche. Human Biol 1971; 43:140.
5. Tanner JM, Whitehouse RH, Hughes PCR, Carter BS. Relative importance of growth hormone and sex steroids for the growth at puberty of trunk length, limb length and muscle width in growth hormone-deficient children. J Pediatr 1976; 89:1000.

6. Van den Bosch JSG, Smals AGH, Kloppenborg PWC, Valk IM. The effect of low-dose estrogens on short-term growth and concomitant biochemical phenomena in girls with tall stature. Acta Endocrinol 1981;98:156.
7. Ross JL, Cassorla FG, Skerda MC, et al. A preliminary study of the effect of estrogen dose on growth in Turner syndrome. New Engl J Med 1983; 309:1104.
8. Valk IM. Accurate measurement of the length of the ulna and its application in growth measurement. Growth 1971;35:297.
9. Ross JL, Long LM, Cassorla F, et al. The effect of low-dose estradiol on 6-month growth rates in patients with Turner's syndrome. J Pediatr 1986; 109:950.
10. Roche AF, Wainer H, Thissen D. The RWT method for prediction of adult stature. Pediatrics 1975;56:1026.
11. Bayley N, Pinneau SR. Tables for predicting adult height from skeletal age: Revised for use with the Greulich-Pyle hand standards. J Pediatr 1952; 40:432.
12. Valk IM, Langhout Chabloz AME, Smals AGH, et al. Accurate measurements of the lower leg length and the ulnar length and its application in short term growth measurement. Growth 1983;47:53.
13. Cutler GB, Jr, Cassorla FG, Ross JL, et al. Pubertal growth: Physiology and pathophysiology. Recent Prog Horm Res 1986;42:443.

DISCUSSION

DR. DOUGLAS FRASIER: I am very concerned about what appeared to be the long duration of unopposed estrogen administered to these young women. What can you tell us about cycling, and what can you tell us about the addition of a progestational agent?

DR. JUDITH ROSS: As soon as there is any evidence of breakthrough bleeding, we plan to commence cycling with an estrogen–progesterone combination.

DR. PATRICK WILTON (STOCKHOLM): Did your ethical committee have any questions about giving growth hormone placebo injections three times a week from 7 to 17 years of age?

Dr. Douglas Frasier is at Olive View Medical Center, Sylmar, California. Dr. Judith L. Ross is at Hahnemann University, Philadelphia, Pennsylvania. Dr. Patrick Wilton is at Kabi Vitrum, Stockholm, Sweden. Dr. James Tanner is at the University of Texas Health Center, Houston, Texas. Dr. Michael B. Ranke is at the Children's Hospital, University of Tübingen, Tübingen, Federal Republic of Germany.

DR. ROSS: No, they did not. They did not have any trouble passing it at several institutions.

DR. WILTON: Did they read the Declaration of Helsinki?

DR. JAMES TANNER: Just for absolute clarification, they are getting a placebo?

DR. ROSS: They are.

DR. MICHAEL RANKE: I think it is very difficult to follow all of the details of such a proposed protocol. I think there are several questions, but I only want to make one. Why do you not increase the dose of growth hormone when you induce puberty?

DR. ROSS: I think that there are so many variables, as you said, in this study that to try and compare between the groups, we had to keep some things fixed and vary others.

30

Estrogen Treatment in Turner Syndrome

Knud W. Kastrup and Turner Study Group*

Glostrup Hospital, University of Copenhagen
Copenhagen, Denmark

INTRODUCTION

In a review of estrogen use in children and adolescents by Conte and Grumbach (1) 10 years ago, it was stated that studies were necessary to determine the effect of a low-dose, early estrogen replacement therapy on growth in girls with Turner syndrome. Such therapy has not yet been demonstrated to increase final height, but we know from an increasing number of studies that a pubertal growth spurt can be induced.

Ross (2) has clearly demonstrated the growth-promoting effect of low doses of estrogens on ulnar growth and, later, in the same patients, on total growth for a period of 6 months (3).

Longer studies over a period of more than 4 years have been reported by Demetriou (4), our group (5), and Bohnet (6). It appears from these studies that growth velocity increased significantly during the first year of treatment, with a decrease in the following period. The growth response was more pronounced in the younger age groups than in older patients. It can be concluded from the findings that estrogens do have a significant effect on growth, at least in some girls with gonadal dysgenesis.

*B. Brock Jacobsen, S. Krabbe, P. E. Lebech (Departments of Obstetrics and Gynecology, Frederiksberg Hospital), B. Peitersen, K. E. Petersen, E. Thamdrup, and R. Wichmann

It is still a matter of debate by which mechanism estrogens induce the growth response observed. It has been suggested that somatomedin C (Sm-C) is the mediating factor, either directly or indirectly through a priming effect on growth hormone secretion. A decline in levels of Sm-C and sleep-related spontaneous GH secretion, after a bone age of 10, was found in the study of Ranke (7). The function of the Sm-C/GH axis appeared to be normal, but the level of function was altered due to absent activation from gonadal hormones. Diminished 24-hour secretion of GH may be explained by the absence of stimulatory influence of ovarian steroids.

A direct effect of estrogens on bone growth cannot be excluded. The relationship between somatomedin C and osteocalcin was followed throughout puberty in a group of girls. The findings by Johansen (14) reveal an earlier increase in osteocalcin followed by the pubertal rise in somatomedin C. This suggests a synergistic effect of estradiol on these two parameters. A direct effect of 17-beta-estradiol on osteoblasts has been demonstrated by Ernst (8).

Normal development of secondary sexual characteristics in Turner syndrome may be of even greater importance, not only from a physical standpoint but also from a psychological one. While treatment previously was postponed to a higher age, it is now the object to keep the patient in line with the development of the peer group (9).

This can be accomplished by the application of low doses of estrogen, but the question of the optimal time for start is not yet definitively answered.

We have tried to establish a regimen where a low dose of 17-beta-estradiol was started at an early age, when ovaries begin to secrete estrogens, and gradually increased this dose over a longer period to induce pubertal development. We aimed at an increase in growth velocity and an eventual increase in final height.

MATERIAL AND METHODS

Thirty-five girls with ovarian dysgenesis participated in a prospective study of the effect of early therapy with a low dose of estrogen. Initial results from this study have been reported by us previously (5).

The natural estrogen 17-beta-estradiol was administered in micronized capsules. Levels of serum estradiol were measured every 3 months. Tentative upper limits for estradiol concentrations were established for various bone-age groups, and the dose was adjusted according to this.

Bone age was determined by the method of Greulich and Pyle (10) by the same observer. The growth chart and tables for untreated girls with Turner syndrome produced by Ranke (11) and Lenko (12) were used as standards for growth variables and for height prediction. When withdrawal bleeding occurred, cyclic treatment was given. This was followed by sequential treatment including a progestin.

Table 1 Bone Age and Characteristics in Two Groups

	Group I (n = 13)	Group II (n = 22)
Height (cm)	121.4 ± 7.1	136.1 ± 7.0 (mean ± SD)
Chronological age (yr)	10.9 ± 1.7	14.3 ± 1.8 (mean ± SD)
Bone age (yr)	8.8 ± 0.9	12.1 ± 1.0 (mean ± SD)
Duration of treatment	1.8–6.3	2.5–4.8 range
(yr)	4.8	4 median
Duration of treatment	5.3 ± 0.6	3.9 ± 0.7 (mean ± SD)
completed (yr)	(n = 6)	(n = 20)

Bone age was less than 10 years in 13 girls (group I) and more than 10 years in the remaining 22 girls (group II). The characteristics of the two groups are given in Table 1.

RESULTS

Pubertal Development

Pubic hair at Tanner stage II was present at the start of treatment in 2 of 13 girls in group I, and in 10 of 22 girls in group II. Two girls in group I and 9 girls in group II entered stage III during the first year of treatment. Stage IV was passed by 5 girls in group I and by 16 girls in group II during the third year.

Breast development was at stage II in 4 girls in both groups at start of treatment. After 1 year, 3 girls in group I and 17 girls in group II had passed stage III. Three girls in group I and 12 girls in group II had passed stage IV after 3 years, and at this time 2 girls in group I and 10 girls in group II had passed stage V.

All girls noted that they found the appearance and development of their pubic hair normal. Some girls found that breast development was too fast and were embarrassed by the size of their busts. The tempo of the pubertal development was within normal limits for the duration of the different stages.

Menarche occurred in 5 girls from group I after a period of 5.2 ± 0.8 years (mean ± SD) and in 16 girls from group II after 1.9 ± 0.5 years. The average bone age at menarche was 16.6 ± 0.6 years in group II and 14.5 ± 0.7 years in Group I.

Growth and Bone Maturation

Growth velocity increased during the first year of treatment from 3.8 ± 0.8 cm (mean ± SD) to 7.9 ± 0.9 cm in group I and from 3.1 ± 0.7 cm to 4.9 ± 1.3 cm

Table 2 Growth Velocity and Standard Deviation During Estrogen Therapy in Turner Syndrome

Year	Group I		Group II	
	cm/yr	SDS	cm/yr	SDS
1	7.9 ± 0.9	4.4 ± 1.4 (13)	4.9 ± 1.3	3.5 ± 2.1 (22)
2	4.8 ± 1.4	1.6 ± 1.4 (13)	2.6 ± 1.2	0.3 ± 1.6 (22)
3	2.8 ± 1.3	0.5 ± 1.1 (11)	1.3 ± 0.9	0.5 ± 1.5 (16)
4	1.8 ± 1.0	-1.4 ± 1.3 (9)	0.5 ± 0.5	-2.3 ± 1.2 (15)

Number in parentheses indicates number of patients.

in group II. The growth velocities and corresponding standard deviations are given in Table 2. It is seen that a waning response was found during the following years with SD below 2 after 5 years of treatment in group I and after 4 years in group II. The growth response was within the range of normal pubertal growth spurt in group I and just below normal range for late limits of age in group II.

The rate of bone maturation was accelerated after the first year in group I ($\Delta BA/\Delta CA = 2$), less in group II ($\Delta BA/\Delta CA = 1.3$). The actual values in months per 12 months and ratio for the following years are given in Table 3.

Table 3 Bone Maturation During E_2 Treatment in Turner Syndrome

Group I:

Year	ΔBA (months)	$\Delta BA/\Delta CA$	
1	24.0 ± 10	2.0	(13)
2	18.0 ± 9	1.5	(13)
3	15.0 ± 9	1.3	(11)
4	13.3 ± 9	1.1	(10)
5	8.5 ± 4	0.7	(4)

Group II:

Year	ΔBA (months)	$\Delta BA/\Delta CA$	
1	15.2 ± 6.2	1.3	(22)
2	18.5 ± 6.3	1.5	(22)
3	14.3 ± 6.4	1.2	(16)
4	15.0 ± 7.5	1.3	(15)

Final height in 6 girls from group I and 20 girls from group II who have finished treatment was 142.7 ± 3.5 cm and 145.6 ± 5.3 cm, respectively, which is within the limits for predicted height in both groups.

Endocrine Parameters

Somatomedin C was within normal range at the onset of treatment and did not change during treatment.

No change in prolactin values was found during therapy in any of the groups. Androstendione values did increase within normal range for bone age during treatment. Gonadotropins (FSH) were elevated in all girls except 1 in group II. A suppression of FSH during therapy was noted in 10 of the girls, but with an escape from suppression after an average period of 12 months. In group I FSH values were elevated in 8 girls. Escape from initial suppression occurred after 18 ± 6 months in 5 girls. Low, suppressed levels were persistent in 1 and no suppression was observed in 2 girls. The findings in group I may represent the onset of a rise in gonadotropins found at this age but may also represent a change in the set point for feedback regulation. It is well known that gonadotropins rise to adult castrate levels by a bone age of 10-11 years in girls with gonadal dysgenesis. This reveals a functioning negative feedback mechanism. The set point of this mechanism is modulated by estrogens. The escape phenomenon may represent a maturational event in the hypothalamic-hypophysial system. These perturbations in the feedback sensitivity are discussed in more details by Maruca and coworkers (13).

CONCLUSIONS

Our findings thus support the results from the short- and long-term studies, but a direct comparison of the effect of different estradiol preparations is difficult.

The natural 17-beta-estradiol preparation used by us has not been applied in any of the previous studies. The micronized preparation used in the study has been shown to be well absorbed and to give reproducible serum levels of estradiol. It is also presumed to have lesser side effects. Metabolic clearing rate, receptor binding, and intracellular effect of this preparation is different from preparations commonly used. The dosage was therefore monitored by serum levels, but initial doses may have been too high, considering the rate of bone maturation. We have therefore reconsidered the timing and dosage in the younger age group in future regimens. The advancement in bone maturation may have had a negative influence on final height, but we have found no significant reduction in predicted height so far.

A growth spurt similar to that found in normal girls can be induced by therapy with estradiol in a low dose at bone age 10. There is no evidence that final height can be increased by this therapy.

A combined therapy with estrogens, according to this regimen, and growth-promoting agents may prove to be useful in this connection.

Estrogen therapy can be adjusted to induce pubertal development at a tempo comparable to normal girls. A lack or postponement of treatment can be a serious threat to normal personality development. Absence of adolescence may have a negative influence on the patient's relations with family and peers. This dimension of therapy will need more consideration in future studies.

REFERENCES

1. Conte FA, Grumbach MM. Estrogen use in children and adolescents: A survey. Pediatrics 1978; 62 (suppl 6):1091–1097.
2. Ross JL, Cassorla FG, Skerda MC, Valk JM, Loriaux DL, Cutler GB. A preliminary study of the effect of estrogen dose on growth in Turner's syndrome. N Engl J Med 1983; 309:1104–1106.
3. Ross JL, Myerson Long L, Skerda M, Cassorla F, Kurtz D, Loriaux DL, Cutler GB. Effect of low doses of estradiol on 6-month growth rates and predicted height in patients with Turner syndrome. J Pediatr 1986; 109: 950–953.
4. Demetriou E, Jean Emans S, Crigler JF. Final height in estrogen-treated patients with Turner syndrome. Obstet Gynecol 1984; 64:459–464.
5. Kastrup KW. Growth and development in girls with Turner's syndrome during early therapy with low doses of estradiol. Acta Endocrinologica (Copenh) 1986; suppl 279:157–163.
6. Bohnet HG. New aspects of oestrogen/gestagen induced growth and endocrine changes in individuals with Turner syndrome. Eur J Pediatr 1986; 145:275–279.
7. Ranke MB, Blum WF, Haug F, Rosendahl W, Attanasio A, Enders H, Gupta D, Bierich JR. Growth hormone, somatomedin levels and growth regulation in Turner's syndrome. Acta Endocrinologica (Copenh) 1987; 116: 305–313.
8. Ernst M, Schmid Ch, Froesch ER. 17-Beta-estradiol but not 17-alpha stimulates proliferation of osteoblasts in vitro. First European Congress of Endocrinology, Copenhagen, 1987; Abstract 156.
9. Brook CGD. Turner syndrome. Arch Dis Child 1986; 61:305–309.
10. Greulich WW, Pyle SJ. Radiographic Atlas of Skeletal Development of the Hand and Wrist. Stanford University Press, 1950.
11. Ranke MB, Pflüger H, Rosendahl W, Stubbe P, Enders H, Bierich JR, Majewski F. Turner's syndrome: spontaneous growth in 150 cases and review of the literature. Eur J Pediatr 1983; 141:81–88.
12. Lenko HL, Perheentupa J, Söderholm A. Growth in Turner's syndrome: spontaneous and fluoxymesterone stimulated. Acta Paediatr Scand 1979; suppl 277:57–63.
13. Maruca J, Kulin HE, Santner SJ. Pertubations of negative feedback sensi-

tivity in agonadal patients undergoing estrogen replacement therapy. J Clin Endocrinol Metab 1983; 56:53-59.

14. Johansen, JS et al., Serum bone Gla-protein. J. Clin Endocrinol Metab 1988; 67:273-278.

DISCUSSION

DR. ROBERT ROSENFIELD: I was very pleased to see the work. It really supports the kind of results we have seen with long-term use of systemic estradiol, in that we get a final outcome of height very similar to predicted height. I do want to make a comment about your statement that this is a physiologic form of treatment. For clarification, when one gives oral estradiol, the predominant estrogen in the blood is estrone. These patients get very high concentrations of estrone, so I would dispute the physiologic nature of the treatment. Similarly, when one uses oral ethinyl estradiol, one does not get estradiol in the blood, either. One gets ethinyl estradiol, which is, on the other hand, an extremely potent estrogen. So these different forms of treatment, although they may sound similar, are really quite different.

DR. KNUD KASTRUP: I agree with you.

DR. PAUL SAENGER: You showed some data on high osteocalcin levels during male puberty. Do you think this is because testosterone is aromatized? If that were so, then I am still puzzled by the fact that we saw the highest osteocalcin levels in those Turner girls that were treated with growth hormone and oxandrolone, which surely cannot be aromatized. How do you explain the rise in the boys?

DR. KASTRUP: For the boys we think it is testosterone. We have studies that are now going to be published of boys with precocious puberty, and we have clearly demonstrated a similar phenomenon.

DR. LESLIE PLOTNICK: I wonder if Dr. Ross feels as comfortable about the long-term use of estrogen treatment in these children. It seems from the data presented that estrogen plus growth hormone does not give as much acceleration

Dr. Robert L. Rosenfield is at the University of Chicago Pritzger School of Medicine, Chicago, Illinois. Dr. Knud W. Kastrup is at the University of Copenhagen, Glostrup, Denmark. Dr. Paul Saenger is at the Montefiore Medical Center/Albert Einstein College of Medicine, Bronx, New York. Dr. Leslie P. Plotnick is at the Johns Hopkins Medical Institutions, Baltimore, Maryland.

in growth as oxandrolone plus growth hormone. The estrogen treatment group did not have augmented adult heights. I am concerned about so many things that I am just wondering where to put the focus. First of all, I am concerned that we are treating children 5 to 10 years of age with estrogen. Some of these children are growing at a normal rate. We are complicating their lives with a lot of medical intervention, and I am not sure we are doing the right thing by them psychologically or medically with all of the therapies proposed. I particularly feel upset about placebo injections for multiple years and wonder what is being done to support these children psychologically throughout all this.

31

Effect of Gonadal Steroids on
Growth and Adult Height in Turner Syndrome

Jaakko Perheentupa

University of Helsinki and University Children's Hospital
Helsinki, Finland

Therapies with androgen (1-6) and estrogen (2,6-13) increase the height velocity of girls with Turner syndrome, but the effects on adult height have been unclear. There are reports that after androgen therapy, adult height was increased (1,3-5) or unchanged (2,14). Estrogen replacement therapy was earlier recommended to be postponed as long as possible, to avoid compromising adult height (15). But according to recent reports (8,11), low-dose estrogen therapy should be started at the average age at which puberty normally appears, being beneficial not only psychologically (16) but also for growth. We have recently analyzed the height velocities and adult heights of our 76 patients treated with androgen, estrogen, or both (6).

These patients were born from 1954 through 1972, and we followed them to adult height. We measured height with a Harpenden stadiometer. The heights of the parents were known for 70 of the patients.

In peripheral blood lymphocytes, 44 of the patients had the 45,X karyotype, five 45,X/46,XX, six 46,X,i(Xq), five 45,X/46,X,i(Xq), three 45,X/47,XXX, and 13 other mosaics.

For androgen therapy fluoxymesterone (1.25-5 mg daily per os, dose increasing with age to an average of 0.1 mg/kg) was given to 32 girls during 0.3-3.4 years, starting at ages of 5.6 (four girls were <10 years) to 17.5 years. Of this group, 24 then continued on fluoxymesterone with added estrogen. For 15 other girls fluoxymesterone was introduced with estradiol valerate and continued until the end of growth.

For ovarian hormone replacement therapy we used conjugated estrogens in 1969-1970, an average of 1.5 mg daily, starting at age 15 at the earliest, and changing to cyclic therapy after a breakthrough bleeding: estrogen on days 1-24 and a progestin on days 18-24 each month. Since 1974 we have used estradiol valerate (0.5-1 mg daily, starting at ages of 12.4-18.9 and increasing gradually to 2-4 mg by age 15 at earliest), changing to cyclic therapy at latest when the dose reached 2 mg. This replacement therapy without androgen was given to 20 girls.

From 1977 the 35 girls reaching the age of start of therapy were randomized to receive estradiol valerate, half with and half without fluoxymesterone.

Six girls had no estrogen therapy, because their spontaneous pubertal development and menstruation were adequate; one of them received fluoxymesterone from age 10.2 to age 13.0.

Standard deviation scores (SDS) of height and height velocity were calculated from our reference data on growth between ages 8 and 18 years in untreated Finnish girls with Turner syndrome; mean height and mean height velocity were expressed as equations, and SD as 2.3% of mean height and 27% of mean height velocity (4). Allowance was made for parental height by adding to each girl's height SDS her parents' mean height SDS divided by 2. We used standard statistical methods, and compared groups with the aid of Student's t test (two-tailed).

HEIGHT VELOCITY

Height velocity increased in almost every case after institution of steroid therapy. In the first therapy year, height velocity SDS was calculated only for those patients who were <16 years at the start of therapy (Fig. 1). The therapy groups were similar in age with mean (SD) age of 14.0 (1.2) years for the estrogen-only group, 13.9 (1.1) years for the androgen-estrogen-simultaneously group, and 14.3 (1.2 and 1.5) years for the two last groups. The androgen-only group had a lower mean age and wider dispersion: 12.7 (2.3) years. All (except one) of them later received estrogen, and these are also included in the last two groups of Fig. 1.

Relative height velocity was highest (mean SDS 7.6) during therapy with androgen and estrogen started simultaneously and next highest (4.6) during androgen therapy alone. Even estrogen alone caused a marked acceleration (2.7). Previous androgen therapy reduced the growth-accelerating effect of estrogen alone but, after approximately a year of androgen therapy, addition of estrogen to it maintained a higher relative height velocity (4.2) than that achieved during the first years of estrogen therapy alone in previously untreated patients. During the second year of the therapies, relative height velocities decreased; we have no exact data, because the groups were then small.

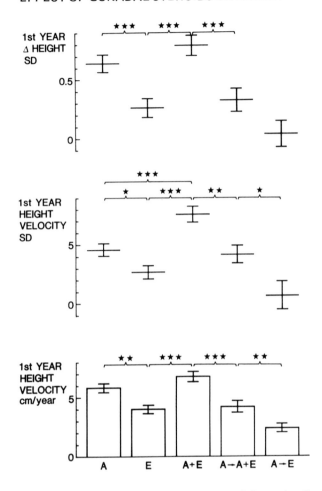

Figure 1 Height velocities (mean ± SEM) in cm/yr (bottom panel) and in SD score (middle panel), and increment in height SD score (top panel) during the first year of therapy with estrogen (with androgen for the androgen-only group) for the different therapy groups. A, androgen alone; E, estrogen alone; A + E, androgen and estrogen started simultaneously; A → A + E, androgen + estrogen after preceding androgen therapy; A → E, estrogen alone after preceding androgen therapy. The numbers of patients with these data were 27, 18, 14, 15, and 9, respectively. Only those patients are included who were <16 years at the start of therapy and were on the therapy for at least a year.

ADULT HEIGHT

The mean adult height was 145.5 ± 5.7 (SD) cm for all patients. Patients with the 45,X karyotype were taller than the others, 146.7 ± 5.8 cm vs. 143.6 ± 5.0 cm (p = 0.02). There was no significant difference between patients born in 1955–1959 (147.0 ± 5.9 cm) and patients born in 1965–1969 (144.8 ± 5.4 cm). The present height of young Finnish adult women is 165.3 ± 5.4 cm.

There was no significant difference between the therapy groups: The mean (SD) height was 147.1 (6.2) cm for the 20 patients of the estrogen-only group, 145.6 (5.3) cm for the 15 patients of the androgen-estrogen-simultaneously group, 145.1 (5.6) cm for all the 32 patients who received estrogen after androgen therapy, and 145.6 (2.6) cm for the six spontaneously developed patients who had received no estrogen therapy. No significant differences appeared even when height was corrected for parental height.

Adult height did not correlate with age at onset of estrogen therapy. Of the patients whose estrogen therapy was started between the ages of 12.5 and 13.5 years, those 10 who received estrogen alone grew 9.8 ± 2.9 cm (over 2.6 ± 0.9 years), those six started on estrogen and androgen simultaneously grew 14.2 ± 2.9 cm (3.1 ± 0.4 years), and those eight who had received androgen previously grew 9.7 ± 2.0 cm (2.5 ± 0.9 years); these differences are not significant.

The patient's adult height correlated with the midparent height: r = 0.49, $p < 0.001$; height of patient = 0.56 × midparent height + 52.0.

COMMENT

With regard to growth and physical development of girls with Turner syndrome, the ideal treatment should achieve two goals. First, at pubertal age the appearance of a great lag behind age-mates in height and pubertal maturation should be avoided, because such a lag carries a serious risk to mental health [16]. That is to say, a treatment which accelerates growth is of great importance even if its effect is only temporary. The second goal, more difficult to achieve and probably less important, is to bring adult height closer to normal. This means that therapies which accelerate growth at puberty are valuable provided that they do not compromise adult height.

Our data show beyond doubt that pubertal acceleration may be achieved by therapy with gonadal steroids, and most effectively with simultaneous introduction of both estrogen and androgen in small doses. Pubertal age girls with Turner syndrome have a deficiency of both [17]; hence the combination is to be regarded as replacement therapy.

That the accelerating effect of estrogen therapy [2,6–13] has not been observed in some studies [18] probably depends on dosage. There is evidence to suggest that the most effective dose for promoting growth is a very small one [8], the larger doses needed to induce feminization and to increase the subnormal plasma somatomedin C levels in these girls (19-20) having little growth-promoting effect (8) and probably strongly accelerating bone maturation in contrast to the small doses. We believe that it is best to adjust the dosage so as to reproduce a slow variant physiologic increase of plasma estradiol level (11).

It is more difficult to suggest why the accelerating effect of androgens has not been observed in some studies (21). Here again it is important to keep the dosage small. Probably androgen may be discontinued after 2-3 years of combined therapy, to allow the full feminizing effect of the estrogen.

Our study may be criticized for being partly retrospective (for other than the subseries randomized to receive estradiol valerate either alone or with fluoxymesterone) and therefore heterogeneous in the dosage and exact nature of the steroids used. Furthermore, we have made no analysis of bone age. To the first criticism we would reply that the hormone dosages used were uniformly small for androgen, and in the initial years for estrogen, though not quite as small as suggested by the data of the group at NIH (8). An analysis of bone age would have given only very approximate information in contrast to our analysis of adult heights.

Interestingly and in contrast to other reports, we confirmed our previous finding (4) of greater adult height in the patients with the 45,X karyotype vs. all other karyotypes combined. The overall adult height in our series, 145.5 ± 5.6 cm, was significantly greater than the mean adult height of 138 untreated patients collected from the literature, 142.9 ± 5.3 cm. This is probably due to a genetic difference between the general populations. We again (4) showed a very strong correlation between the height of adult patients and their midparent height. This has been found repeatedly (22), although not in less detailed studies (14).

The availability of human growth hormone may change the prospects of growth in girls with Turner syndrome. However, until the value of growth hormone is defined, we shall start replacement therapy at the age of 12-13 years with 2.5 mg fluoxymesterone and 0.25 mg estradiol valerate daily, change to cyclic therapy with this estrogen and a progestin 4 to 6 months later, and slowly increase the estrogen to a full replacement dose within 2-3 years, discontinuing the androgen at the same time. This will not significantly increase the adult height but is essential for the development of a healthy self-esteem.

REFERENCES

1. Johanson AJ, Brasel JA, Blizzard RM. Growth in patients with gonadal dysgenesis receiving fluoxymesterone. J Pediatr 1969; 75:1015-1021.
2. Lev-Ran A. Androgens, estrogens and the ultimate height in XO gonadal dysgenesis. Am J Dis Child 1977; 131:648-649.
3. Urban MD, Lee PA, Dorst JP, Plotnick LP, Migeon CJ. Oxandrolone therapy in patients with Turner syndrome. J Pediatr 1979; 823-827.

4. Lenko HL, Perheentupa J, Söderholm A. Growth in Turner's syndrome: Spontaneous and fluoxymesterone stimulated. Acta Paediatr Scand 1979; Suppl 277:57–63.

5. Joss E, Zuppinger K. Oxandrolone in girls with Turner's syndrome: A pair-matched controlled study up to final height. Acta Paediatr Scand 1984; 73:674–679.

6. Lenko HL, Söderholm A, Perheentupa J. Turner syndrome: Effect of hormone therapies on height velocity and adult height. Acta Paediatr Scand 1988; 76:699–704.

7. Lucky AW, Marynick SP, Rebar RW, Cutler GB, Glen M, Johnsonbaugh RE, Loriaux DL. Replacement oral ethinyloestradiol therapy for gonadal dysgenesis: Growth and adrenal androgen studies. Acta Endocrinol (Copenh) 1979; 91:519–528.

8. Ross JL, Cassorla FG, Skerda MC, Valk IM, Loriaux DL, Cutler GB. A pre-liminary study of the effect of estrogen dose on growth in Turner's syndrome. N Engl J Med 1983; 309:1104–1106.

9. Lyon AJ, Preece MA, Grant DB. Growth curve for girls with Turner syndrome. Arch Dis Child 1985; 60:932–935.

10. Bohnet HG. New aspects of oestrogen/gestagen-induced growth and endocrine changes in individuals with Turner syndrome. Eur J Pediatr 1986; 145:275–279.

11. Kastrup KW and Turner Study Group. Growth and development in girls with Turner's syndrome during early therapy with low doses of estradiol. Acta Endocrinol (Copenh) 1986; Suppl 279:157–163.

12. Ross JL, Long LM, Skerda M, Cassorla F, Kurtz D, Loriaux DL, Cutler GB. Effect of low doses of estradiol on 6-month growth rates and predicted height in patients with Turner syndrome. J Pediatr 1986; 109: 950–953.

13. Martinez A, Heinrich JJ, Domené H, Escobar ME, Jasper H, Montuori E, Bergadá C. Growth in Turner's syndrome: Long term treatment with low dose ethinyl estradiol. J Clin Endocrinol Metab 1987; 65:253–257.

14. Sybert VP. Adult height in Turner syndrome with and without androgen therapy. J Pediatr 1984; 104:365–369.

15. Van Wyk JJ. Disorders of the ovaries. In Current Pediatric Therapy, Gellis SS, Kagan BM, ed., 5. ed. WB Saunders Co, Philadelphia, 1971.

16. Perheentupa J, Lenko HL, Nevalainen I, Niittymäki M, Söderholm A, Taipale V. Hormonal therapy in Turner's syndrome: Growth and psychological aspects. Proc XIV Internat Congr Pediatr, Buenos Aires 1974; 5: 121–127.

17. Apter D, Lenko HL, Perheentupa J, Söderholm A, Vihko R. Subnormal pubertal increases of serum androgens in Turner's syndrome. Hormone Res 1982; 16:164–173.

18. Ranke MB, Haug F, Blum WF, Rosendahl W, Attanasio A, Bierich JR. Effect on growth of patients with Turner's syndrome treated with low estrogen doses. Acta Endocrinol (Copenh) 1986; Suppl 279:153–156.

19. Ranke MB, Blum WF, Haug F, Rosendahl W, Attanasio A, Enders H, Gupta

D, Bierich JR. Growth hormone, somatomedin levels and growth regulation in Turner's syndrome. Acta Endocrinol (Copenh) 1987; 116:305–313.

20. Cuttler L, Van Vliet G, Conte FA, Kaplan SL, Grumbach MM. Somato-medin-C levels in children and adolescents with gonadal dysgenesis: Differences from age-matched normal females and effect of chronic estrogen replacement therapy. J Clin Endocrinol Metab 1985; 60:1087–1092.

21. Prader A. The influence of anabolic steroids on growth. Acta Endocrinol (Copenh) 1961; 39:Suppl 163:78.

22. Brook CGD, Mürset G, Zachmann M, Prader A. Growth in children with 45,XO Turner's syndrome. Arch Dis Child 1974; 49:789–795.

DISCUSSION

DR. FREDERICK HOLLAND: Thank you. I would like to touch on some issues, in particular the influence of birth weight on final height, and also the influence of spontaneous menarche when normal estrogen is entering the situation and what influence that makes on final height.

To do this I would like to take the information from a longitudinal and cross-sectional study on height, growth, and sexual maturation in 116 patients followed in our hospital in Toronto over the last 20 years.

These patients were ascertained both retrospectively and prospectively, and for most of the prospective information, most of the height measurements and bone age measurements were done by one person. These are the data of Elizabeth Park and John Bailey of our hospital.

Seventy-one patients were XO, and 33 patients had some form of mosaicism. Twelve patients had some structural aberration of the X chromosome.

As with the findings in most other studies, the chief reason for ascertainment in these patients was short statue. Virtually all of our patients were short, i.e., less than 2 standard deviations below the mean for age.

Dr. Frederick Holland is at the Hospital for Sick Children, Toronto, Canada. Dr. Felix Conte is at the University of California at San Francisco, San Francisco, California. Dr. Barbara MacGillivray is at the University of British Columbia, Vancouver, Canada. Dr. Michael Preece is at the Institute of Child Health, London, England. Dr. Gordon B. Cutler is at National Institute of Child Health and Human Development, Bethesda, Maryland. Dr. Melvin Grumbach is at the University of California at San Francisco, San Francisco, California. Dr. Joseph Gertner is at New York Hospital, New York, New York. Dr. Patrick Wilton is at KabiVitrum, Stockholm Sweden. Dr. Itsuro Hibi is at the National Children's Hospital, Tokyo, Japan. Dr. Douglas Frasier is at the Olive View Medical Center, Sylmar, California. Dr. James Tanner is at the University of Texas Health Center, Houston, Texas.

In answer to some questions asked earlier, we did find hypertension in some of these patients, but I cannot separate those out from those that have known congenital cardiac abnormalities. Our findings of 30% of renal and cardiac abnormalities match those of others.

Of the 116 patients followed, 13 children had spontaneous menarche. Two of these apparently had XO cell lines only. The remaining had non-XO cell lines comprised of a number of both structural deletions and mosaic types.

The mean age of onset of natural menarche in these patients was 13.4 years. Thirty-eight other agonadal patients received conventional cyclical estrogen therapy, using 20 to 40 μg of mestranol along with a progestational agent, with therapy commencing at a mean chronological age of 17 years. This translated into a bone age of approximately 13½ years at the time of ascertainment.

Where possible, those groups identified as having spontaneous menarche or treated with estrogen had growth velocities ascertained 2 years prior to that event and 2 years afterwards to examine the impact of menarche or estrogen therapy on growth velocity both before and after. I would like to review some of the results of this group of patients.

Of our 116 patients, 99 provided data on birth age and gestational duration. The mean duration of gestation in all of our patients was 39 ±1.7 weeks, and this did not differ between XO patients and non-XO patients. In full-term babies, the birth weight of XO and non-XO groups were almost identical and were significantly lower than that in published reports in normal, full-term female infants.

An important piece of information from this study was the correlation of birth weight with adult height and with height and weight at different chronological and bone ages.

For example, for bone ages from 9 through 17 years, there was a strong correlation between the height and weight and birth weight, with r values between 0.75 and 0.95.

The girls are shorter at all ages of ascertainment. Growth velocity was in the lower range of normal until after a bone age of approximately 12½ years, when there is a definite fall-off in growth velocity as a function of bone age.

The final heights of these patients at a bone age of 17 years was 142 ± 7.6 cm with a range of 131 to 167. This mean height is equivalent to a height age of a 10- to 11-year-old normal child.

There is no difference in the growth velocities between those that have an XO karyotype and those who are non-XO in their karyotype. Although numbers were small, growth did not appear to be influenced by the presence of an XX cell line. For example, at a bone age of 13 years, 9 patients with an XO genotype had a mean height of 140.6 cm compared to 139.4 centimeters in 8 patients with a 45,X/46,XX cell line; they were indistinguishable.

Similarly, we could detect no differences between patients monosomic for the short arm of P or disomic for the short arm of P in terms of their growth velocity as a function of bone age.

At all ages, bone ages were significantly retarded for chronological age, particularly for chronological age beyond 12 years. Extrapolation of these data suggested that complete epiphyseal fusion occurred at a mean chronological age of about 19 years.

Finally, we wanted to look at the influence of either spontaneous menarche or conventional estrogen therapy on the final heights of these patients. Thirty-eight patients were treated with estrogen, while 13 patients had spontaneous menarche. If we take time 0 as time of the initiation of this event, that is, either spontaneous menarche or the beginnings of treatment, we can look at growth velocity 1 or 2 years prior to this event and 1 and 2 years post this event.

In patients requiring replacement estrogen therapy, growth velocity was constant in the 1 or 2 years prior to the initiation of treatment and did not change significantly in a positive manner with the onset of conventional estrogen therapy.

Although the numbers are small, there seems to be a small increase in growth velocity in patients with spontaneous menarche, which fell significantly with the onset of menarche.

DR. FELIX CONTE: We have been interested in the effect of estrogens on development of secondary sexual characteristics and final height. The study was done by Ron Alexander, Klaus Rodens, Mel Grumbach, Selna Kaplan, and Felix Conte, University of California.

We looked at 56 patients with Turner syndrome and divided them into six groups based on treatment regimen and age at onset of therapy.

Group 1 included 12 patients who were treated at the age of 12.9 years (early) with a dose of ethinyl estradiol of 140 ng/kg/day for the first 21 days of that month—so-called low-dose estrogen treatment.

Group 2 was treated with conjugated estrogens at 12.8 years (early) at a dose of 9 ± 2.3 μg/kg of conjugated estrogens.

Group 3 included 14 patients treated at a chronologic age of 15 years (late) with the same dose of conjugated estrogens, 9.3 ± 3.1 μg/kg.

Group 4 (6 patients) was treated at a chronologic age of 15 (late) with a *large* dose of conjugated estrogens, greater than 40 μg/kg/day, equivalent to 2.5 mg of Premarin per day.

Group 5 are 6 patients were *untreated* because they had normal gonadal function. Group 6 includes 8 patients who were historical patients from Columbia University who were never treated with estrogens or androgens until at least 18 years of age.

In the Group 1 and 2 patients (low-dose early estrogen treatment), 18 of the 23 had developed Tanner II breasts by one year posttreatment. Twelve of the 23 had developed menarche or withdrawal bleeding after 2 years of therapy. If you look at the effect on growth, you will see that both Group 1 and Group 2 patients had a growth spurt which was significant in the first year but thereafter declined significantly to below the pretreatment growth rate.

Mean final height in the low-dose early estrogen-treated group was 141 ± 5.2 cm. In the early low-dose conjugated estrogen-treated patients, mean height was 141 ± cm. In the low-dose late conjugated estrogen-treated patients, final height was 144.3 cm. In the high-dose conjugated estrogen-treated patients final height was 140.5 ± 5.8 cm. For patients who had normal puberty with no treatment, final height was 142.4 ± 5.8 cm. In Group 6, which includes Turner girls not treated before 18 years of age, final height was 145.5 ± 6.1 cm.

There is no statistical difference in these numbers. There is no statistical difference in the midparental heights of the first three groups.

We also looked briefly at the literature prior to 1969, 1969 to 1980, and 1980 to 1987. These include all the Turners reported from the United States. The mean final height is 143 cm. These included patients treated with estrogens, androgens, and whatever, and the final height was the same as in our patients, i.e., 143 cm.

We looked briefly at the effect of growth velocity on final height and were not able to see a significant difference in growth velocity in the first year of therapy. We also looked at the effect of bone age on final height and did not see a significant difference, although attained height as far as midparental height is concerned in the girls treated less than 11 years of age, with a bone age less than 11, appeared to be somewhat less than the girls treated with a bone age over 11 years of age.

In conclusion, low-dose estrogen therapy of ethinyl estradiol 97–219 ng/kg per day for the first 21 days of the month or conjugated estrogens, 5.8–12 ng/kg day administered before 14 years of age prompted a significant increase in linear growth velocity during the first year of therapy, which was not sustained, despite continuing therapy.

Low-dose estrogen therapy initiated at 12-14 years of age did not result in a significant change in final height when compared to final height in patients untreated or treated with similar or higher doses of estrogen after 14 years of age.

Low-dose estrogen therapy given in a cyclical manner evoked the development of secondary sexual characteristics and withdrawal bleeding.

DR. BARBARA MAC GILLIVRAY: We have been listening to the various treatments this afternoon, where it has been argued that on the basis of psychological advantage, different kinds of treatment are being given to Turner syndrome patients. I think we should be very much aware that we are lacking a prospective, well-controlled study to really argue this point. We do not have that kind of study, and while it may make good clinical sense for some patients, that even a temporary increase in height may be of an advantage, whether that would be true in a well-controlled study is just not known at this point. When it comes to injections, then I must say I have really grave concern about giving placebo injections for a prolonged time to children. I have seen quite a few children who were severely bothered by sustained injections, and if they really needed it, physiologically, one would argue and support them to continue with injections. When it comes to placebo injections, I have great concern. Also, I would raise the question of informed consent by the child in that situation. I am really quite amazed that that would pass any kind of ethical committee at a hospital or at a university.

DR. MICHAEL PREECE: I want to take on that theme a little further, if I may. I think that there are obvious concerns about up to 10 years of placebo. But additionally, I think there are actually some invalid statistical presumptions. The whole point of a double-blind, randomized, placebo-controlled study is that it remains blind throughout the whole experiment, and that compliance is broadly similar in all groups or limbs of the study. There is enough published information in existing growth hormone studies, particularly in the Genentech study. Many of the results are available in the professional and lay media. Any child or any family of any child receiving a double treatment program, of a tablet and injection, who shows no response in the first 6 to 12 months is going to smell a rat. They are going to feel fairly convinced of what they are having. You cannot constrain the child to stay in the study at that point, and I would lay money that compliance in that limb will wither away over quite a short period of time. I think there is also another point concerning placebo . . . and I support placebo-controlled studies in the short term and went out on a limb about this some years ago. A short-term placebo effect I find very easy to accept and understand. However, studies have already shown that a placebo-induced growth effect actually does not happen, or if it happens it is trivial. How you can suspect that there will be a long-term placebo effect on mature height, when there is no short-term effect, I find impossible to imagine.

DR. GORDON B. CUTLER: Let me just respond to Dr. Preece, because I think this is important. I have actually never had the chance to discuss his study with a 6-month placebo, but I do not find it so inconceivable that after 10 years of treatment there may be a significantly different effect of a certain magnitude at a certain p value. Our studies are usually designed to pick up a difference of 4 cm at a $p = 0.05$ level. That is the kind of magnitude that we look for. Now let us just imagine that there is a drift between an untreated control group and a placebo group, and that it takes 10 years to see a 4-cm difference at $p = 0.05$

level. I can imagine some difference between an untreated control group and a placebo group. You are giving injections, injections hurt, there is endorphin, growth hormone, whatever. If it takes 40 patients, for example, to see a 4-cm difference after 10 years, then you have to ask what would be the statistical power needed to be able to exclude the possibility of a placebo effect of that magnitude within, say, a year? And if you propose that this drift is occurring at a similar rate, it would be 0.4 cm in a year. To exclude an effect of 0.4 cm with 1 year of placebo versus 1 year of untreated control is difficult because the statistical power goes with the inverse of the size. So you would need to pick up 1/10 the effect in a short-term study of this sort, which would require 100 times the patients. Until a study is done with 4000 patients as untreated controls and 4000 on placebo for a 1-year period, we cannot exclude this difference.

DR. MELVIN GRUMBACH: Now we need to hear what the growth hormone study is going to show on this, but I suspect that it may not be a continuous pattern of growth. So maybe you will find that you accomplish this in 1 year, 2 years, or 3 years, whatever it may be. It does not mean that that increment is going to be maintained or is equally or even well distributed over a 10-year period of time.

DR. JOSEPH GERTNER: The way I have always considered this placebo business is to try and apply a logical analysis to it, and really I would like to ask Gordon Cutler what he thinks about that. The placebo treatment either works to increase growth rate, or it works to decrease growth rate, or it does not do anything at all. If it does nothing at all, then we do not need it. So we only need to consider whether it increases growth rate or decreases growth rate. If it decreases growth rate, then I think that it is a fundamental contradiction of primum no noceri to give somebody 10 years of a treatment which hurts and which decreases growth rate. If it increases growth rate, then it is an inherent part of growth hormone therapy, and what you want to know is not what growth hormone as a chemical substance does to the patient, but what growth hormone therapy does to the patient including the benefit of the placebo effect. So I would really like to know what you think you are going to gain from knowing what the placebo is going to do?

DR. CUTLER: The way I look at it is I want to find out whether a growth hormone or any of these things are beneficial or not. And the null hypothesis, of course, that we should all start out with is that none of these things is beneficial until proven otherwise. The only valid test of the null hypothesis is to make treatment the only variable and find out whether it works or not. That is the scientific method. Anything else is unscientific in terms of a rigid, rigorous application of scientific method. Now if you did this thing, let us just take the point and let us just assume that the benefit were due to a placebo effect. I think it would be a terrible tragedy to spend many untold millions of dollars putting growth hormone in those shots if placebo would have done the same thing. In other words, I want to know whether the growth hormone is effective, not whether this benefit is due to the placebo effect of puncturing the skin.

DR. PATRICK WILTON: Dr. Cutler, I got the impression that you suggested that it works through endorphins. Isn't it time then to do a placebo-controlled study in growth hormone–deficients patients, because perhaps it could be the same substance there and not the growth hormone. I agree, it is a very scientifically good study if it really worked as placebo, but I totally agree that probably it will not be blinded after the first year.

DR. ITSURO HIBI: I believe it could be permitted to make the doctor blind, but it should not be permitted to make the patients blind.

DR. DOUGLAS FRASIER: In general, before instituting a placebo-controlled study in humans, one would hope to have a placebo-controlled study in animals. I just wonder if such a study exists, and if so, if no placebo effect has been shown, why proceed with such a study in humans. These are children and not rats.

DR. JAMES TANNER: Mike, could you give a very brief comment on what you think of Gordon's reply to you?

DR. PREECE: I think I take the point that if you are looking at a 6-month study you may not have seen a powerful enough change to predict what will happen after 10 years. However, the most likely effect of a placebo effect is going to be in the earlier phase rather than in the later phase of the study, I would have thought, although I do not think anyone can prove that one way or another. As far as the actual statistical sums you did, I would have to sit down with a pencil and paper. It did not sound quite right to me. Certainly, I agree it would need far bigger numbers than we looked at, but I suspect they are not quite as big as you were suggesting.

DR. CUTLER: If the magnitude of the effect is 1/10, which, for example, would be 1 vs. 10 years, you need 10^2 times the number of subjects to pick it up at the same level of significance. That is straightforward.

DR. PREECE: No, the variance is the square, the SD is the root of that.

DR. TANNER: I think we will let the statisticians have a go at this.

32

Growth Hormone Therapy in Turner Syndrome

Ron G. Rosenfeld and Raymond L. Hintz

Stanford University School of Medicine, Stanford, California

Ann J. Johanson, Barry M. Sherman, and the Genentech Collaborative Group*

Genentech, Inc., South San Francisco, California

In the 50 years since Henry Turner's (1) original description of a syndrome of infantilism, congenital webbed neck, and cubitus valgus, it has become apparent that growth retardation is one of the most common features of this syndrome. Recent reviews have reported mean adult heights ranging from 140.2 to 146.3 cm (2-7). In a study combining growth data from four major European studies of 366 untreated Turner girls, Lyon et al. (8) reported a mean final adult height of 142.9 cm. Similarly, in a review of the American literature over the last 20 years, combining both untreated Turner girls and patients receiving sex steroids, Conte and Grumbach have reported a final adult height of 143 cm ($n = 563$) (personal communication).

Because of the limited supplies of pituitary-derived human growth hormone (hGH), early experience with GH treatment of Turner syndrome was generally limited to short-term studies of limited numbers of patients (Table 1). Inter-

---

*Investigators in the Genentech Collaborative Group: Jo Anne Brasel, M.D., Stephen Burstein, M.D., Ph.D., Steven Chernausek, M.D., Peter Compton, James Frane, Ph.D., Ronald W. Gotlin, M.D., Raymond L. Hintz, M.D., Ann J. Johanson, M.D., Joyce Kuntze, Barbara M. Lippe, M.D., Patrick C. Mahoney, M.D., Wayne V. Moore, M.D., Ph.D., Maria I. New, M.D., Ron G. Rosenfeld, M.D., Paul Saenger, M.D., Barry Sherman, M.D., and Virginia Sybert, M.D.

Table 1 Growth Hormone Therapy in Turner Syndrome

Number of subjects	Age (yr)	Average dose of hGH/wk[a]	Pre-Rx growth (cm/yr)[b]	On-Rx growth (cm/yr)	Ref.
1	14	35.0 mg	3.8	7.5	9
2	13.9, 11	13.5 mg	3.1	4.3	10
2	12, 15.9	17.0 mg	3.2	5.7	12
2	12.5, 13	35.0 mg	3.2	6.8	13
1	14	10.0 mg	2.7	6.0	14
5		10.0 mg	2.9	3.9	11
1	8	8.0 mg	–	+4.1	15
1	10	7.5 mg	2.3	6.4	16
1	17.4	7.5 mg	2.7	2.7	17
6	12.8 (11–15)	0.25 mg/kg	2.0	3.8 7.6[d]	18
4	11–12.5	11.3 mg	3.3	3.7	19
2	5.6, 12.4	10.9, 8.7 mg/m^2	4.8	9.2[d]	20
3	11–13	0.30 mg/kg	3.4	6.5	21
8	16	6–12 mg	2.6	2.2[e]	22
8	11.8 (9.2–14.8)	0.25 mg/kg (0.09–0.32)	3.3	4.9	23
20	12.3 (8.4–16.1)	0.27 mg/kg (0.20–0.42)	3.7	5.7	24
21[c]	11.5 (7.4–13.8)	0.28 mg/kg (0.11–0.47)	3.6	5.5	25
52	(4.5–14.5)	0.30 mg/kg)	3.2	5.9	26
70	9.3 (4.7–12.4)	0.375 mg/kg	4.2	6.6 9.8[d]	27
16	11.7 (7.9–15.2)	14 mg/m^2	3.4	7.2[f]	28
9	9.8 (4.4–13.4)	6.0 mg	3.7	5.2	29

[a]Determinations of hGH dose are arbitrarily based upon an estimated potency of 2 U/mg. This may not be true for all hGH preparations, especially the earlier ones.
[b]Growth rates are expressed as cm/yr, although actual periods of study may have been as short as 3 months.
[c]16/20 subjects from the immediately preceding study are included in this study.
[d]hGH in combination with oxandrolone or fluoxymesterone.
[e]Stahnke reported that 2/8 Turner patients responded to hGH, with growth rates as high as 7–8 cm/yr. For the 6 nonresponders, the growth rate on treatment averaged 2.2 cm/yr.
[f]Girls >13 years of age were also given ethinyl estradiol (0.1 μg/kg qod).
Source: Adapted from Refs. 30 and 31.

estingly, Henry Turner himself reported in one patient that "anterior pituitary growth hormone, 2 cc. 3 times weekly, was prescribed, and injections were continued for approximately 5 months without any appreciable increase in her height" (1). Presumably, this 18-year-old patient received a crude bovine pituitary extract, and her failure to respond is not surprising.

The short-term studies performed in the 1960s and 1970s gave conflicting results. Earlier studies by Almqvist et al. (32) and Forbes et al. (33) had demonstrated that hGH treatment of patients with Turner syndrome resulted in increased sulfation factor activity, as well as retention of nitrogen, phosphorus, magnesium, sodium, potassium, and chloride. However, both Soyka et al. (10) and Tanner et al. (11) reported increases in annual growth rates of only 1-1.2 cm/yr. While subsequent studies were often more optimistic, variability in patient age, GH dosage, length of therapy, and presence or absence of concomitant sex steroid treatment made results difficult to interpret (Table 1).

Two more recent studies of pituitary hGH in Turner syndrome are worthy of comment. Raiti et al. (26) reported the results of GH treatment of 52 Turner patients ranging in age from 4.5-14.5 years. Pituitary-derived hGH was administered at a dosage of 0.2 IU/kg three times per week (approximately 0.3 mg/kg/ wk), resulting in an increase in growth rate from 3.2 to 5.9 cm/yr. During a subsequent 6-month period off hGH, the growth rate fell to 3.1 cm/yr. Thirty-one subjects were then given a second course of hGH, with a rise in growth rate back to 5.9 cm/yr.

The second study, reported by Buchanan et al. (29), was originally designed as a double-blind, placebo-controlled trial of pituitary-derived hGH. This trial was stopped when pituitary-derived hGH was withdrawn from use in the United Kingdom in May 1985, following reports of Creutzfeldt-Jakob disease in hGH recipients (34). Nevertheless, the 6-month data indicated that hGH recipients increased their Turner growth rate from -0.3 to +1.4 SD, while placebo subjects decreased their Turner growth rate from +1.1 to -0.7 SD.

To date, the use of recombinant DNA-derived hGH in Turner syndrome has been reported in two major prospective studies, the Genentech Collaborative Study (see below) (27,31,35) and the Japanese experience, reported by Takano et al. (24,25). In the first Japanese study, the mean annual growth rate increased from 3.7 to 5.7 cm/yr, based upon 6-month growth data. In the second study, growth rates increased from pretreatment values of 3.6 ± 0.8 cm/yr (range 2.0-5.0) to 5.5 ± 1.2 cm/yr (range 3.4-7.8). All subjects, except one, showed an increase in annual growth rate. During a second year of treatment with hGH, eight subjects demonstrated an average annual growth rate of 5.1 ± 0.6 cm/yr.

GENENTECH COLLABORATIVE STUDY OF GH
THERAPY IN TURNER SYNDROME

This prospective, randomized study was initiated in 1983, and involved a total of 70 patients from 11 medical centers (27,31,35). Chronologic ages ranged from 4.7 to 12.4 years, with a maximal skeletal age of 11.2 years. All had heights at least 1 SD below the mean for normal females of equivalent chronologic age, and documented prerandomization growth rates <6 cm/yr. Additionally, all subjects had provocative GH levels of at least 7 ng/ml. Subjects were excluded if they had received any anabolic agent, sex steroid, or GH within 3 months of entering the study or if they had cumulative past exposure to such agents exceeding 1 month duration.

After an observation period of at least 6 months, to document prerandomization growth rates, subjects were assigned to one of four study arms. Balance was sought with respect to prerandomization growth rate, chronologic age, and karyotype (Table 2). The four study arms are listed in Table 3. After the first phase of the study, which lasted 12-20 months, Groups 1 and 2 (control and oxandrolone, respectively) were placed on combination met-hGH (0.125 mg/kg tiw) and oxandrolone (0.0625 mg/kg/d). Group 3 (met-hGH) remained on GH, alone. Group 4 (combination) remained on combination therapy, but at the lower oxandrolone dose.

Table 2 Comparison of Study Groups at Baseline

	Control	Oxandrolone	Met-hGH	Combina-tion
Age (yr)	9.3 ± 2.3	9.6 ± 2.0	9.1 ± 2.1	8.9 ± 2.5
	(18)	(18)	(17)	(17)
Height (cm)	114.4 ± 10.7	115.3 ± 9.9	114.6 ± 9.5	113.8 ± 10
	(18)	(18)	(17)	(17)
Weight (kg)	23.7 ± 9.3	24.7 ± 7.0	23.6 ± 7.2	23.4 ± 6.2
	(18)	(18)	(17)	(17)
Growth rate	4.2 ± 1.1	4.1 ± 1.0	4.5 ± 0.8	4.3 ± 0.9
(cm/yr)	(18)	(18)	(17)	(17)
Bone age	8.3 ± 2.3	8.5 ± 2.1	7.7 ± 1.9	7.7 ± 2.2
(yr)	(17)	(17)	(17)	(17)
Karyotype				
45,X	15	12	13	13
Other	3	6	4	4

Data are presented as the mean ± SD for each group of (n) subjects. There were no statistically significant differences between groups in the mean age, height, weight, prerandomization growth rate, or bone age.
Source: Ref. 35.

Table 3 Study Arms

Group	Phase 1[a]	Phase 2
1	No treatment	met-hGH, 0.125 mg/kg, 3x/wk + oxandrolone, 0.0625 mg/kg/day
2	oxandrolone, 0.125 mg/kg/day	met-hGH, 0.125 mg/kg, 3x/wk + oxandrolone, 0.0625 mg/kg/day
3	met-hGH, 0.125 mg/kg, 3x/wk	met-hGH, 0.125 mg/kg, 3x/wk
4	met-hGH, 0.125 mg/kg, 3x/wk + oxandrolone, 0.125 mg/kg/day	met-hGH, 0.125 mg/kg, 3x/wk + oxandrolone, 0.0625 mg/kg/day

[a]Phase 1 consisted of a 12- to 20-month period.
Source: Ref. 31.

Table 4 lists the annual growth rates in each of the study arms. The control group (Group 1) experienced the anticipated growth deceleration typical of Turner patients, with a decline in growth rate from 4.2 to 3.8 cm/yr. Met-hGH, both alone (Group 3) and combined with oxandrolone (Group 4), resulted in significant growth acceleration in year 1, to 6.6 cm/yr and 9.8 cm/yr, respectively, Although growth rates fell in years 2 and 3 for both Groups 3 and 4, the rates remained significantly greater than year 1 of the control group, despite the fact

Table 4 Annual Growth Rates[a]

Group	Prerandomization	Year 1	Year 2[b]	Year 3
1 (control)	4.2 ± 1.1 (18)	3.8 ± 1.0 (16)	8.3 ± 1.2 (16)	6.7 ± 1.4 (16)
2 (oxand.)	4.1 ± 1.0 (18)	7.9 ± 1.0 (17)	7.1 ± 1.6 (17)	5.3 ± 2.4 (16)
3 (met-hGH)	4.5 ± 0.8 (17)	6.6 ± 1.2 (17)	5.4 ± 1.1 (17)	4.6 ± 1.4 (17)
4 (comb.)	4.3 ± 0.9 (17)	9.8 ± 1.4 (17)	7.4 ± 1.4 (16)	6.1 ± 1.5 (16)

[a]Growth rates are expressed as cm/yr ± SD for (n) subjects.
[b]Year 2 is the first year of Phase 2 for each group. This phase began 12- to 20-months after the beginning of Year 1.

Table 5 Turner Growth Velocity Z-Score[a]

Group	Prerandomization	Year 1	Year 2[b]	Year 3
1 (control)	+0.2 ± 1.2	−0.1 ± 1.0	+5.3 ± 1.4	+3.9 ± 1.6
2 (oxand.)	+0.2 ± 1.0	+4.3 ± 1.7	+4.0 ± 1.5	+2.3 ± 2.3
3 (met-hGH)	+0.5 ± 0.8	+3.0 ± 1.2	+2.0 ± 1.1	+1.4 ± 1.5
4 (comb.)	+0.2 ± 0.9	+6.6 ± 1.2	+4.2 ± 1.4	+2.9 ± 1.3

[a]Growth velocity Z-scores for untreated Turner patients derived from Ref. 36.
[b]Year 2 is the first year of Phase 2 for each group. This phase began 12–20 months after the beginning of Phase 1.

that the subjects were now 1–2 years older. It is also interesting to note that control subjects (Group 1) grew well when placed on combination therapy, despite receiving a lower oxandrolone dose than the original combination group (Group 4).

In Table 5, the growth velocity data are presented as z-scores (standard deviation scores) for untreated Turner patients, based upon the data of Ranke (36). This method permits one to assess the effect of hormonal therapy upon growth rates, while taking into account the fact that subjects are advancing in age over the 3 years of the study. Thus, while the control group had a growth velocity z-score of −0.1 SD during the year of observation, the group receiving met-hGH (Group 3) had growth velocities of +3.0, +2.0, and +1.4 SD during years 1–3, respectively. Similarly, the original combination group had growth velocity z-scores of +6.6, +4.2, and +2.9 SD in years 1–3.

The effect of therapy on the actual height of the Turner subjects, relative to untreated Turner patients, is presented in Table 6, which expresses the mean z-score for Turner height in each group, using the growth data of Lyon et al. (8). After 3 years of met-hGH therapy (Group 3), the height z-score rose from −0.2

Table 6 Turner Height Z-Score[a]

Group	Prerandomization	Year 1	Year 2[b]	Year 3
1 (control)	−0.3 ± 0.9	−0.3 ± 0.9	+0.6 ± 1.0	+1.0 ± 1.0
2 (oxand.)	−0.2 ± 0.9	+0.5 ± 0.9	+1.4 ± 0.9	+1.6 ± 1.1
3 (met-hGH)	−0.2 ± 0.9	+0.3 ± 0.9	+0.6 ± 1.0	+0.7 ± 1.0
4 (comb.)	−0.1 ± 0.7	+1.0 ± 0.8	+1.7 ± 0.8	+2.0 ± 0.9

[a]Height Z-score for untreated Turner patients derived from Ref. 8.
[b]Year 2 is the first year of Phase 2 for each group. This phase began 12–20 months after the beginning of Phase 1.

Table 7 ΔHeight Age/ΔBone Age Ratios[a]

Group	Year 1	Year 2[b]	Year 3	Cumulative
1 (control)	0.7	1.1	1.4	1.1
2 (oxand.)	0.9	1.2	1.2	1.0
3 (met-hGH)	1.0	0.8	1.8	1.0
4 (comb.)	1.0	0.9	1.3	1.0

[a]Height Age data for normal American females derived from the National Center for Health Statistics (NCHS), Hyattsville, Maryland. Bone age values derived from Ref. 39. Ratios represent median values.
[b]Year 2 is the first year of Phase 2 for each group. This phase began 12–20 months after the beginning of Phase 1.

to +0.7 SD. In the original combination group, the height z-score rose over 2 SD during 3 years of treatment, from −0.1 to +2.0 SD.

A potential complication of growth-promoting therapy is that changes in height may occur at the expense of accelerated skeletal maturation, resulting in compromised final adult height. The relative effects of therapy upon skeletal growth and maturation are reported in Tables 7 and 8. Table 7 shows the ratio of delta height age/delta bone age, using height age data for normal American females (National Center for Health Statistics), which includes the normal pubertal growth spurt. Even when reported in this manner, the ratio is never <1.0, indicating that advancing skeletal maturation is fully compensated for by increased growth. Probably a fairer way to present the data is shown in Table 8, where growth data are expressed as the ratio of Δ Turner height age/Δ bone age, using the Turner height age data for untreated Turner patients, reported by Lyon et al. (8). When analyzed in this manner, 3-year therapy with met-hGH alone (Group 3) or combination (Group 4) results in a ratio of 1.6. These results indicate that treatment resulted in considerable advancement in height relative to untreated Turner patients, and that this height increment exceeded the advance in skeletal maturation.

Table 8 Δ Turner Height Age/Δ Bone Age Ratios[a]

Group	Year 1	Year 2[b]	Year 3	Cumulative
1 (control)	1.1	2.0	2.5	1.7
2 (oxand.)	1.6	1.9	2.9	1.7
3 (met-hGH)	1.7	1.4	2.2	1.6
4 (comb.)	1.6	1.6	2.5	1.6

[a]Turner height age data for untreated Turner patients derived from Ref. 8. Bone age data based upon Ref. 39. Ratios represent median values.
[b]Year 2 is the first year of Phase 2 for each group. This phase began 12–20 months after the beginning of Phase 1.

Table 9 Cumulative Increments in Predicted Adult Height (cm)[a]

Group	1 Year	2 Years[b]	3 Years
1 (control)	1.1	4.9	7.3
	(12)	(11)	(8)
2 (oxandrolone)	2.1	5.0	6.6
	(13)	(12)	(10)
3. (met-hGH)	2.4	2.5	4.7
	(12)	(13)	(12)
4 (combination)	3.6	5.6	8.1
	(11)	(11)	(9)

[a]Predicted adult heights based upon Ref. 37. Data are presented as the mean cumulative increment in predicted adult height (cm) at the end of 1, 2, or 3 years in the study for (n) subjects.
[b]Year 2 is the first year of Phase 2 for each group. This phase began 12–20 months after the beginning of Phase 1.

As this study enters into its fourth year, 65 of the original 70 subjects remain active participants, and all are still growing. Accordingly, it is premature to evaluate the ultimate effect of therapy upon final adult height. Nevertheless, the Bayley-Pinneau method (37) has proven to be a reasonable means for predicting adult height in *untreated* Turner patients (38). When this method is applied to all subjects who had an initial bone age $\geqslant 6$ years, it appears that therapy resulted in significant increases in final adult height. In 12 subjects treated with met-hGH alone (Group 3), 3-year treatment resulted in a 4.7 cm increase in predicted adult height. Similarly, in 9 subjects completing 3 years of combination therapy (Group 4), treatment resulted in an 8.1 cm increase.

The data at the end of 3 (see Table 9) years support the following conclusions:

1. Growth hormone, both alone and in combination with oxandrolone, stimulates linear growth in Turner syndrome over a minimum of 3 years. This acceleration is particularly impressive when the results are compared to the natural history of growth in Turner syndrome.
2. Patients with Turner syndrome do not, however, respond to GH therapy as well as patients with growth hormone deficiency, indicating some level of end organ resistance to either GH or somatomedin. Growth acceleration, while statistically significant, is generally modest, and both patient and physician expectations must be realistic.
3. Acceleration of skeletal maturation appears to be fully compensated for by increases in linear growth.
4. While it is premature to determine the effects of therapy upon final adult height, it would appear that treatment with GH, either alone or in combina-

tion with low doses of oxandrolone, does not compromise ultimate height. Rather, analysis of the data at the end of 3 years suggests a probable increase in mean final height. Whether such treatment will permit a majority of patients with Turner syndrome to attain a normal final height (>150 cm) remains to be seen.

REFERENCES

1. Turner HH. A syndrome of infantilism, congenital webbed neck, and cubitus valgus. Endocrinology 1938; 23:566–574.
2. Palmer CG, Reichmann A. Chromosomal and clinical findings in 110 females with Turner syndrome. Hum Genet 1976; 35:35–49.
3. Park E, Bailey JD, Cowell CA. Growth and maturation of patients with Turner's syndrome. Pediatr Res 1983; 17:1–7.
4. Brook CGD, Murset G, Zachmann M, Prader A. Growth in children with 45,XO Turner's syndrome. Arch Dis Child 1974; 49:789–795.
5. Lev-Ran A. Androgens, estrogens, and the ultimate height in XO gonadal dysgenesis. Am J Dis Child 1977; 131:648–649.
6. Sybert VP. Adult height in Turner syndrome with and without androgen therapy. J Pediatr 1984; 104:365–369.
7. Ranke MB, Pfluger H, Rosendahl W, Stbbe P, Enders H, Bierich JR, Majewski F. Turner syndrome: Spontaneous growth in 150 cases and review of the literature. Eur J Pediatr 1983; 141:81–88.
8. Lyon AJ, Preece MA, Grant DB. Gowth curve for girls with Turner syndrome. Arch Dis Child 1985; 60:932–935.
9. Escamilla RF, Hutchings JJ, Deamer WC, Li CH. Clinical experiences with human growth hormone (LI) in pituitary infantilism and in gonadal dysgenesis. Acta Endocrinol 1960; 35 suppl 51:253 (A).
10. Soyka LF, Ziskind A, Crawford JD. Treatment of short stature in children and adolescents with human pituitary hormone (Raben). N Engl J Med 1964; 271:754–764.
11. Tanner JM, Whitehouse RH, Hughes PCR, Vince FP. Effects of human growth hormone treatment for 1 to 7 years on growth of 100 children with growth hormone deficiency, low birthweight, inherited smallness, Turner's syndrome and other complaints. Arch Dis Child 1971; 46:745–782.
12. Wright JC, Brasel JA, Aceto T, et al. Studies with human growth hormone (hGH). Am J Med 1965; 38:499–516.
13. Hutchings JJ, Escamilla RF, Li CH, Forsham PH. Human growth hormone administration in gonadal dysgenesis. Am J Dis Child 1965; 109:318–321.
14. Tzagournis M. Response to long-term administration of human growth hormone in Turner's syndrome. JAMA 1969; 210:2373–2376.
15. Pena J, Tresanchez J, Suarez M, Osorio C. Growth hormone (hGH) treatment of 7 cases of hyposomatotropism and 1 case of Turner's syndrome. Rev Clin Esp 1972; 126:323–326.

16. Brook CGD. Growth hormone deficiency in Turner's syndrome. N Engl J Med 1978; 298:1203-1204.
17. Bottazzo GF, McIntosh C, Stanford W, Preece M. Growth hormone cell antibodies and partial growth hormone deficiency in a girl with Turner's syndrome. Clin Endocrinol 1980; 12:1-9.
18. Rudman D, Goldsmith M, Kutner M, Blackston D. Effect of growth hormone and oxandrolone single and together on growth rate in girls with X-chromosome abnormalities. J Pediatr 1980; 96:132-5.
19. Butenandt O. Growth hormone deficiency and growth hormone therapy in Ullrich-Turner's syndrome. Klin Wochenschr 1980; 58:99-101.
20. Lenko HL, Leisti L, Perheentupa J. The efficacy of growth hormone in different types of growth failure. Eur J Pediatr 1982; 138:241-249.
21. Dolan LM, Khoury B, Parker MW, Johanson AJ. Accelerated growth in Turner's syndrome (TS) treated with human growth hormone (hGH). Clin Res 1983; 31:23 (A).
22. Stahnke N. Human growth hormone treatment in short children without growth hormone deficiency. N Engl J Med 1984; 310:925-926.
23. Singer-Granick C, Lee PA, Foley TP, Becker DJ. Growth hormone therapy for patients with Turner's syndrome. horm Res 1986; 24:246-250.
24. Takano K, Hizuka N, Shizaume K. Treatment of Turner's syndrome with methionyl human growth hormone for six months. Acta Endocrinol (Copenh) 1986; 112:130-137.
25. Takano K, Hizuka N, Shizume K. Growth hormone treatment in Turner's syndrome. Acta Paediatr Scand (Suppl) 1986; 325:58-63.
26. Raiti S, Moore WV, Van Vliet G, Kaplan SL. Growth-stimulating effects of human growth hormone in patients with Turner syndrome. J Pediatr 1986; 109:944-949.
27. Rosenfeld RG, Hintz RL, Johanson AJ, et al. Methionyl human growth hormone and oxandrolone in Turner syndrome: Preliminary results of a prospective randomized trial. J Pediatr 1986; 109:936-943.
28. Rongen-Westerlaken C, Wit JM, Drop SLS, et al. Methionyl growth hormone (met-hGH) in a dosage of 4 IU/m² day promotes growth in Turner syndrome. 26th Annual Meeting of the European Society for Paediatric Endocrinology 1987; 128 (A).
29. Buchanan CR, Law CM, Milner RDG. Growth hormone in short, slowly growing children and those with Turner's syndrome. Arch Dis Child 1987; 62:912-961.
30. Wilton P. Growth hormone treatment in girls with Turner's syndrome. Acta Paediatr Scand 1987; 76:193-200.
31. Rosenfeld RG, Hintz RL, Johanson AJ, et al. Growth hormone therapy in Turner syndrome. In Bercu BB (ed), Basic and Clinical Aspects of Growth Hormone, Plenum Press, New York, 1988, 331-337.
32. Almqvist S, Hall K, Lindstedt S, et al. Effects of short term administration of physiological doses of human growth hormone in three patients with Turner's syndrome. Acta Endocrinol 1964; 46:451-464.

33. Forbes AP, Jacobsen JG, Carroll EL, Pechet MM. Studies of growth arrest in gonadal dysgenesis: Response to exogenous human growth hormone. Metabolism 1962; 11:56–75.
34. Powell-Jackson J, Weller RO, Kennedy P, et al. Creutzfeldt-Jakob disease after administration of human growth hormone. Lancet 1985; 2:244–246.
35. Rosenfeld RG, Hintz RL, Johanson AJ, et al. Results from the first 2 years of a clinical trial with recombinant DNA-derived human growth hormone (somatrem) in Turner's syndrome. Acta Paediatr Scand (Suppl) 1987; 331: 59–66.
36. Ranke MB. Spontanes Wachstum beim Turner-Syndrom. Der Kinderarzt 1985; 16:1205–1208.
37. Bayley N, Pinneau SR. Tables for predicting adult height from skeletal age: Revised for use with the Greulich-Pyle hand standards. J Pediatr 1953; 40:423–441.
38. Zachmann M, Sobradillo B, Frank M, et al. Bayley-Pinneau, Roche-Wainer-Thissen, and Tanner height predictions in normal children and in patients with various pathologic conditions. J Pediatr 1978; 93:749–755.
39. Greulich WW, Pyle SI. Radiographic Atlas of Skeletal Development of the Hand and Wrist. Stanford University Press, Stanford, CA, 1950.

DISCUSSION

DR. DAVID BAYLINK: Why were the somatomedin C levels higher in the growth hormone plus the androgen group when the androgen group alone did not seem to have any effect?

DR. RON G. ROSENFELD: I think that it is true that there was a significant elevation in somatomedins in the group receiving growth hormone alone and growth hormone in combination with oxandrolone, but there was no significant difference between those two groups. So as far as we could tell, oxandrolone had no additive effect or no significant additive effect to growth hormone in terms of raising somatomedin C levels. The whole question of why oxandrolone stimulates short-term growth is an interesting one, because we now know from some of the data published from Virginia that testosterone replacement does increase somatomedin C levels, whereas oxandrolone, whether you use it for treatment of constitutional delay or, in this case, for Turner syndrome, does not. Whether that means that testosterone and oxandrolone are stimulating growth through different mechanisms or through some common mechanism that has nothing to do with the growth hormone-IGF axis, remains to be established.

DR. DOUGLAS FRASIER: You have presented now two groups of patients receiving the combination therapy, the difference being the dose of anabolic steroid. It looked to me as though those responses were the same, but I do not know that you presented mean data. Could you do that please?

DR. ROSENFELD: The original combination group using the higher dosage of oxandrolone grew 9.8 cm during their first year. The control group, which at the end of 12 to 20 months of observation was put on growth hormone plus the lower dose of oxandrolone, grew 8.8 cm, so a centimeter a year less. On the other hand, they were 12 to 20 months older. So if you express the growth rates in terms of Z-score for chronological age, there is no significant difference between the group receiving higher dose oxandrolone or lower dose oxandrolone.

DR. ITSURO HIBI: I have two questions. The first one, have you measured the skeletal maturation of each group? The second point, what percentage of your patients with combination therapy have manifested spontaneous puberty?

DR. ROSENFELD: If you express the bone age data as Δheight age/Δbone age ratio using height age for normal females, at the end of 3 years of therapy the median Δheight age/Δbone age ratio for both the growth hormone-alone group and the combination group was almost exactly 1. If you express the Δheight age/Δbone age as the ΔTurner height age/Δbone age ratio, then it was 1.7 at the end of 3 years for the combination group and 1.6 for the growth hormone-alone group. Regarding the second question, I know of at least two girls who have entered into spontaneous puberty in the combination group and at least one girl in the growth hormone-alone group.

DR. JUDITH L. ROSS: I just wanted to know if you factored in any way midparental height in looking at the two groups that you carried out the furthest.

DR. ROSENFELD: We have not yet done that. We need to go back and do that.

DR. JAMES TANNER: We will go on to Dr. Frane, who will talk about the prediction of adult height in these same patients.

Dr. David Baylink is at the Loma Linda University School of Medicine and the Jerry L. Pettis Memorial Veterans' Hospital, Loma Linda, California. Dr. Ron G. Rosenfeld is at the Stanford University School of Medicine, Stanford, California. Dr. Douglas Frasier is at the Olive View Medical Center, Sylmar, California. Dr. Itsuro Hibi is at the National Children's Hospital, Tokyo, Japan. Dr. Judith L. Ross is at Hahnemann University, Philadelphia, Pennsylvania. Dr. James Tanner is at the University of Texas Health Center, Houston, Texas.

33

Predicted Adult Height in Turner Syndrome

James W. Frane, Barry M. Sherman,
and The Genentech Collaborative Group

Genentech, Inc.
South San Francisco, California

INTRODUCTION

Four methods for predicting adult height were evaluated for their ability to predict adult height of untreated girls with Turner syndrome: Bayley-Pinneau (1,2), Roche-Wainer-Thissen (3), Tanner-Whitehouse (4,5), and Lyon-Preece-Grant (6). The first three methods are based on data from normal girls, and the authors do not advocate their use for Turner girls. Nevertheless, it has been thought that it might be possible to use one or more of these methods to predict the adult height of untreated or treated Turner girls.

We used results from the literature as well as our own experience to show that the Bayley-Pinneau (BP) method might be useful in predicting adult height of untreated Turner girls, but that the Roche-Wainer-Thissen (RWT) and Tanner-Whitehouse (TW) methods give unrealistically high predictions of adult height in Turner syndrome and are unlikely to be of value.

The fourth method, Lyon-Preece-Grant (LPG), is based on untreated Turner patients. We find that this method also provides estimates of adult height for untreated Turner girls consistent with the ranges of expected heights based on historical records.

STATURE OF UNTREATED TURNER PATIENTS

Table 1 summarizes results from a number of studies of adult height of Turner patients. Lyon et al. (6) pooled the results of three European studies and showed that untreated adult Turner women have a mean height of approximately 143 cm and a standard deviation of 6.7 cm. The results from Lyon et al. include those from Ranke et al. (7).

Results from a survey of 13 studies in the United States are also summarized in Table 1 and show a mean adult height of 143.3 cm, essentially the same as for European girls summarized by Lyon (6). Details from the American survey are provided in Table 2 (8–20) and in even greater detail in Rodens et al. (20). Patients in the American survey generally received some kind of therapy such as estrogen or oxandrolone. Since the mean adult stature of the American and European girls is so similar, it is doubtful whether any of these treatments had any effect on adult height.

These two summaries establish a normative range for untreated adults with Turner syndrome in the range of 129 to 156 cm (95% confidence interval) and suggest that secular influences or national differences are not important determinants of stature.

THE LYON-PREECE-GRANT PREDICTED ADULT HEIGHT

The LPG method predicts adult height based on the height percentiles for Turner patients derived from data summarized by Lyon et al. (6), incorporating the earlier summary of Ranke et al. (7). To obtain the LPG predicted adult height, one first computes the girl's current percentile for age. The adult percentile is predicted to be the same as the current percentile. One can also obtain the same predicted adult height from the current height standardized for age (also called height z-scores or height SDS). For example, if an untreated Turner

Table 1 Observed Adult Heights for Turner Patients

	Sample size	Mean (cm)	Standard deviation
Lyon et al. survey of adult height from 4 European studies (untreated patients) (6)	188	143.0	6.7
Survey of adult height from 13 American studies (treated and untreated patients) (8–20)	563	143.3	5.8

Table 2 Adult Turner Heights

n	Approx. mean	Approx. standard deviation	Ref.
24	142		8
25	140.9	6.4	9
46	141.2		10
30	140.2	5.2	11
18	144.0	7.1	12
24	144.2		13
46	143.8	5.6	14
109	143.6		15
54	143.3	5.0	16
28	142.0	7.6	17
66	147.0		18
7	142.6	4.8	19
56	142.7	5.9	20

Data compiled by F.A. Conte and M.M. Grumbach.

girl has a standardized height of 1.0 then her predicted adult height (cm) would be

$$143.0 + (1.0 \times 6.7) = 149.7$$

where 143 is the mean Turner adult height and 6.7 is the standard deviation. Since the standard deviation is estimated by Lyon et al. to be 0.047 times the mean height for age, the formula simplifies to merely

$$143 + (\text{current height } z\text{-score}) \times (0.047 \times 143)$$
$$= \frac{143 \times (\text{current height of patient})}{\text{mean Turner height for age of patient}}$$

Using half-year increments in age, the above formula is used to obtain the scaling factors in Table 3 for easy computation of LPG predictions. For example, for a girl 10 years old, her LPG predicted adult height is simply 1.197 times her current height.

Partial validation of the LPG method is provided by Lyon et al. (6). Twenty-nine girls with Turner syndrome were first seen between the ages of 3 and 12 and last seen between the ages of 19 and 24 years. These 29 patients were not among those used to establish the percentiles for untreated Turner patients. For these girls, the correlation between initial and final height standardized heights was 0.95. The average initial standardized height for these girls was approximate-

408   FRANE ET AL.

Table 3 Scaling Factors for Lyon-Preece-Grant
Predicted Turner Adult Height

Age (yr)	Scaling factor
3.0	1.696
3.5	1.631
4.0	1.570
4.5	1.473
5.5	1.429
6.0	1.387
6.5	1.360
7.0	1.333
7.5	1.308
8.0	1.284
8.5	1.261
9.0	1.239
9.5	1.217
10.0	1.197
10.5	1.179
11.0	1.163
11.5	1.146
12.0	1.130
12.5	1.117
13.0	1.104
13.5	1.091
14.0	1.078
14.5	1.066
15.0	1.055
15.5	1.043
16.0	1.032
16.5	1.022
17.0	1.016
17.5	1.010
18.0	1.004
18.5	1.002
19.0	1.000

ly -0.63, and their final average was approximately -0.51, an increase of only 0.12, which translates to approximately 0.8 cm. The standard deviation of the observed adult height about the LPG prediction was 2.1 cm, i.e., the majority (actually 21 of 29) of the adult heights were within 2.1 cm of the predicted adult height.

These data show that Turner girls do not tend to experience notable changes in height percentiles over long periods of time. For example, a Turner girl in the tenth percentile for Turner girls age 8 is likely to be in the 10th percentile of adult Turner women if left untreated. This is due in part to a lack of a pubertal growth spurt.

This conclusion is reinforced by examination of the pretreatment heights of 17 (out of 71) Turner patients from a Genentech clinical trial described by Rosenfeld et al. (21) for whom at least 3 years of pretreatment heights were available (Fig. 1). These trajectories are plotted on a background containing estimates of the 10th, 50th, and 90th percentiles for untreated Turner girls based on the data of Lyon et al. There is a remarkable tendency for these untreated patients to remain at more or less the same Turner percentile over long periods of

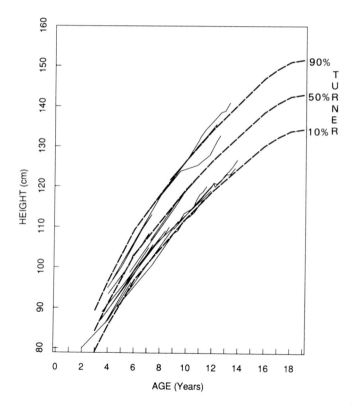

Figure 1 Pretreatment heights for 17 Turner syndrome patients with at least 3 years of pretreatment data.

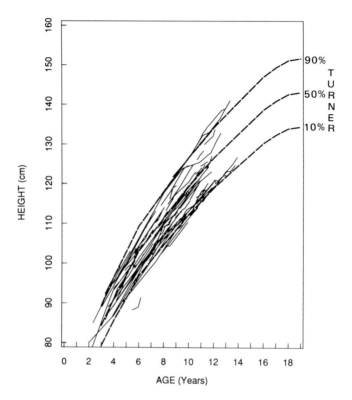

Figure 2 Pretreatment heights for 71 Turner syndrome patients.

time. Figure 2 shows all of the pretreatment heights for the 71 patients in the same Genentech clinical trial and reinforces the impression that untreated girls remain in the same percentile.

The use of the LPG prediction has been challenged on the grounds that it depends on the mean of 143 cm and that the true mean for Turner girls may be different, e.g., as a result of a possible trend over time to attain greater adult heights. A detailed discussion contained in Appendix I shows that the basic validity of the LPG estimate for a given patient's adult height does not depend on the accuracy of the mean height estimate of 143 cm.

A more detailed technical discussion contained in Appendix II shows that the LPG method can be refined further by taking into account the bone age of the patient.

BAYLEY-PINNEAU, ROCHE-WAINER-THISSEN, AND TANNER-WHITEHOUSE PREDICTED ADULT HEIGHT

The BP estimate of adult height is obtained by multiplying the current height by an appropriate factor. The multiplicative factor is tabulated according to sex, current Greulich-Pyle bone age, and current age. The RWT estimate is obtained from multiple linear regression using sex, parental height, and current age, weight, recumbent length, and the Roche-Wainer-Thissen bone age. The TW estimate is obtained from multiple linear regression using sex and current age, height, menarcheal status, and the Tanner-Whitehouse bone age. It also makes use of current growth rate and current rate of change in bone age if available.

Although these methods use different definitions of bone age, the differences do not seem to be substantial. See Appendix III for a detailed discussion.

COMPARISON OF METHODS OF PREDICTING ADULT HEIGHT

Table 4 summarizes the predicted adult heights using each method for 90 Turner patients (age 4 to 12) enrolled in two clinical studies sponsored by Genentech, Inc., the first of which is described by Rosenfeld et al. (21) and the second of which began in 1987. (Only those patients are included for whom all four methods of predicting adult height were computable.) The LPG and BP methods give average predicted adult heights similar to each other and to the adult heights from the European and American surveys (Table 1). (In addition, the mean standardized heights at the time of enrollment in the studies were 0.16 and -0.03, i.e., very close to zero.) This shows that the patients from the Genentech studies were similar to the European and American surveys.

Table 4 Predicted Adult Heights Before Treatment for Genentech Turner Patients

	Sample size	Mean (cm)	Standard deviation
Bayley-Pinneau	53	143.6	4.7
Predicted adult height	37	146.2	5.2
Roche-Wainer-Thissen	53	153.8	3.5
Predicted adult height	37	154.4	3.5
Tanner-Whitehouse	53	151.4	4.1
Predicted adult height	37	151.9	3.9
Lyon-Preece-Grant	53	141.9	5.5
Predicted adult height	37	142.8	5.8

The average RWT and TW predicted adult heights for the same patients are substantially greater than the European and American historical averages (Table 1). This observation is consistent with Zachmann et al. (22) who found that RWT and TW provide estimates of adult height that are too large and found the BP method to be more accurate on average than RWT and TW, although there were only six patients.

Additional information on predicted adult heights in general is given by Roche (26).

PARENTAL HEIGHT AND KARYOTYPE

Parental height is known to be a determinant of adult height. This influence seems to be evident in the first years of life and it is possible that parental height would be an important variable in predicting adult height of Turner patients. The pretreatment standardized height of girls in the Genentech clinical trials had a small but statistically significant correlation with mother's height ($n = 134$, $r = .43$, $p < 0.05$), consistent with other observations (19-24). (The father's heights were not measured by the investigators.)

Results regarding the effect of karyotype are mixed, e.g., Park et al. (17). We found no correlation between karyotype and pretreatment standardized height, which suggests that the specific karyotype is not an important determinant of stature.

PREDICTED ADULT HEIGHTS FOR TREATED PATIENTS

Although the BP and LPG estimates may be appropriate for untreated patients, they would not be appropriate for predicting adult height of patients undergoing any therapy to increase adult height. Since the RWT and TW methods provide estimates notably larger than the historical averages for untreated patients, they might be useful in predicting adult height for patients receiving optimal therapy or could prove to be an upper bound of what might be accomplished by optimal therapy.

To date, we have seen significant increases in the average BP and RWT estimates as the result of growth hormone treatment while the average TW estimate has remained essentially unchanged. Once a significant number of these patients have reached adult height, we will be able to rigorously interpret this increase in the BP estimate. In the mean time, the increase in BP provides a note of optimism about the effect of growth hormone treatment. It is not clear whether either RWT or TW may be useful or whether one is any better than the other as far as predicting adult height of optimally treated Turner girls.

CONCLUSIONS

The Lyon-Preece-Grant method and perhaps the Bayley-Pinneau method may be useful for estimating the adult height of a Turner girl assuming no treatment. For girls undergoing treatment, comparison of the height percentile during therapy with the pretreatment percentile may be a way of monitoring progress in the course of treatment. Bayley-Pinneau estimates might also be a useful way of monitoring progress. Roche-Wainer-Thissen and Tanner-Whitehouse should not be used to estimate adult height of untreated Turner patients although, in the future, RWT and TW may prove to be useful in estimating adult height of optimally treated patients.

ACKNOWLEDGMENTS

Results of the American survey of Turner studies were obtained from Felix Conte and Melvin Grumbach at the University of California at San Francisco. The conduct of the Genentech studies have involved a very large number of clinical investigators and Genentech staff. Data handling and statistical presentation have been handled primarily by Kerry Nemo and Peter Compton of Genentech.

APPENDIX I—INSENSITIVITY OF LPG TO MEAN ADULT HEIGHT

The use of the LPG prediction has been challenged on the grounds that it depends on the mean of 143 cm and that the true mean for Turner girls may be different, e.g., as a result of a possible trend over time to attain greater adult heights. The validity of LPG, however, does not overly depend on the estimated mean of 143 cm. To see that this is so, suppose, for example, that the real mean adult height is 147 cm (the highest mean reported among the studies in Table 3). This represents an increase of 2.8%. It would be natural to assume that the mean at each age would also increase by about 2.8% and that the standard deviation would be about 0.047 times the mean as for LPG. Under these assumptions, the modified LPG estimate becomes

$$\frac{147 \times (\text{current height of patient})}{\text{modified mean Turner height for age of patient}}$$

$$= \frac{1.028 \times 143 \times (\text{current height of patient})}{1.028 \times (\text{mean LPG Turner height for age of patient})}$$

where the modified mean Turner height is 1.028 times the LPG mean Turner height for the age of the patient in question. This reduces, then, to exactly the same formula as was given previously since the factor of 1.028 appears in both the numerator and denominator. Thus, the basic validity of the LPG estimate for a given patient's adult height does not depend on the accuracy of the mean adult height estimate of 143 cm.

In fact, the LPG predicted adult height can be obtained more simply as

$$\frac{\text{(current height)}}{\text{(\% of adult height attained by average Turner girl of this age)}}$$

The simplest way, however, is just

(current height) $\times$ (scaling factor for age)

where the scaling factor for age is just the reciprocal of the percent of adult height attained by average Turner girl of the same age as the girl in question. To facilitate these computations, the scaling factors for ages 3 to 19 are listed in Table 3.

APPENDIX II—USE OF BONE AGES IN LPG

The LPG method can be refined further by taking into account the bone age of the patient. The average bone age deficit is approximately 1.3 years for Turner girls between the ages of 3 and 14 (7), similar to the deficit of 1.2 years was found in the patients in the first Genentech clinical trial. The mean height for a given bone age, x, is equal to the mean height for age $x + 1.3$. Using data from the Genentech clinical trial, the standard deviation is 0.85 $\times$ 0.047 times the mean height for bone age. (To obtain the 0.85 adjustment, a preliminary standardization was first obtained by using 0.047 times the mean height for bone age, as would be done for standardizing height for chronological age. The standard deviation of these scores was 0.85 times the standard deviation of the heights standardized for age.) The most important use of the bone age is, of course, when the girl in question has an advanced bone age or a bone age that is unusually delayed. As for the ordinary LPG estimate, the bone age adjusted estimate could be simply obtained as

(current height) $\times$ (scaling factor for bone age)

More normative data are needed to firmly establish the scaling factors for bone age.

APPENDIX III—BONE AGES USED IN PREDICTING ADULT HEIGHT

The BP predicted adult height uses the detailed version of the Greulich and Pyle (GP) method of estimating bone ages (24). The RWT and TW predicted adult heights use their own corresponding bone age determinations. However, for our computations, the GP bone ages (determined by Dr. Alex Roche's group at the Fels Institute) were used not only for the BP estimate but also for the RWT and TW equations. It is not believed that the use of GP bone ages has had a substantial effect on the average RWT or TW predicted adult height.

A partial validation of the use of GP for the purposes at hand was obtained by having the TW bone ages of 66 X-rays determined by Dr. Leslie Cox at the Institute of Child Health in London. The mean GP bone age from the Fels Institute for these patients was 9.0 years while the mean TW bone age was 9.1 years. The correlation of the GP and TW bone ages was 0.97.

One of the problems with using BP, RWT, and TW for Turner girls is that bone ages of Turner girls are more difficult to determine accurately than the bone ages of normal girls.

REFERENCES

1. Bayley N, Pinneau S. Tables for predicting adult height from skeletal age. J of Pediatrics 1952; 50:423–441.
2. Post E, Richman R. A condensed table for predicting adult stature. J of Pediatrics 1981; 98:440–441.
3. Roche AF, Wainer H, Thissen D. Predicting Adult Stature for Individuals. S. Karger, Basel, 1975.
4. Tanner JM, Landt KW, Cameron N, Carter BS, Patel J. Prediction of adult height from height and bone age in childhood. Arch Dis Child 1983; 58: 767–776.
5. Tanner JM, Whitehouse RM, Marshall WA, Healy MJR, Goldstein H. Assessment of skeletal maturity and prediction of adult height (TW2 method). Academic Press, London, 1975.
6. Lyon AJ, Preece MA, Grant DB. Growth curve for girls with Turner syndrome. Arch Dis Child 1985; 60:932–935.
7. Ranke MB, Pfluger H, Rosendahl W, Stubbe P, Enders H, Bierich JR, Majewski F. Turner syndrome: spontaneous growth in 150 cases and review of the literature. Eur J Pediatrics 1983; 141:81–88.
8. Heskel M, Haddad HM, Wilkens L. Congenital anomalies associated with gonadal aplasia. Pediatrics 1959; 23:895.
9. Engel E, Forbes AP. Cytogenetic and clinical findings in 48 patients with congenitally defective or absent ovaries. Medicine 1965; 44:135–164.
10. Goldberg MB, Sailly AL, Solomon IL, Steinbach HL. Gonadal dysgenesis in phenotypic female subjects: a review of 87 cases with cytogenetic studies in 53. Amer J Med 1968; 45:529–543.
11. Johanson AJ, Brasel JA, Blizzard RM. Growth in patients with gonadal dysgenesis receiving fluoxymesterone. J Pediatrics 1969; 75:1015–1021.
12. Snider ME, Solomon IL. Ultimate height in chromosomal gonadal dysgenesis without androgen therapy. Amer J Dis Child 1974; 127:673–674.
13. Moore DC, Tattoni DS, Ruvalcaba RHA, Limbeck GA, Kelly VC. Studies

of anabolic steroids VI: Effect of prolonged administration of oxandrolone on growth in children and adolescents with gonadal dysgenesis. J Pediatrics 1977; 90:462–466.

14. Urban MD, Lee PA, Dorst JP, Plotnick LP, Migeon CJ. Oxandrolone therapy in patients with Turner syndrome. J Pediatrics 1979; 94:823–827.

15. Conte FA, Grumbach MM. Estrogen use in children and adolescents: a survey. Pediatrics 1978; 62:supp. 1091–1097.

16. Lippe BM. In Ovarian Failure in Clinical Pediatrics and Adolescent Endocrinology, Kaplan SA (ed). W.B. Saunders, Philadelphia, 1982, p. 280.

17. Park E, Bailey JD, Cowell CA. Growth and maturation of patients with Turner's syndrome. Ped Res 1983; 17:1–6.

18. Sybert VP. Adult height in Turner syndrome with and without androgen therapy. J Pediatrics 1984; 99:365–369.

19. Demetriou D, Emans SJ, Crigler JF. Final height in estrogen-treated patients with Turner syndrome. Obst Gyn 1984; 64:459–464.

20. Rodens KP, Alexander RL, Conte FA, Grumbach MM, Kaplan SL. The effects of initiating estrogen treatment in adolescence in the syndrome of gonadal dysgenesis. In preparation, 1988.

21. Rosenfeld RG, Hintz RL, Johanson AJ, Brasel JA, Burstein S, Chernausek SD, Clabots T, Frane J, Gotlin RW, Kuntze J, Lippe B, Mahoney PC, Moore WV, New MI, Saenger P, Stoner E, Sybert V. Methionyl human growth hormone and oxandrolone in Turner syndrome: preliminary results of a prospective randomized trial. J of Pediatrics 1986; 109:936–943.

22. Zachmann MB, Sobradillo B, Frank M, Frisch H, Prader A. Bayley-Pinneau, Roche-Wainer-Thissen, and Tanner height predictions in normal children and in patients with various pathologic conditions. J of Pediatrics 1978; 98:749–755.

23. Roche AF. Adult stature prediction: a critical review. Acta Med Auxol 1984; 16:5–28.

24. Greulich WW, Pyle SI. Radiographic atlas of skeletal development of the hand and wrist, ed 2. Stanford Univ. Press, Stanford, CA, 1959.

DISCUSSION

DR. JAMES TANNER: It makes a lot of sense that the RWT and the TW predictions are wrong in this situation. Also, it makes sense that you would expect Bailey-Pinneau to be wrong, because what they are really doing is adjusting the situation for whether you are into an early or a later adolescent growth spurt, and they use the bone age to cope with that situation, but there ain't no adolescent growth spurt. There is, however, a more subtle point, perhaps, and that is that, if under treatment, you alter the shape of the curve that is being traced out and turn the thing into a steeper sort of parabola, you do not quite know what you are turning it into, then you may have some problems in the evolving changes in the predicted adult height. I think all I am saying is that if you impose a sort of iatrogenic spurt on the kids, then you may perhaps depart from the nonspurt predictions. That could, it seems to me, be something of a problem. What is your reaction to that?

DR. JAMES FRANE: We noticed over a period of time during which the girls were treated that there was very little change in the Roche-Weiner-Theissen estimate, but there was a modest increase in the Tanner-Whitehouse estimate. And, as Dr. Rosenfield pointed out, there was quite a bit of change in the Bailey-Pinneau.

DR. MICHAEL PREECE: Through the last couple of days I have steadily seen everything I was going to say tomorrow said by somebody else. I have got one thing left, but I will leave that for tomorrow. There is one other item, just to complete that comment, about the bone age. We did look at our 29 patients for validity of the prediction and tried putting bone age into the system directly and it did not improve the prediction one iota. The only thing it did do was that the two worst predicting children were ones with very unusually delayed bone ages. And they were sort of whipped into line a little bit, not completely but a little bit. So it may be with a larger database and that is something we need to look at (maybe you have already done that too), we could actually really look at whether bringing in the bone age we can further refine the prediction.

DR. TANNER: Dr. Preece, did you look at putting in the mean parent height, or is that redundant, given their height now?

Dr. James Tanner is at the University of Texas Health Center, Houston, Texas. Dr. James W. Frane is with Genentech, Inc., South San Francisco, California. Dr. Michael Preece is at the Institute of Child Health, London, England. Dr. Robert Blizzard is at the University of Virginia at Charlottesville, Charlottesville, Virginia. Dr. Felix Conte is at the University of California at San Francisco, San Francisco, California.

DR. PREECE: I have the suspicion that that is the case, but in the data set we were using we did not have adequate numbers of individuals with good measured parental data. I am very keen to revalidate this method with the new data set with extra information, because what we have not done now is to have gone back and, having used our own patients for cross-validation, incorporated them back into the whole prediction system and refined the coefficient slightly. We now need a whole new data set to actually fully test that, the parental heights being one of the things. So if there are any offers . . .

DR. TANNER: In the Genentech combined study I trust and hope we have got measured parental heights on everybody. I think for the most part we have measured maternal heights, but in general we have very few, if any, paternal heights that have been measured.

   The points Dr. Preece made about how much does the bone age help? Well, in general, for all of these variables where there is just a little bit of correlation, it tells us something about the extreme patients and I think it is important. If you have the child who is especially retarded or who happens not to be retarded, then that girl is not exactly where you think she is. And the same sort of thing goes for the parent heights, that for the most part the big value is taking into account the extraordinarily tall or short parents. For the kids whose parents are more or less normal, it squeezes the estimate down a little bit, but it is not something that is very spectacular.

DR. ROBERT BLIZZARD: A couple of questions that require clarification first. In the Ranke data, these patients were untreated as I have understood the last couple of days, and the American data, if I heard correctly, is a hodgepodge, and that certainly would have to be taken into consideration because that means that there must be patients in there who were treated with estrogen 20 years ago and in doses that were a bit excessive. In the Preece data, I am totally unclear as to whether these patients had any interference in respect to their growth.

DR. FRANE: I believe that the ones that were used to establish the norms were all reputedly untreated. The 29 patients who were used to cross-validate, most of them probably were treated with estrogen. The reason that I include all of those American patients in illustrating the average is that we have heard over and over again that the estrogens have had no effect on the average.

DR. BLIZZARD: But that is low dose, not high dose and in the days of the "giants" the dosages that were used were significant. They were not always low dose.

DR. FRANE: You are saying that you believe then that the children ended up shorter than they would have been if they had not been treated?

DR. BLIZZARD: They may have. Now, in respect to the data that you showed of the various groups through the years, there were some phenomenal figures in respect to the range of individual heights, if I read the slide right. Something like as high as 167 cm, is that it? Now I wonder about those particular patients and you may not have any way to ferret that out, but I suppose it is possible that there are patients in there that might be pure gonadal agenesis.

DR. FRANE: I think there is a real possibility there. I think that there is a lot of dirt and noise associated with all of these data dealing with the heights and the effects of treatment. I think that what we are getting here is not any kind of a definitive prediction equation or that definitive answer to the average height, but a fairly good ballpark estimate as to what these girls look like.

DR. FELIX CONTE: Data that was extracted came basically from the old data of Haddad, at Johns Hopkins, and from Engels' and Forbes' data. Now when we go through the chart or the paper, you can compare karyotypes and final heights. No patient with XY gonadal dysgenesis or XX gonadal dysgenesis was included in that calculation. It is true that the "giants" treated late, and they treated with rather large doses of estrogen. The mean heights in those patients before 1969 were basically Engle's and Forbes' and Haddad's from Hopkins, and were 141.5 cm. All you can do is look at what is reported and their karyotype vs. final height. I have a feeling that in all reports they did not measure them that well. But that is what we have to work with when we look at retrospective data.

DR. TANNER: Dr. Preece, could you answer that previous question: In your group, were they untreated or treated?

DR. PREECE: The group that everything was standardized on were untreated.

34

Clinical Trials of Human Growth Hormone Therapy in Turner Syndrome in Japan

Kazue Takano and Kazuo Shizume

Tokyo Women's Medical College, Tokyo, Japan

Itsuro Hibi

National Children's Hospital, Tokyo, Japan

The members of the committee for the treatment of Turner's Syndrome

The Foundation for Growth Science in Japan, Tokyo, Japan

INTRODUCTION

Turner syndrome is a genetic disorder with many physical abnormalities. Short stature is one of them. For treatment of short stature, anabolic steroids, low doses of estrogen, and/or human growth hormone (hGH) have been used (1-5). Since the success of hGH synthesis by recombinant DNA technology (6), clinical trials of hGH treatment have been systematically employed in United States and Japan. Recently, Rosenfeld et al. (7) reported the effectiveness of hGH treatment in American patients with Turner syndrome. We previously reported the biological effects of met-hGH in 20 patients with Turner syndrome. This chapter will present preliminary data of clinical trials of human growth hormone therapy in Turner syndrome in Japan.

PATIENT SELECTION AND STUDY DESIGN

One hundred and forty-eight patients with Turner syndrome were accepted from endocrinologists from multiple centers within Japan. The criteria for acceptance into the study are listed in Table 1. At the beginning of the study, they submitted to the following: growth hormone stimulation test, oral glucose tolerance test, LH-RH-test, hand and wrist X-ray examination, and other routine chemistries.

Table 1 Criteria of Turner Syndrome for the Acceptance of Clinical Trials of Recombinant hGH Treatment

1. Sex chromosome analysis suitable for Turner syndrome
2. Birth body weight more than 2000 g
3. Chronological age more than 5 years old
4. Body height less than −2.0 SD of age-matched normal girls
5. Bone age less than 11 years old
6. No previous therapy

Clinical trials were performed with methionyl hGH (m-hGH) the first time (started June 1986) and methionine-free hGH (mf-hGH) the second time (started September 1986). Thirty-two patients were treated with m-hGH 0.5 IU/kg/week divided two to four times per week, and 25 patients with a combination of m-hGH (0.5 IU/kg/week) and anabolic steroid (stanozolol, 1 mg/day). Forty-five patients were treated with mf-hGH 0.5 IU/kg/week, and 46 patients with mf-hGH 1.0 IU/kg/week divided two to six times per week. The patients' heights were measured once a month. Blood count, urinalysis, routine chemistries, HbA_1, hormones (T_3, T_4, TSH, somatomedin C), and antibody against hGH were measured every 2 months. Bone age was evaluated using the method of Tanner et al. (TW2 method) (1975) by one specialist every 6 months.

Informed consent was obtained from each patient and her parents, and the experimental protocol was approved by the Human Subjects Investigation Committee of each department. Clinical findings or these patients are shown in Table 2. There was no difference between the two groups of the first trial by m-hGH treatment and between the two groups of the second trial by mf-hGH treatment, respectively.

Table 2 Clinical Findings in Patients with Turner Syndrome

	First trial (from June 1986)		Second trial (from Sept. 1986)	
	Somatonorm 0.5 IU/kg/wk	Somatonorm 0.5 IU/kg/wk + anabolic H	SM-9500 0.5 IU/kg/wk	SM-9500 1.0 IU/kg/wk
Case	32	25	45	46
Chr. age (yr)	10.7 ± 2.8	10.8 ± 3.2	11.1 ± 3.0	11.1 ± 2.9
Chr. age (yr)	8.5 ± 2.4	8.7 ± 2.5	9.4 ± 2.2	9.1 ± 2.5
Height (SD)	−3.9 ± 1.0	−3.7 ± 1.0	−3.6 ± 0.9	−3.8 ± 1.2

Table 3 Growth Rate in Patients with Turner Syndrome Treated by Recombinant hGH for 6 Months

		Growth rate (cm/year)			
		Before		During	
Treatment	Cases	M ± SEM	Range	M ± SEM	Range
First clinical trial					
Somatonorm (0.5)	32	3.7 ± 0.2	1.5–6.0	5.1 ± 0.3	1.4–8.0
Somatonorm (0.5) + anabolic H	25	3.8 ± 0.2	2.0–5.9	6.9 ± 0.4	2.6–10.4
Second clinical trial					
SM-9500 (0.5)	45	3.8 ± 0.1	1.6–6.1	5.4 ± 0.2	1.8–9.9
SM-9500 (1.0)	46	3.5 ± 0.1	1.0–5.9	6.1 ± 0.2	3.0–9.6

Synthetic methionyl hGH (m-hGH; Somatonorm) and methionine-free hGH (mf-hGH, SM-9500) were kindly provided from KabiVitrum AB, Stockholm, Sweden.

CLINICAL RESULTS

We show here the results of 6-month treatments. The growth rates before and during hGH treatment are shown in Table 3. The growth rate before treatment was an actual growth rate prior to the treatment, and the growth rate during hGH treatment was calculated from the 6-month treatment. The mean growth rates before treatment ranged between 3.5 to 3.8 cm/year. During the 6 months of treatment, the mean growth rates increased between 5.1 and 6.9 cm/year. The numbers of patients who grew 1.5 cm more than the pretreatment value were 19 of 32 (59.4%), 20 of 25 (80.0%), 25 of 45 (55.6%), and 35 of 46 (76.1%), re-

Table 4 Change of Bone Age (TW2 method) Before and 6 Months After hGH Treatment in Patients with Turner Syndrome

Treatment	Cases	Before	After	Change
First clinical trial				
Somatonorm (0.5)	17	8.2 ± 0.6	8.7 ± 0.6	0.4 ± 0.1
Somatonorm (0.5) + Anabolic H	16	9.4 ± 0.5	9.9 ± 0.5	0.5 ± 0.1
Second clinical trial				
SM-9500 (0.5)	37	9.1 ± 0.4	9.4 ± 0.4	0.3 ± 0.0
SM-9500 (1.0)	39	9.0 ± 0.4	9.4 ± 0.4	0.4 ± 0.0

spectively. The bone age did not accelerate during the treatment with hGH, as shown in Table 4.

Antibody against hGH appeared in 64.3% of m-hGH treated patients and in 4.5% of mf-hGH treated patients, respectively.

DISCUSSION

We investigated the effect of recombinant-hGH on growth in 148 patients with Turner syndrome for 6 months. Ninety-nine patients increased the growth rate

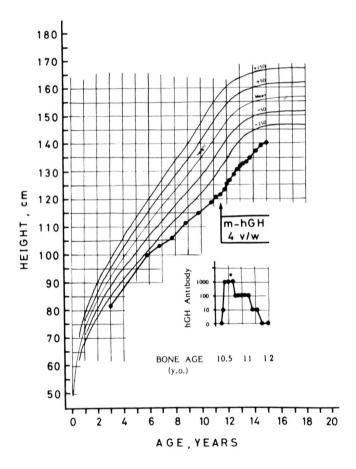

Figure 1 Effect of m-hGH treatment on height increase and the production of anti-hGH antibody in a patient with Turner syndrome. At the age of 12.2 years (*), the m-hGH preparation was changed from batch No. 82412 to 81000. ECP contents in these batches were 220 and 3 ng per vial, respectively.

Table 5 Effect of hGH in Turner Syndrome Reported in Literature

Ref.	n	Duration	Dose	Effect
(1)	3	2 X 2 days	40–120 μg/kg	anabolic response (+)
(2)	2	4 months	5 mg/day	3.2 → 6.8 cm/yr
(3)	5	12 months	20 IU/wk	2.9 → 3.9 cm/yr
(5)	8	6 months	12 IU/wk	2.6 → n = 2, 6–8 cm/yr
				→ n = 6, 2.2 cm/yr
(10)	35	6 months	0.6 IU/kg/wk	3.2 → 6.6 cm/yr
	22	12 months	0.6 IU/kg/wk	3.2 → 5.9 cm/yr
(9)	20	6 months	16 IU/wk	3.7 → 5.7 cm/yr
(7)	17	0–12 months	0.75 IU/kg/wk	4.5 → 6.6 cm/yr
		12–24 months	0.75 IU/kg/wk	→ 5.4 cm/yr

more than 1.5 cm as compared to the pretreatment value. The mean growth increase was similar to that reported earlier by us in another study (9). Eight out of 20 patients reported in 1986 had been treated with m-hGH for more than 3 years, and the mean growth rates (m ± SD) of years 1, 2, and 3 were 6.3 ± 1.3, 5.3 ± 1.9, and 3.8 ± 1.6 cm/year, respectively. Figure 1 shows one such patient who has been treated with m-hGH for more than 3 years. Her growth rate for years 1, 2, and 3 was 7.4, 4.3, and 5.5 cm/year, respectively. Table 5 summarizes the effect of hGH in Turner syndrome reported in the literature.

Further study will be required to conclude the effect of hGH treatment on both physical and psychological functions in patients with Turner syndrome.

ACKNOWLEDGMENTS

The authors are very grateful to Sumitomo Pharmaceutical Co., Ltd. (Osaka, Japan) and KabiVitrum AB (Stockholm, Sweden) for supplying methionyl- and methionine-free hGH preparations. This report was supported by a research grant from the Foundation for Growth Science in Japan.

REFERENCES

1. Almqvist S, Hall K, Lindstedt S, Lindsten J, Luft R, Sjöberg HE. Effects of short term administration of physiological doses of human growth hormone in three patients with Turner's syndrome. Acta Endocrinol (Copenhagen) 1964; 46:451–464.
2. Hutchings JJ, Escamilla RF, Li CH, Forsham PH. Li human growth hormone administration in gonadal dysgenesis. Am J Dis Child 1965; 109:318–321.
3. Tanner JM, Whitehouse RH, Hughes PCR, Vince FP. Effect of human growth hormone treatment for 1 to 7 years on the growth of 100 children, with growth hormone deficiency, low birthweight, inherited smallness,

Turner's syndrome and other complaints. Arch Dis Child 1971; 46:754–782.

4. Ross JL, Lauren M, Lynn DL, Cutler GB. Growth hormone secretory dynamics in Turner syndrome. J Pediatr 1985; 106:202–206.
5. Stahnke N. Human growth hormone treatment in short children without growth hormone deficiency. N Engl J Med 1984; 310:925–926.
6. Goeddel DV, Heyneker HL, Hozumi T, Arentzen R, Itakura K, Yansura DG, Ross MJ, Miozzari G, Crea R, Seeburg PH. Direct expression in Escherichia coli of a DNA sequence coding for human growth hormone. Nature 1979; 281:544–548.
7. Rosenfeld RG, Hintz RL, Johnson AJ, Sherman B, the Genentech Collaborative Group. Results from the first 2 years of a clinical trial with recombinant DNA-derived human growth hormone (Somatonorm) in Turner's syndrome. Acta Poediatr Scand (suppl) 1987; 331:59–66.
8. Tanner JM, Whitehouse RH, Marchall WA, Healy MJR, Goldstein H. Assessment of Skeletal Maturity and Prediction of Adult Height (TW2 method). Academic Press Inc., London, 1975.
9. Takano K, Hizuka N, Shizume K. Treatment of Turner's syndrome with methionyl human growth hormone for six months. Acta Endocrinol 1986; 112:130–137.
10. Raiti S, Kaplan SL, August GP. Growth-stimulating effects of human growth hormone therapy in Turner's syndrome. A preliminary report. In Raiti S, Tolman RA (ed). Human growth hormone. Plenum Medical, New York, 1986; pp. 109–113.
11. Rauch HL, Butenandt O. Prospektive Endgröße bei 28 Patientinnen mit Ullrich-Turner-Syndrom. Mschr. Kinderheilkunde 1988; 136:703.
12. Brook CDG, Mürset G, Zachmann M, Prader A. Growth in children with 45 XO-Turner's syndrome. Arch Dis childh 1974; 49:789.

DISCUSSION

DR. OTFRID BUTENANDT: In 1988 it will be 60 years that research started in our house on children with gonadal dysgenesis. When Ullrich presented his first case, he stated that this is a typical entity and the cause must be in the same drawer as was the cause for Down's syndrome and should be found. He was right, those were chromosomal disorders. At noontime today, it only came into

Dr. Otfrid Butenandt is at the Children's Hospital, University of München, München, Germany. Dr. Wayne Moore is at the University of Kansas Medical Center, Kansas City, Kansas. Dr. David Rimoin is at the Cedars-Sinai Medical Center, Los Angeles, California. Dr. Jaako Perheentupa is at the University Children's Hospital, Helsinki, Finland.

my mind that actually Ulrich has followed the line of logic in looking at lymphatics for the malformations.

Now to the topics I would like to address. You have heard that prediction of height cannot be really done using the three methods, and these methods are based on observations of healthy girls. However, if you wanted to know how good they were, you would start to evaluate a cohort of girls who have reached final height and recalculate their predictions from the original X-rays. We have done this from our files.

Using the method of Roche-Weiner-Theissen, there is a high overprediction of height, and this cannot be used at all (Fig. 2). Using the method of Tanner-Whitehouse with three variables, in the younger age group there are only six patients, but there is 5% confidence so these are two different numbers (Fig. 3).

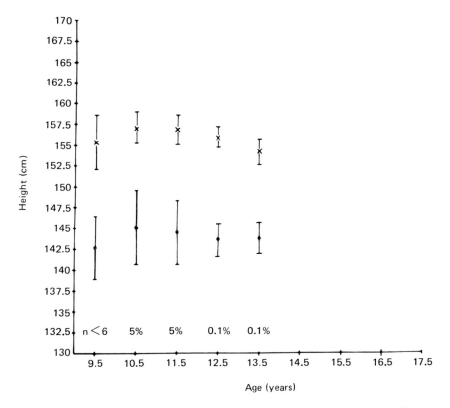

Figure 2 Determination of final height using the method of Roche-Wainer-Thissen (1975). · Attained final height. x estimated final height. (I 95 percent confidence intervals.

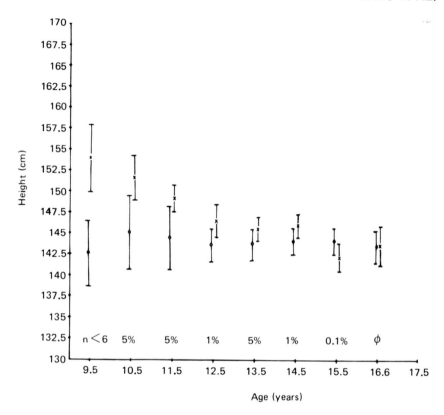

Figure 3 Determination of final height using the method of Tanner-Whitehouse II (1975). •–Attained final height. x–estimated final height.

There is a big difference between the prediction and the actual attained height of these girls, and it's already stated earlier that the closer you come to final height, the more precise your predictions will be. Increasing the numbers of variables does not help too much.

Now, when you come to Bailey-Pinot, then you really find quite a practical way to predict final height, but still there is some discrepancy in a group of only six children. It is remarkably well done to age 13, 14, then there is a discrepancy until the end (Fig. 4).

Now taking this into account, we took our data and compiled some data from untreated patients from the literature to recalculate the percentage of reached final height. The original Bailey-Pinot curve does not fit the Ulrich-Turner girls as well. I must admit that the database is still too small to say this is definite, and this should be done with a bigger database, too.

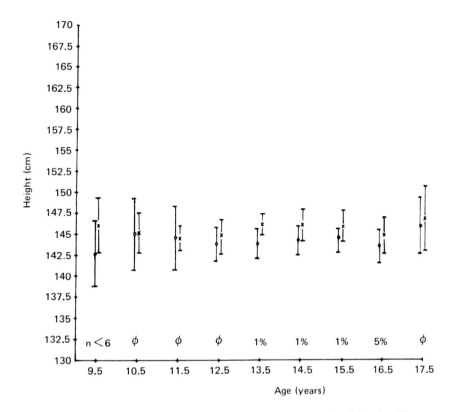

Figure 4 Determination of final height using the method of Bayley-Pinneau (1952). •-Attained final height. x-estimated final height.

Now you can see that Brook's data fit very well onto this curve, but this must be because some of this data are in the calculations (Fig. 5) (Ref. 11, 12). But there is another thing. Some girls have received anabolic steroids during approximately this age, and later on low or higher dosages of estrogen. Again these values fit very well to the curve. And we suggest to use a curve like this may be better with more data for the prediction in Ulrich-Turner syndrome.

DR. WAYNE MOORE: I want to make a comment about the overnight growth hormone secretory profiles. We have done sequential overnight profiles on two consecutive nights in about 30 children, and we find significant variation between the nights as far as the overnight secretory mean growth hormone profiles are concerned. I, therefore, question whether any of the overnight profiles are evaluable without objective sleep data such as EEG monitoring. The other thing

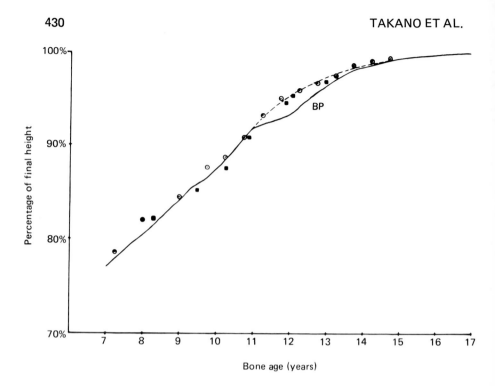

Figure 5 Percentage of final height in Ullrich-Turner-syndrome at a given bone age. BP = Bayley-Pinneau-Dates. ⊙ = own values. ■ = values from Brook et al. 1974.

I wanted to show is one case of a child that we treated with Turner syndrome. We initially started her on oxandrolone therapy at about 9 years of age because we did not have anything else to treat her with, and you can see she was treated with oxandrolone until 16 years of age. At about 14 years of age her growth rate started decreasing as is typical with the girls that have received oxandrolone. We then started her on growth hormone (Protropin), and we have gotten an additional 5, almost 6 cm of growth after cessation of growth with the oxandrolone therapy. I present this as a possible alternative form of therapy for girls with Turner syndrome that would be less expensive in terms of growth hormone cost. Maybe the accomplishment of the same result is possible, as far as adult height is concerned.

DR. DAVID RIMOIN: Before this conversation on growth promotion ceases, I just thought I would let this audience know about the experience in various centers in Europe now with leg length lengthening for skeletal dysplasias. In

Russia, Italy, and Spain there have been some very active groups of orthopedic surgeons who have been using percutaneous techniques to lengthen bones. Instead of getting growth rates of 7 cm, they are getting growth rates of 30 cm a year. And actually some of these, especially the group in Barcelona, that of Dr. Bill Arubius, has increased length of achondroplastic dwarfs by over 30 cm, with two days in hospital on two different occasions. He claims very little vascular/ neurologic effect. Obviously these have not been well studied yet in terms their physiological effects, but he has done a number of Turner syndrome patients as well and claims that he has good results with them. I know that there are several of these people that are coming to a symposium here sometime during this year and I am sure that you will be hearing about this from your orthopedic colleagues.

We are going to be starting a trial of certain of these techniques and try to control for some of the adverse effects that might happen, but with personally seeing the kids who are a foot larger in height than they were the year before, I think we are all going to have to pay some attention to this technique.

DR. JAAKKO PERHENTUPA: This in direct reply to what you said, Dr. Rimoin. I think a foot or 30 cm is a little bit exaggerated because you would have to stretch the nerves and everything else, which does not work out. As far as I have heard, and this is something that is discussed, 10 cm, at the most, over one year is a more realistic figure.

DR. RIMOIN: Well, I think you can get all stages. The ones that I have seen have achieved 30 cm in a little over a year and this, I think, because they were achondroplastic dwarfs and achondroplastic dwarfs have excess soft tissues. But certainly it is possible. Now the Wagner technique that has been used for years has involved open reduction and a lot of complications. These are all percutaneous techniques. The Russians have a lot of foot drop after this. There are a lot of questions that have to be answered, but I think you are going to be hearing a lot more about this technique.

35

Effects of Growth Hormone and Oxandrolone on Carbohydrate Metabolism in Turner Syndrome

Darrell M. Wilson, Raymond L. Hintz, and Ron G. Rosenfeld

Stanford University School of Medicine, Stanford, California

James W. Frane, Barry M. Sherman, Ann J. Johanson, and The Genentech Turner's Collaborative Group*

Genentech, Inc., South San Francisco, California

INTRODUCTION

Many patients with Turner syndrome have impaired glucose tolerance (1-10). Since therapies to increase adult height may further impair carbohydrate metabolism, we evaluated the effect of methionyl human growth hormone (GH) (Protropin) and oxandrolone (Anavar), alone and in combination, on glucose metabolism in girls with Turner syndrome (11).

METHODS

Seventy-one girls with Turner syndrome, 4.7 to 12.4 years of age, were studied at 11 medical centers. The details concerning these subjects and their growth response to the various therapies have been reported (12) and appear elsewhere in this book. The subjects were randomly allocated to four groups: no therapy; oxandrolone (0.125 mg/kg body weight, adjusted to the nearest half pill, po daily); GH (0.125 mg/kg body weight, IM three time weekly); and a combination of both therapies. GH was given daily (0.125 mg/kg) for the first 4 days of the study. Subjects receiving therapy had standard oral glucose tolerance tests

---

*See Appendix for full list of collaborators.

(OGTT) (1.75 g/kg-maximum 75 g) with measurement of plasma glucose and serum insulin concentrations before therapy and at 5 days, 2 months, and 12 months while control subjects had OGTTs at baseline and 12 months. The laboratory determinations were performed separately at each of the 11 clinical centers.

Integrated glucose and insulin levels were calculated (after subtracting the baseline concentration from the concentration obtained at each subsequent time point) using the trapezoidal method. National Diabetes Data Group criteria for children (13-14) were used to define impaired glucose tolerance (fasting glucose < 140 mg/dl and a 2-hr value > 140 mg/dl).

Between-group comparisons were made using the two-sample t-test. Within-group changes over time were evaluated using paired t-test. P-values less than 0.05 were considered significant.

RESULTS

Baseline

Fasting plasma glucose concentrations among the Turner subjects at baseline were normal (88 ± 13 mg/dl). Prior to any therapy, however, 11 of 71 (15%) subjects had impaired glucose tolerance. Integrated glucose levels at baseline were similar in each group and were not correlated with age. There was a significant positive correlation between age and integrated insulin concentrations ($r = 0.5$, $p < 0.001$). Integrated insulin levels were similar in each group (ANOVA, $p = 0.08$).

Treatment

The mean fasting plasma glucose concentration did not rise in any of the treatment groups. Mean integrated glucose concentrations, however, increased significantly among those receiving oxandrolone at 2 months and 12 months and for those receiving combination therapy at 5 days (Fig. 1, paired t-test, $p < 0.05$).

Mean fasting insulin levels increased significantly only in the combination group at 5 days and 2 months. Integrated insulin concentrations rose significantly among the subjects who received oxandrolone, either alone or in combination (Fig. 2). There were significant increases in the mean integrated insulin concentrations at 2- and 12-month visits for the group receiving oxandrolone alone. The group receiving combination therapy had significant increases in integrated insulin concentrations at all three follow-up OGTTs. There were no sig-

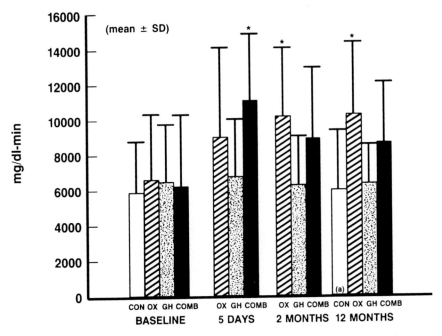

Figure 1 Effect of therapy on mean (± 1 SD) integrated glucose concentrations at 5 days, 2 months, and 12 months. * indicates a significant difference from baseline (a) Data from one control subject with a clearly abnormal OGTT (peak glucose, 624 mg/dl) has been removed from the 12 months data in this figure. (Reprint with permission from Ref. 11.)

nificant increases in integrated insulin in the GH only group through the first year.

The proportion of subjects with impaired glucose tolerance reached a maximum of 53% in the combination group 5 days following the initiation of therapy, significantly higher than the pretreatment value of 16% (Table 1, $p < 0.005$). Despite the increased incidence of impaired glucose tolerance in the subjects receiving oxandrolone, there was no significant difference between the control group and any of the treatment groups in glycosylated hemoglobin levels obtained at the end of one year of treatment. There was no glycosuria during the study.

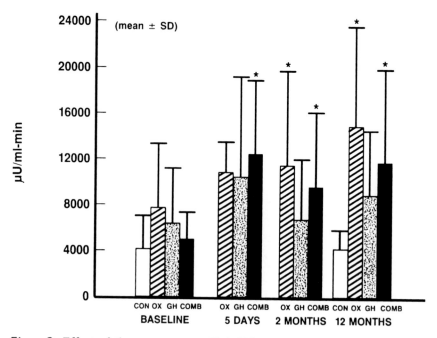

Figure 2 Effect of therapy on mean (± 1 SD) integrated insulin concentrations at 5 days, 2 months, and 12 months. * indicates a significant difference from baseline. (Reprint with permission from Ref. 11.)

Table 1 Number of Subjects with Impaired Glucose Tolerance (National Diabetes Data Group Criteria)

	All subjects	CON	OX	GH	COMB
Baseline	11/71	3/18	3/19	4/17	1/17
	15%	17%	16%	24%	6%
5 days			3/19	5/17	9/17
			16%	29%	53%*
2 months			5/18	2/16	4/16
			28%	13%	25%
12 months		2/15	7/16	1/16	4/14
		15%	44%	6%	29%

Number of subjects with impaired glucose tolerance/Total number of subjects in group.
Changes in the percent of subjects with impaired glucose tolerance within each group were evaluated using McNemar test of symmetry; * $p < 0.05$.
CON = control group; OX = oxandrolone group; GH = methionyl human growth hormone group; COMB = combination methionyl human growth hormone and oxandrolone group.

DISCUSSION

Growth hormone has significant effects on carbohydrate metabolism, and many studies have examined the effect of GH on carbohydrate metabolism in Turner syndrome (10,15-18). In our subjects, there was no significant change in mean fasting glucose or insulin concentration, mean integrated glucose or insulin concentration, or the proportion of subjects with impaired glucose tolerance following OGTT in subjects treated with GH alone. These findings are consistent with those reported earlier (10,15,17-19). Insulin concentrations were not reported in any of these studies.

The mean integrated insulin concentration for the GH group after five daily injections of GH was nearly twice that of the baseline concentration ($p = 0.06$) and equal to the mean value of the oxandrolone group. During this phase of the study, the subjects were receiving nearly twice as much GH per week as they did during the rest of the study. These data suggest that doses of GH in excess of 0.375 mg/kg per week may result in impaired glucose tolerance in girls with Turner syndrome. Alternatively, the impaired glucose tolerance during the first 4 days of GH therapy may merely reflect an acute metabolic response which is eventually compensated for during chronic therapy.

While a number of investigators have studied the growth effects of anabolic steroids in girls with Turner syndrome (20-23), no data regarding the effect of these agents on glucose tolerance in Turner syndrome are available. Our data demonstrate that oxandrolone, either alone or in combination with GH, has effects on carbohydrate metabolism. These effects were much greater than those seen when only GH is used. Both integrated glucose and insulin concentrations increase substantially to nearly twice those seen at baseline with 44% of the subjects receiving oxandrolone alone having impaired glucose tolerance at the end of the first year of the study. Despite these abnormal OGTT responses, both fasting glucose and glycosylated hemoglobin concentrations remained within the normal range.

The clinical importance of increased glucose intolerance associated with oxandrolone therapy in girls with Turner syndrome is unknown. Since both the fasting glucose concentrations and glycosylated hemoglobin remained normal, short-term complications from this degree of impairment of glucose tolerance seem highly unlikely. The long-term risk of impaired glucose tolerance is less clear. Despite the preexisting carbohydrate abnormalities and the relatively high dose of GH, we did not detect significant changes in glucose and insulin concentrations when girls with Turner syndrome were treated with GH alone. Oxandrolone, either alone or in combination with GH, had significant effects on carbohydrate metabolism in these subjects. The long-term consequences of impaired glucose tolerance or isolated hyperinsulinemia in Turner syndrome are unknown. Since the long-term efficacy of oxandrolone therapy on ultimate height remains unclear, physicians should carefully consider the risk/benefit ratio before undertaking this mode of therapy.

APPENDIX

The Genentech Turner's Collaborative Group consists of Jo Anne Brasel, MD, Harbor-UCLA Medical Center; Stephen Burstein, MD, University of Chicago Medical Center; Steven D. Chernausek, MD, Children's Hospital Medical Center, Cincinnati; Ronald W. Gotlin, MD, University of Colorado Medical School; Joyce Kuntze, Genentech Inc., South San Francisco; Barbara M. Lippe, MD, UCLA School of Medicine; Patrick C. Mahoney, MD, The Mason Clinic, Seattle; Wayne V. Moore, MD, University of Kansas Medical Center, Maria I. New, MD, Cornell Medical Center; Paul Saenger, Montefiore Hospital, New York; Virginia Sybert, Children's Orthopedic Hospital and Medical Center, Seattle.

REFERENCES

1. Forbes AP, Engel E. The high incidence of diabetes mellitus in 41 patients with gonadal dysgenesis and their close relatives. Metabolism 1963; 12:428.
2. Saenger P, Schwartz E, Wiedemann E, Levine L, Tsai M, New MI. The interaction of growth hormone somatomedin and oestrogen in patients with Turner syndrome. Acta Endocrinol 1976; 81:9.
3. Rasio E, Antaki A, Van Campenhout J. Diabetes mellitus in gonadal dysgenesis. Studies of insulin and growth hormone secretion. Europ J Clin Invest 1976; 6:59.
4. Polychronakos C, Letarte J, Collu R, Ducharme JR. Carbohydrate intolerance in children and adolescents with Turner syndrome. J Pediatr 1980; 96:1009.
5. Zinman B, Kabiawu SIO, Moross T, et al. Endocrine, cytogenetic and psychometric features of patients with X-isochromosome 46, X,i(Xq) Turner's syndrome. A preliminary study in nine patients. Clin Invest Med 1984; 47:135.
6. AvRuskin TW, Crigler Jr JF, Soeldner JS. Turner's syndrome and carbohydrate metabolism. Amer J Med Sci 1979; 277:145.
7. Van Campenhout J, Antaki A, Rasio E. Diabetes mellitus and thyroid autoimmunity in gonadal dysgenesis. Fertil Sertil 1973; 24:1.
8. Nielsen J, Johansen K, Yde H. The frequency of diabetes mellitus in patients with Turner's syndrome and pure gonadal dysgenesis. Acta Endocrin 1969; 62:251.
9. Jackson IMD, Buchana KD, McKiddie MT, Prentice CRM. Carbohydrate metabolism and pituitary function in gonadal dysgenesis (Turner's syndrome). J Endocrin 1966; 34:289.
10. Van Vliet G, Styne DM, Kaplan SL, Grumbach MM. Turner's syndrome and

human growth hormone. Biochemical studies. In Raiti S, Tolman RA (eds). Human Growth Hormone. Plenum, New York, 1986.

11. Wilson DM, Frane JW, Sherman B, Johanson AJ, Hintz RL, Rosenfeld RG. Carbohydrate and lipid metabolism in Turner syndrome: The effect of therapy with growth hormone, oxandrolone, and a combination of both. J Pediatr 1988; 112:210.

12. Rosenfeld RG, Hintz RH, Johanson AJ et al. Methionyl human growth hormone and oxandrolone in Turner syndrome. Preliminary results of a prospective randomized trial. J Pediatr 1986; 109:936.

13.–14. The National Diabetes Data Group. Classification and diagnosis of diabetes mellitus and other categories of glucose intolerance. Diabetes 1979; 28:1039.

15. Raiti S, Moore WV, Van Vliet G, Kaplan SL, et al. Growth-stimulating effects of human growth hormone therapy in patients with Turner syndrome. J Pediatr 1986; 109:944.

16. Tzagournis M. Response to long-term administration of human growth hormone in Turner's syndrome. JAMA 1969; 210:2373.

17. Singer-Granick C, Lee PA, Foley TP, Becker DJ. Growth hormone therapy in Turner's syndrome. Hormone Res 1986:24:246.

18. Takano K, Hizuka N, Shizume K. Growth hormone treatment in Turner's syndrome. Acta Paediatr Scand [Suppl] 1986; 325:58.

19. Wilton P. Growth hormone treatment in girls with Turner's syndrome. Acta Paediatr Scand 1987; 76:193.

20. Moore DC, Tattoni DS, Ruvalcaba RHA, Limbeck GA, Kelley VC. Studies of anabolic steroids. VI. Effects of prolonged administration of oxandrolone on growth in children and adolescents with gonadal dysgenesis. J Pediatr 1977; 90:462.

21. Johanson AJ, Brasel JA, Blizzard RM. Growth in patients with gonadal dysgenesis receiving fluoxymesterone. J Pediatr 1969; 75:1015.

22. Lev-Ran A. Androgens, estrogens, and ultimate height in XO gonadal dysgenesis. Am J Dis Child 1977; 31:648.

23. Lenko LL, Perheentupa J, Soderholm A. Growth in Turner's syndrome. Spontaneous and fluoxymesterone stimulated. Acta Paediatr Scand [Suppl] 1979; 277:57.

DISCUSSION

DR. ANDREW HOFFMAN: Were there any changes in adiposity in these kids? Are they gaining more weight or mass index?

DR. DARRELL WILSON: I did not look at that directly. There was no correlation that we could find between BMI and any of the glucose tolerance data. Of interest, there was a slight positive correlation between age and integrated insulin levels which suggests that they were making progressively more insulin as they were getting older, but again this group only went up to 12 years of age.

DR. HOFFMAN: When large doses of androgens are given to adults, or the body builders, they have also developed glucose intolerance, so it is not totally surprising.

DR. WILSON: Some of the adult literature on oxandrolone suggests that when given to Type II diabetics there is an improvement in glucose tolerance, so it is a very fuzzy field. A lot of people make hypotheses about it, but many of them are trying to explain an apparent decrease in blood sugar.

DR. DOROTHY BECKER: I just want to show a little bit of data that we have on glucose tolerance from a small cohort of patients that we studied in Pittsburgh about 6 or 7 years ago and then try and extrapolate to what we are doing (Table 2).

There were 15 girls with Turner syndrome who were untreated, and they were divided into groups of less than 13 years of age and more than 13 years of age. The reason for doing this is that there is little normal glucose or insulin data in the literature, and you cannot use much of the literature data because there is a large age and sex variation with both glucose and insulin levels during glucose tolerance tests. Unless one subdivides, one really cannot compare with normals or pubertal status.

These patients were relatively glucose intolerant. Fifty percent of them had what we call non-normal glucose tolerance tests. There are differences in the adults and the pediatric criteria for diagnosing diabetes. American standards are

---

Drs. Andrew Hoffman and Darrell Wilson are at Stanford University, Stanford, California. Dr. Dorothy Becker is at the Children's Hospital, Pittsburgh, Pennsylvania. Dr. Michael Preece is at the Institute of Child Health, London, England. Dr. Barbara Lippe is at the University of California at Los Angeles Hospitals and Clinic, Los Angeles, California. Dr. Inger Hansen is at the Medical University of South Carolina, Charleston, South Carolina. Dr. G. Van Vliet is at the Hospital Universitaire Saint-Pierre, Brussels, Belgium.

Table 2 Body Mass Index, Glucose Area, Insulin Area, and 15-Minute Insulin for Girls with Turner Syndrome and Controls

	BMI	GA (mg/min)	IA (μU/min)	15 min I (μU/mL)
		Age 7–12.9 years		
TS	21.3 ± 2.1 *	172 ± 34 ***	196 ± 48 *	63 ± 10 *
C	16.7 ± 0.3	68 ± 4.2 **	95 ± 8	40 ± 3
BMI-C	17.9 ± 0.3	69 ± 6	110 ± 10	46 ± 4
		Age 13–17 years		
TS	21.3 ± 1	141 ± 12 **	172 ± 13	87 ± 13 **
C	20.7 ± 0.4	78 ± 8	137 ± 8	47 ± 3

$*p < 0.05$; $**p < 0.01$; $***p < 0.001$.

higher than European ones. You do not need to have fasting hypoglycemia before you get elevation of glycosylated hemoglobins.

In these particular patients we looked at Turner syndrome girls compared to 114 age- and sex-matched girls because there is a difference between males and females although it is not very striking at this stage.

Glucose area is the glucose incremental glucose area during glucose tolerance tests, and IA is the insulin area. The 15-minute insulin is analogous to early insulin release. Decrease in first basal early insulin release is thought to be the first sign of insulin-dependent diabetes. Glucose area above the curve is markedly higher, almost three times higher than age-matched controls without any treatment. The insulin area is about twice as high as normal and these are statistically different. But it is interesting that the 15-minute insulin level is higher than controls suggesting that they are able to release insulin very early.

However, the body mass index of the Turner's girls compared to the controls at this age is much higher. When we tried to match the body mass index of Turner girls, we got a nonstatistical difference, 21.3 compared to 17.9, but we did not have as many obese normal girls. They were normal sibs of diabetics.

The glucose area in the sibs was not very different from the other controls and still different from the Turner's. The insulin area was slightly higher, but not statistically different from the Turner girls because of the large standard error,

48 compared to 10, and the 15-minute not very different. So this is age 7 to 13, where much of the glucose intolerance and hyperinsulinism may be explained by the increased body mass index.

The question is, what is the chicken and what is the egg? In other words, is the obesity causing the hyperinsulinism or is hyperinsulinism making them eat more and therefore become obese?

When you look at the older children who by now have "caught down" or the controls have "caught up" to them as far as body mass index goes, glucose area is double, so again there are higher glucose levels. Insulin area is higher, and not different significantly this time. But look how high the 15-minute insulin value there is. That is extremely high. That is way out of the range of normal suggesting that we are dealing with insulin resistance. Insulin resistance has also been suggested by some glucose clamp studies.

The reason that I am presenting this data is that I am very concerned about what we are doing to these patients when treating with growth hormone or oxandrolone. We know that acromegaly, which is large amounts of growth hormone, results in insulin resistance, it results in hypertension, it results in atherosclerosis, it results in cardiomegaly, all the things that we worry about in patients with Turner syndrome.

It is possible that the short-term studies that we have heard about today do not show huge changes, but I would like to remind you that the insulin values that you saw were done in their own labs, every lab being different, and I can assure you that insulin assays are just as variable as growth hormone assays.

Fifty percent of our children had hypocholesterolemia. And I was quite surprised actually to see very little changes in cholesterols and triglycerides because I had anticipated bigger ones. Cholesterol assays vary as much as growth hormone assays and insulin assays across labs. And so, I would like to make a plea that before we advocate growth hormone or oxandrolone treatment—oxandrolone as you heard causes hyperlipidemia as well—that we are careful with what we are doing to these patients.

At this stage hyperinsulinism seems to be the major epidemiologic associate of atherosclerosis. It is the bad guy when it comes to hypertension and I think we need to look a little bit further than just height and growth in our patients.

I am not saying that we should not treat them, I think we should be looking very hard at what we are doing. Other than in growth, look for side effects and try and decide if a few more centimeters in height or getting there a little faster is worth potential deleterious effects. And whether we like it or not, the popularity of growth hormone treatments with the results we have heard today has made it universal therapy for Turner's children around the world. At the moment there are many girls being treated who are not in studies, who are not being followed.

I would like to ask that we use this opportunity that Genentech has given us of a large cohort of patients to look at what we are doing, that we do not stop looking at 1 year or 2 years, but we follow these patients into adulthood and find out what we are doing.

DR. MICHAEL PREECE: I agree with an awful lot of what Dr. Becker just said, but one thing that struck me from the data was that in every case, for every measured variable, the most striking difference between the Turner's and the control was the vastly increased variance. Doing some quick F tests in my head, I think every one of them would have been significant. And that to me suggests there is something very funny about the population. Have you looked at whether there is bimodal distribution amongst them and whether there are subgroups which we might be able to identify?

DR. BECKER: I think we need large populations to do that. Ours is only 15, and that is why we have not done any more with it over the years because in one center none of us have enough patients to assess age, body mass index, and sex. We have got to do it together. We cannot do it individually.

DR. BARBARA LIPPE: We did that a few years ago and never published it for other reasons, but in over 100 oral glucose tolerance tests done in the same lab with insulin by the same methods, it was totally bimodal. You could divide the patients up into two groups. One group was completely normal, independent of their body mass index and one group was very abnormal. That was the same whether they were thin or heavy. Now I think it is interesting and I am going to back and look at them again.

DR. PREECE: What percentage broke off?

DR. LIPPE: It was almost 50/50, so much so that I started to do this business about one chromosome and the other and thinking about which X it was and what their parents were like and who they inherited things from because it was almost exactly 50/50.

DR. BECKER: I think there is little doubt that there is abnormal glucose tolerance and hyperinsulinism in Turner's. I do not think we can explain it yet. My concern is what else are we doing to all this with the treatment that we are advocating right now.

DR. INGER HANSEN: I would like to reecho what Dorothy says in terms of looking at insulin sensitivity in patients with chronic elevated growth hormone concentrations in acromegalic subjects. For example, whether or not they have very, very elevated growth hormone concentrations: Even in the patients with only minimal elevations of growth hormone, when Dr. Rizza and I looked at them using the insulin-glucose clamp, they still were profoundly insulin-resistant so that we may be causing a secondary defect.

DR. G. VAN VLIET: Could you comment on glycosylated hemoglobins in these patients, or can this be done?

DR. BECKER: No, I really feel very strongly that in a study like this, glycosylated hemoglobin is not the screening method. Proteins and hemoglobin glycosylate very late. On the benchtop you need an ambient or mean serum glucose of well above 200 before you get glycosylation, and you can have really major abnormalities in glucose tolerance and diabetic glucose tolerance tests before you get glycosylation. We do not know whether glucose toxicity, hyperinsulinism, or anything else is what is bad for you. There is no doubt that we have major hyperinsulinism in these patients, and if we are going to increase that, maybe that is the thing that we should worry about the most and not glycosylation of tissues.

DR. WILSON: In the first year of the Turner study there were a couple of things. At the end of the year glycosylated hemoglobins were done all in the same lab, and there was absolutely no difference among the four groups. In addition if you look at fasting insulin levels throughout treatment, there were only two times on those glucose tolerance tests where there was any significant rise. It was fairly minor and fasting insulin is the only one up in the combination group at 5 days and at 2 months.

DR. BECKER: I would like to suggest that unless you have good assays, you can't really tell.

DR. WILSON: I think there is a question certainly about comparing people to historical controls. But on the other hand, subjects were run in the same assay at the same center. So the paired data are really pretty good. I think while you can argue what the baseline was, the effect of treatment is substantially more robust and there was not much effect on fasting insulins.

DR. VAN VLIET: I certainly share your concern about aggravating the hyperinsulinemia. Now a few years ago there were some claims that a so-called 20K variant of growth hormone could still have the growth-promoting effect of the full molecule but not its diabetogenic effect. I do not know if there is any further information on that and whether it has been confirmed.

DR. BECKER: I do not know of any.

DR. WILSON: In answer to your question, in our initial studies of methionyl growth hormone in human adult volunteers using pure 22K recombinant growth hormone, we saw all the diabetogenic effects that have been ascribed to pituitary growth hormone. So certainly the 22K classical growth hormone is fully diabetogenic. I just wanted to make one other comment before we left the issue of growth hormone, which is a piece of information which just recently became known to me. That is that the first person to treat a Turner patient with growth hormone was Henry Turner. If you look in his 1938 article, he in fact did treat one of his original patients with bovine pituitary extract and it did not work.

DR. BECKER: We are using relatively large doses of growth hormone that I think most of us are not used to using, and using them per kilo body weight. We have a group of patients who are relatively obese. We are not using surface area. And as Dr. Prader said to me this morning, most things we do have a dose effect, and I wonder if anybody knows what kind of circulating thresholds we are producing in these overweight girls. When I get up to 8 to 19 units per injection, I have cold shivers running up my spine. That is the dose if you really have some pretty overweight children.

Summary of Part IV

James Tanner

University of Texas Health Science Center, Houston, Texas

In this session we examined the effects of various treatments designed to increase the stature of children with Turner syndrome; we discussed how best to decide whether it was likely that a treatment was going to increase final adult height over what it would have been in the absence of treatment; and we looked at the side effects of those treatments that seemed most efficacious.

The treatments were anabolic steroids, chiefly oxandrolone, growth hormone, and estrogen, chiefly ethinyl estradiol, and some combinations of them.

In the short term the results are really quite clear. Oxandrolone, best at a fairly small dose, growth hormone, and estrogen at a dose of 4 μg/day will increase the rate of growth in height in most patients over at least the first year. This they mostly do without increasing bone age velocity, at any rate in this first year. In the biggest study, that reported by Dr. Rosenfeld, the height velocity rose from 4.2 cm/yr to 6.6 cm/yr on growth hormone; on oxandrolone to 7.9 cm/yr, and on both combined to 9.8 cm/yr. The untreated group had a velocity of 3.8 cm/yr.

This is already something worth while to do for Turner patients. But the bigger hope is that final height will be increased (in spite of a feeling that the basic lesion is one of the physiology of the growth plate). The difficulty is to know whether or not a treatment is really altering final height. Change in the prediction of final height based on normal children is clearly untrustworthy. Change in predictions based on standards for untreated Turner patients, in other words, showing that the treated patient has departed from the centile for Turner girls that she was previously on, is better. But it is still illogical to use untreated girls' curves to predict what will be the endpoint of the possibly quite differently shaped curves produced by the treatment. There is no substitute for waiting; if and when a patient reaches a height above that projected from her initial centile on the Turner chart, that is evidence, subject to sampling error, of the treatment's success. The chief strength of Dr. Rosenfeld's report is that by the end of 3 years of treatment, 10 out of the 16 girls on the combined treatment had exceeded this point, and all were still growing. So the prospect looks good.

Primum, however, non nocere. Do we pay for the extra few centimeters with an increased risk of atherosclerosis in adult life? There is evidence of induced hyperinsulinism in some at least of these patients, and the reports of Drs. Wilson and Becker will be read with care and perhaps some apprehension. Dr. Rimoin mentioned that it was said that percutaneous surgical intervention could now lengthen the legs of Turner patients by perhaps some 10–15 cm with, it seemed, little risk or gross inconvenience: Here clearly is another and differently timed treatment that may be adjunctive.

Finally, the reader will find some discussion of the ethical problems of clinical trials. It seems that the NIH is conducting a 10-year-long trial in which some of the children will receive, over this whole period, approximately one thousand injections of growth hormone carrier fluid to determine the effect of a placebo. Many members of the symposium were horrified: One invoked the Helsinki Declaration. A calmer voice pointed out that no child would be stupid enough to undergo such a thing unless the effects of placebo were of the same order as those occurring in the other, non–placebo-treated members of the group. The trial would self-destruct. Perhaps Dr. Hibi had the wisest word: The doctors should be blinded in such a trial, he said, but not the patients.

Part V

Intellectual and Psychosocial Development

INTRODUCTION

Dr. Raymond Hintz, Stanford University, Stanford, California

Over the last 2 days we have heard a lot of information about Turner syndrome, everything from its history, to genetics, to insights into the pathophysiology. What is missing is the human aspect of that.

None of the therapies that are being tested or are proposed would make much sense if we did not address the human issues that these young ladies have in dealing with their world and interacting with their peers in a way that makes them feel like successful human beings. And so it is these issues about their intellectual and psychosocial development in the future that we are going to try to address here.

36

Mental Aspects of Turner Syndrome and the Importance of Information and Turner Contact Groups

Johannes Nielsen

Cytogenetic Laboratory, Psychiatric Hospital in Århus
Risskov, Denmark

INTRODUCTION

In 1938, Turner (1) described a syndrome in women characterized by the triad:
1. short stature with undeveloped secondary sexual characteristics. 2. webbing of the neck. 3. cubitus valgus. The only one of these signs invariably present in women with Turner's syndrome is short stature, while webbing of the neck is only found in approximately 30% and cubitus valgus in approximately 60%.

The most common karyotype in Turner syndrome is 45,X, which is found in approximately half of these women. The other half comprises women with a great variation of different chromosome aberrations, such as 45,X/46,XX, 45,X/46,X,i(Xq), 45,X/46,X,r(X), 46,X,i(Xq), 46,X,del(Xq), 46,X,del(Xp), other X deletions and translocations, as well as mosaics with Y chromosome material (2,3).

Lack of X chromosome material in individuals with female phenotype is the criterion for inclusion in our studies of girls with Turner syndrome.

With a few exceptions, such as the recent study by Søderholm (4), studies of the mental development of girls with Turner syndrome have often been based on quite small and selected groups with the main emphasis on more or less sophisticated psychological test results and with fairly little emphasis on behavior in general, school performance and social adjustment, the importance of information, as well as on the many positive aspects of the mental development of Turner girls.

The rapid increase in the use of prenatal examinations from 8 cases in Denmark in 1970 to 6,700 in 1986 with induced abortion of 71% of those with sex chromosome aberrations, including Turner syndrome (5), makes it extremely important for those of us working in behavior genetics to procure thorough information concerning the development of children with sex chromosome aberrations, including Turner syndrome. Geneticists giving information to parents in relation to prenatal examination need this information, and prospective parents need to be able to read about it. Such information is further of great value for Turner girls, Turner parents as well as for everybody who gets into contact with Turner girls in a professional capacity.

In the Risskov group, we believe that the lack of sufficiently good studies of large, unselected groups of girls with Turner syndrome has led to the fact that in certain countries the great majority of prenatally diagnosed fetuses with Turner syndrome are aborted. In Denmark, 32 of the 38 cases of Turner syndrome diagnosed prenatally till 1980 were aborted, i.e., 84% (5). Due to an increasing amount of Turner information during recent years (2,3,8) the frequency of induced abortion of Turner fetuses has, however, decreased from 100% during the 1970s to 64% in 1985–1987. With even better information and improved treatment possibilities, I believe it will decrease further in the years to come.

In the present study we have mainly focused on the mental aspects of girls with Turner syndrome: how they manage at home, at school, at work, and in their relationships with family and other people.

We have also focused on the importance of early diagnosis and thorough information to parents, physicians, and educators of children with Turner syndrome, as well as to the girls themselves as they grow up. We have further paid attention to the importance of establishing Turner contact groups.

We have previously published two monographs about Turner syndrome (2,3) comprising a total of 150 Turner women. The present data are mainly from one of these studies comprising 115 unselected girls with Turner syndrome found among the 460,000 Danish girls born between 1955 and 1966; they comprise 85% of the expected number of Turner girls in Denmark in this age group.

A complete examination with interviews of the girls and their parents, as well as information from schools, family physicians, and hospitals, has been made of 82 of the 115 Turner girls, and I am presenting some mental aspects of these 82 girls. There is no indication that the 82 Turner girls deviated from the rest as far as mental or other aspects are concerned. Fifty-seven percent have the karyotype 45,X, and the rest have other karyotypes with lack of X chromosome material.

MENTAL ASPECTS OF TURNER SYNDROME

Motor and Speech Development

Motor development was delayed in 24% of the Turner girls with 45,X compared with only 3% in those with other karyotypes and 4% in controls. Delayed speech development was found in 18% of the Turner girls with 45,X, 9% of those with other karyotypes, and 16% in controls. Delay in motor development might, to a certain extent, be associated with edema of the back of hands and feet, as the frequency of delayed motor development in girls with such edema was as high as 73%. In such girls there is thus a need for special stimulation of motor function during early childhood.

Behavior

Crying and disturbed behavior as babies were recorded in 41% of those with karyotype 45,X during the first year of life, but only in 26% of those with other karyotypes. After the first year of life the great majority of the Turner girls were, however, described as quite similar to their sisters in this respect. It might, however, be mentioned that 71% had shown only very weak or hardly any defiance during their assertive age.

School Level

Distribution of school level was found to be no different from that of their sisters and what would be expected in an unselected group of Danish girls. Only 7% were in special teaching groups, and a total of 22% received extra teaching in one or more subjects. These figures correspond with what is expected in Danish schools.

Twenty-six percent of those in the age group 17 years and above were in college, and 10% were apprentices; this is not significantly different from their sisters and what is expected. It is remarkable that only one was unemployed, as the average unemployment frequency among youngsters in Denmark is approximately 20%.

The school level was quite similar to that of their sisters, which is in accordance with a previous study made from our laboratory of 45 women with Turner syndrome, compared with their sisters and a control group of girls with primary amenorrhea and short stature but normal karyotype. We found no significant difference in school level between these three groups (2).

School Statement

Most of the Turner girls were described as being average at school. They were usually very diligent and had a good relationship with teachers and schoolmates.

In most cases the teachers answered our requests in a very comprehensive and apparently also reliable way. A rather typical answer in an abbreviated form is: "Grethe has worked with interest at school. She has shown great care with her work, and she has had both good will and energy to solve the tasks and to work in groups. She has had a good influence on her group due to her quiet, friendly, and healthy interests for human problems."

As a supplement to this statement made when Grethe left school, it was said that she had always been hard-working with her homework. She did, however, work somewhat slowly, but very thoroughly. Her self-confidence level was rather low, and she always needed to be completely sure before she gave any answers. Her energy and stubbornness helped her to get a very good exam. Arithmetic and mathematics in general were the subjects with which she had the most difficulties. She was always very positive towards the school and school work. She was well accepted in her group, but she was somewhat quiet and reticent.

School Achievement and Diligence

Seventy-six percent of the Turner girls were average or above average at school, but 40% had special difficulties in mathematics, compared with only 20% of their sisters. The difficulties in mathematics are most probably due to the specific difficulties in solving spatial problems and difficulties in nonlinguistic tasks in general.

Seventy-six percent were above average at school as far as diligence is concerned and only 9% below, and there are many examples in the case histories of diligence and conscientiousness definitely more pronounced than in their sisters and in girls in general.

Relationship with Schoolmates and Teachers

Good or extremely good relationship with schoolmates was found in 78% and with teachers in 98%, a remarkably high percentage. As they are often hard-working and conscientious concerning their homework and often lack interest in outdoor activities, they rarely have many friends. In many cases, however, they prefer to enjoy a cozy time at home with their books, needlework, or together with their parents. Early social stimulation in day institutions for children and encouragement to group activities are of great importance for Turner girls.

It might, however, be mentioned that the Turner girls we have diagnosed at birth and follow regularly with information and counseling are much more active than those diagnosed later in life.

Personality Traits and Behavior

Personality traits, which were underlined by the parents and teachers, were extroversion, good and stable mood, diligence, and conscientiousness. Carefulness and sense of order in appearance and dressing were also characteristic.

Eighty-five percent of those who had an authoritative, strict, or overprotective type of upbringing had emotional maturity below average, compared with only 42% among those with an average or especially stimulating, consistent, and sensible type of upbringing. We found parental overprotection to be associated with a tendency to psychopathology in these girls.

It is understandable that parents of girls with Turner syndrome who are short of stature tend to treat them in an overprotective way, more according to stature than according to age. This is, however, very inappropriate, as it tends to fixate the girls in their emotional immaturity and dependency instead of stimulating them to become mature and independent.

Treatment with very small doses of estrogen from the age of 11-12 years will most probably speed up the mental maturity process as well as increase growth velocity in Turner girls during treatment.

Mental State

The evaluation of mental state was made on the basis of parents' descriptions, information from schools and other anamnestic information, as well as on the examiner's evaluation at the time of the examination; 73% of the girls were considered to be mentally well functioning by the parents, the school, and the examiner, i.e., girls who, apart from some emotional immaturity, did not present any problems.

The designation "mental problems" has been used in a very broad sense from the presence of very mild symptoms to manifest mental illness. Girls who on account of emotional immaturity have difficulties in getting along with others the same age and suffer on account of this, girls who are extremely passive and aggression-repressed or have poor concentration, attention-diversion, or concrete and perseverating thinking are included under the description "mental problems." According to this definition, mental problems had been or were present in only 27%.

Normal intelligence level was recorded in 94%. None of the girls had been admitted to psychiatric hospitals or treated for mental illness. The 27% with mental problems—most of them minor problems—and no cases of actual mental

illness as found in the present study is certainly not above the expected frequency in the general Danish population, where prevalence studies of actual
mental illness have revealed figures from 20 to 30%.

Upbringing

There was a significant association between the results of evaluation of mental
state and childhood environment with only 18% of those with a normal mental
state having a poor or very poor type of childhood environment, compared with
66% of those with mental problems ($X^2 = 11.31, p < 0.001$).

Forty-seven percent of those who grew up with different persons had mental
problems or emotional immaturity, compared with only 24% of those who grew
up with both parents ($p < 0.05$).

Only 18% of the girls, who had an especially authoritative, overprotecting,
or laissez-faire type of upbringing, were evaluated as having a completely normal
mental development at the age of the examination, compared with 63% of the
Turner girls who had an especially warm, realistic, consistent, and stimulating
upbringing ($p < 0.01$), and 42% of those who had what we have called an
ordinary type of upbringing ($p < 0.01$).

THE IMPORTANCE OF INFORMATION AND
TURNER CONTACT GROUPS

Here we will discuss the importance of Turner contact groups and information
concerning Turner syndrome to Turner girl parents, Turner girls, the public, and,
last but not least, Turner fetus parents.

Fifty-seven percent of the Turner girls 15 years and above had been given
complete information about their chromosome, hormone, fertility, and growth
conditions, 32% were only partly informed, and 11% were not informed at all.
That is, of course, far from a satisfactory level of information (6), which ought
to be 100% at 15 years of age.

Should parents of newborn Turner girls be told all the facts concerning the
development of their daughters with Turner syndrome? The answer is definitely
yes.

It is our experience from investigation of a considerable number of newborn
girls with Turner syndrome and adults not diagnosed till rather late in life that
it is extremely important for parents to know as much as possible about their
daughter with Turner syndrome as early as possible in order to be able to provide the best possible conditions for a Turner girl with maximal stimulation in
all aspects, but especially stimulation to independence and avoidance of overprotection. A Turner girl should be treated according to age and not according
to stature.

It is thus essential that the diagnosis of Turner syndrome be made during early childhood in all cases, preferably at birth, so that information can be given to the parents. In Denmark with fairly good cytogenetic and pediatric service, only 60% of the Turner girls are, however, diagnosed before the age of 17, with variations from 10 to 100% in the different counties.

Chromosome examination should be made of all girls with one or more signs of Turner syndrome at birth or later and all growth-retarded girls with a stature 2 standard deviations or more below normal mean irrespective of Turner signs. This would lead to diagnosis of practically all Turner girls at an early age and early enough for both information and relevant growth hormone oxandrolone and estrogen therapy.

Early and good information to parents of Turner girls also gives them the possibility of providing information to their daughter with Turner syndrome as she grows up and wants to know why she differs from other girls her age in stature and other aspects.

The information should be given by a person with good knowledge and a lot of experience concerning Turner syndrome in children, as well as adults, a person to whom the parents can return at any time for further information, a person with sufficient time and patience to listen to and answer questions from the parents.

If these conditions are fulfilled, the reaction of the parents to full and early information is extremely positive and appreciative. Parents do in general know how to handle information and counseling in a constructive way. They are spared a lot of anxiety and worries about why their daughter with Turner syndrome develops somewhat differently from her siblings and friends, and first and foremost they are given the knowledge how to bring her up in the best possible way for a girl with Turner syndrome.

Should girls with Turner syndrome be told all the facts about the syndrome, including karyotype, hormone conditions, etc.? As in the case of the parents, the answer according to our experience in Risskov is definitely yes.

To protect a girl with Turner syndrome by telling her that nothing is wrong, that she should not be worried at the same time that she is taken from one examination to another, can only be disturbing and cause anxiety as well as decrease her confidence in her parents, physicians, and adults in general. There are still many examples of this.

It is our experience that adult girls with Turner syndrome, like persons with other types of sex chromosome aberrations, have as a rule been informed too poorly and too late. They have often made their own impression and guesses and get their own ideas about what is wrong with them, and this is usually much worse than the facts.

At the Cytogenetic Laboratory in Risskov, we have excellent results in giving full information in close cooperation with the parents to girls with Turner syndrome at a very early age. We have primary school girls with Turner syndrome who have sufficient knowledge to give lectures about Turner syndrome at the school, mainly based on a small book published by the National Society of Turner Contact Groups in Denmark (7). Such lectures always stop any previous teasing concerning, for instance, short stature. It is important that information about Turner syndrome be available in a form that can be read and understood by Turner girls and parents as well as everybody else who needs such information.

When Turner syndrome is diagnosed at a later age, full information is always appreciated, and the Turner girls' reaction to full information is nearly always that they would very much have preferred to have had this information and knowledge much earlier. This would have spared them a lot of anxiety and concern about why they were short of stature, late in developing breasts and secondary sex characteristics, etc. Information helps the Turner girls accept the fact that they have Turner syndrome, and such acceptance is of great value for them.

It is very important for Turner girls to be informed about their rather late pubertal development at an age when girls with normal chromosomes enter puberty or, preferably, earlier. It is also essential that they be fully informed about their rather scanty chance of having children, and at the same time they should be given information about their good chance of adopting a child, which is equal to that of others, as well as the fact that to adopt a child can be as rewarding as is biological parenthood.

All the positive aspects of adoption should also be presented, and they should be promised assistance if difficulties in obtaining permission to adopt a child should turn up on account of short stature or the chromosome aberration. It should also be stressed that a normal sex life and married life definitely are as common for Turner women as for others.

The question of fertility should always be presented in the context of probability. Approximately 15% of Turner girls have spontaneous menstruation, and during spontaneous menstruation there is usually a chance of becoming pregnant. It should further be mentioned that it may be possible to obtain in vitro fertilization for some Turner women (8). At the same time that Turner women are told about some of the negative results of the chromosome aberration, it is very important that they are also told about the many positive aspects and the available treatment possibilities for further growth and development of normal secondary sexual characteristics and menstruation.

A key word in professional relationship with girls with Turner syndrome is *information*, and not only superficial information given in a hurry by a busy physician with little experience concerning Turner syndrome.

Information should be given by persons with extremely good knowledge and experience concerning Turner syndrome and plenty of time, and I believe that information should also be given by the members of a local Turner contact group.

In this connection it might be mentioned that during the last 5 years we have in Denmark had great success with establishing Turner contact groups. They now exist in all areas of Denmark, and a national society of Turner contact groups in Denmark was established 3 years ago. These groups have been of great benefit to the Danish Turner girls, and the national Turner society plays an important role in initiating, promoting, and participating in Turner research as well as in procuring Turner information and counseling. Turner girls from the society participate in teaching medical students about Turner syndrome, and on a couple of occasions Turner girls have travelled with me to scientific Turner meetings in Belgium and Canada to talk about Turner syndrome and Turner contact groups. At present the national Turner society is lobbying for legal permission for ovum donation for in vitro fertilization in Turner women and others in need of this, and the society is planning to hold an international seminar in Denmark in 1988 with participants from Turner contact groups around the world.

The parents of a fetus with Turner syndrome diagnosed prenatally should be given all the previously mentioned information as well as information about the physical aberrations and the reduced growth velocity during childhood and reduced final height. However, at the same time they should also be told that those with a severe physical disorder such as aortic stenosis can be treated successfully, and that growth velocity and, to a certain extent, also final height can be increased with growth hormone, oxandrolone, and probably also with small doses of estrogens.

The many positive aspects in the mental development of girls with Turner syndrome should be stressed, that is to say that they have normal intelligence, they have good and positive personality traits, these girls are active, open, and extroverted with good contact with others. They are usually diligent, happy, and have a very good social adaptability in general. They have a remarkable ability to cope with stress and adversity.

To hint at or have the attitude that fetuses with Turner syndrome should be aborted is a clear discrimination against women with Turner syndrome around the world, women who are usually mentally and physically healthy and as intelligent and well adjusted as their siblings (9-14).

Information about Turner's syndrome should also be given to the public, preferably in close cooperation with Turner contact groups and professionals with a good knowledge about Turner syndrome. In Denmark we have had a great success with a radio program about Turner syndrome and with a number of interviews on radio and television, in newspapers, and weekly magazines by members of Turner contact groups. The previously mentioned book about Turner syndrome and Turner contact groups was written in close cooperation with a number of Turner girls aged 10 to 40 years, all members of different Turner contact groups. It might be mentioned that this book has recently been published in English and French (15,16). It will soon appear in German and Japanese, and translation into Italian, Spanish, and Swedish is considered. Thanks to a donation from KabiVitrum and no profit for the authors and translators, these books can be distributed free of charge.

Better public knowledge about Turner syndrome as well as about other sex chromosome aberrations will tend to decrease discrimination and teasing, which to a great extent is due to lack of knowledge.

We physicians have been, and still are, far too poorly trained to give full information to the public. We are, actually, to a great extent trained to conceal information with the purpose of protecting the patient. But it is my experience that in most cases we have done, and still do, a lot of harm by being secretive, and this is definitely the case when we talk about Turner syndrome as well as other sex chromosome aberrations.

CONCLUSION

Girls with Turner syndrome usually manage quite well at home, at school, and at work if diagnosed early, preferably at birth, if the parents are given good information at the time of birth of their daughter with Turner syndrome, and if the girls grow up under good conditions, that is, if they are stimulated to independence and activity, treated according to age, and not overprotected and infantilized.

Turner contact groups should be available, and all Turner girls and their parents should be encouraged to join such groups. It is furthermore very important to give sufficient realistic and thorough information to the parents and, at suitable age levels, to the girls themselves, to treat them with growth hormone, estrogens, and most probably also oxandrolone started at the appropriate age and continued for an appropriate number of years.

REFERENCES

1. Turner H. A syndrome of infantilism, congenital webbed neck, and cubitus valgus. Endocrinology 1938; 23:566–574.
2. Nielsen J, Nyborg H, Dahl G. Turner's syndrome. A psychiatric-psychological study of 45 women with Turner's syndrome, compared with their sisters and women with normal karyotypes, growth retardation and primary amenorrhoea. Acta Jutlandica XLV, Medicine Series 21, Århus, 1977.
3. Nielsen J, Sillesen I. Turner's syndrome in 115 Danish girls born between 1955 and 1966. Acta Jutlandica LIV, Medicine Series 22, Århus, 1981.
4. Söderholm A. Turners syndrom. En psykosocial och somatisk undersökning

av 62 kvinnor. Helsingfors Universitetscentralsjukhus I pediatriska kliniken, 1985.

5. Mikkelsen M, Philip J, Therkelsen AJ, Nielsen J, Hansen J, Wolf E. Praenatale undersøgelser i Danmark 1985. Report from the Danish Cytogenetic Central Register, 1987.

6. Nielsen J, Stradiot M. Transcultural study of Turner's syndrome. Clin Genet 1987; 32:260-270.

7. Nielsen J og medlemmer af Turner-kontaktgrupperne i Danmark. Turners syndrom. Turner-kontaktgrupper. En orientering. Udgivet af Turner-kontaktgrupper i Danmark, 1985.

8. Navot D, Laufer N, Kopolovic J, Rabinowitz R, Birkenfeld A, Lewin A, Granat M, Margalioth EJ, Schenker JG. Artificially induced endometrial cycles and establishment of pregnancies in the absence of ovaries. N Engl J Med 1986; 314:806-811.

9. Rosenfield RL. Toward optimal estrogen-replacement therapy. N Engl J Med 1983; 309:1120-1121.

10. Kastrup KW & Turner study group. Growth and development in girls with Turner's syndrome during early therapy with low doses of estradiol. In Illig R & Visser HKA (eds). Paediatric Endocrinology 1986. Acta Endocrin, 1986, Suppl. 279, 157-163.

11. Ranke MB, Haug F, Blum WF, Rosendahl W, Attanasio A, Bierich JR. Effect on growth of patients with Turner's syndrome treated with low estrogen doses. In Illig R & Visser HKA (eds). Paediatric Endocrinology 1986. Acta Endocrin, 1986, Suppl. 279, 153-156.

12. Ross JL, Myerson Long L, Skerda M, Cassoria F, Kurtz D, Loriaux DL, Cutler GB. Effect of low doses of estradiol on 6-month growth rates and predicted height in patients with Turner's syndrome. J Pediat 1986; 109: 950-953.

13. Rosenfeld RG, Hintz RL, Johanson AJ, Brasel JA, Burstein S, Chernausek SD, Clabots T, Frane J, Gotlin RW, Kuntze J, Lippe BM, Mahoney PC, Moore WV, New MI, Saenger P, Stoner E, Sybert V. Methinol human growth hormone and oxandrolone in Turner syndrome: Preliminary results of a prospective randomized trial. J Pediat 1986; 109:935-943.

14. Rosenfeld RG, Hintz RL, Johanson AJ, Sherman B, and the Genetech Collaborative Group. Results from the first 2 years of a clinical trial with recombinant DNA-derived human growth hormone (somatrem) in Turner's syndrome. Acta Paediatr Scand (suppl.) 1987; 331:59-66.

15. Nielsen J and members of Turner Contact Groups in Denmark. Turner's syndrome. Turner contact groups. An orientation. Published by The National Society of Turner Contact Groups in Denmark, 1987.

16. Nielsen J et des membres des groupes d'amitie-Turner. Le syndrome de Turner. Les groupes d'amitie-Turner. Une information. Publie par l'Association Nationale des Groupes d'Amitie-Turner du Danemark, 1987.

DISCUSSION

DR. ROBERT L. ROSENFIELD: We have not heard anything about psychological studies addressed to the issue of short stature generally. I would like to know what the current status of that is.

DR. ANKE EHRHARDT: In terms of growth hormone–deficient children or constitutionally delayed children, there are a number of studies in the literature which have shown a reasonably consistent picture that the social maturation is very much correlated with how a child is treated by the environment. There were a number of studies, years ago, with growth hormone–deficient children in Buffalo done with Drs. McGillivray and Aceto, which showed the beneficial effect of growth hormone treatment on social maturity. We also could establish at that time that IQ was not negatively affected in hypopituitary dwarfism. We did not show a specific pattern of deficit, as in Turner syndrome. In the newer studies, there has not been much of a focus on the kinds of new treatments that are available. We really are lacking good controlled studies. I do not know at this point, Margaret, whether there is any study which you have been doing with the psychoendocrine program at Children's Hospital in terms of induction of puberty, whether you want to add something to that.

DR. MARGARET MC GILLIVRAY: Dick Klopper and Tom Mazur are doing a study looking at psychosexual adjustments in hypopituitary young men who lack gonadotropin treatment and are on an HCG Pergonal treatment program. The treatment as much as possible is blinded. There is medication given, but I have to tell you, the patients know when they are not getting the therapy. There is a period with testosterone and there is a no-treatment period. I cannot tell you the results of the study at this time, except that there is a lot of psychological data and there are also sleep studies.

Dr. Robert L. Rosenfield is at the University of Chicago Pritzger School of Medicine, Chicago, Illinois. Dr. Anke A. Ehrhardt is at the Columbia University College of Physicians and Surgeons, and the New York State Psychiatric Institute, New York, New York. Drs. Margaret McGillivray is at the Children's Hospital, Buffalo, New York, and Judith G. Hall is at the University of British Columbia, Vancouver, British Columbia, Canada. Dr. Patrick Wilton is at KabiVitrum, Stockholm, Sweden. Dr. Johannes Nielsen is at the Psychiatric Hospital in Århus, Risskov, Denmark. Dr. G. Van Vliet is at the Hospital Universitaire Saint-Pierre, Brussels, Belgium. Drs. Ron G. Rosenfeld and Raymond L. Hintz are at the Stanford University School of Medicine, Stanford, California. Dr. Arthur Robinson is at the University of Colorado Health Science Center, and the National Jewish Center, Denver, Colorado. Dr. Annlis Söderholm is at the Social Service Center, Helsinki, Finland.

DR. PATRICK WILTON (STOCKHOLM): Dr. Ehrhardt, you presented so very many interesting data, so I probably missed some of them. What about children? Do they have children? Do you think it is very important for these girls to have children, and if so, do you think it is most important to have egg donation compared to adoption? I am perhaps a little bit biased, because I think you can create problems with all these three situations—not having children, adoption, and egg donation. I see one problem with egg donation that you do not find in the adoption situation. That is that you are really equal as husband and wife or man and woman, I should say, in the adoption situation and not in the egg donation, where it is just the husband who is the parent, so to say. It is a complicated question.

DR. EHRHARDT: Yes, I share your reservations—more from the studies on women who do not have Turner syndrome and in terms of coping with the new reproductive technologies. I do not have personal experience with any Turner woman who has had a child by egg donation. I can tell you in terms of adoption that many Turner women who are married are very eager to have a child. At Hopkins and Buffalo and Columbia I have worked with couples to adopt a child, and I have not seen that it was difficult. It depends very much as a medical professional how we present it to them. If we are very positive about adoption, and I am very positive about adoption, then I think to have a child by adoption is as good as going through a lot of complicated, at this point, often still experimental, technologies with a whole other host of the problems you alluded to. It may change in the future certainly. At this point, the answer is yes. Many of them want to have children. Among families I have followed, Turner women who have either adopted children or have married a widower with children have done very well as mothers.

DR. JOHANNES NIELSEN: To the last question of adoption or in vitro fertilization, I think we should ask the Turner women themselves, actually, and not speculate too much about what they should choose. We should present the possibilities, and we have discussed this very much in the Turner contact groups in Denmark. We have given them all the facts, and I do believe that a great majority of the Danish women would prefer in vitro fertilization. Who are we to say they should not. I think probably adoption would be better, but it is very important to present it to them and to write about it, and they can study it. So I think they will choose anyway. It may be very frustrating, certainly. Now in some Turners you can get their own eggs. This is a possibility, especially the mosaics. There is no doubt, you can stimulate even a few and find them. But donor eggs would be their best choice.

Now the question of stature. Also, this has been discussed very much in the Danish Turner contact group. Now we do so much about growth hormone, oxandrolone, and everything. We have a huge study running. And we always end up asking them, do you really want all this?

Because we know from the Danish study, and they know it, there is no correlation between how tall a Turner girl is and how well she manages, not in the Danish study, not in any study. But always they end up saying it is a stress to be so short. So, you must go on, but there is no scientific background for it that they manage better socially in any way by getting a few centimeters taller. We have to keep it a little in mind if we add drug after drug. Now it is three drugs that probably help growth. But still we have to go back to the Turner girls and ask them what do you want, and they want it. So we have to go ahead.

Now we compared also Turner girls with a group of women with short stature, primary amenorrhea and *normal* karyotypes. The group with normal karyotypes and short stature, they were more similar to the sisters in this group than to the Turner girls. The Turner girls have specifics due to the chromosome examination, chromosome aberration, and not so much to the stature, I think.

DR. G. VAN VLIET: There have been about 12 cases, I think, in the literature of Turner syndrome and anorexia nervosa. I assume that there must be a bias of reporting there, because this is the kind of combination that fascinates psychiatrists and endocrinologists alike. In the large-scale surveys from the Scandinavian countries, is there any evidence that anorexia nervosa is any more frequent than in the normal female population?

DR. NIELSEN: Yes, I believe it is slightly higher.

DR. RON G. ROSENFELD: I think we have actually heard some mixed experiences about the psychological outcome of girls with Turner syndrome. And I just want to voice a word of caution, rather than present any data, because I do not have any data. I think we should be very careful that we do not fall into the same trap which we have fallen into with the growth hormone-deficient children in whom it has turned out that their long-term outcome psychosocially as adults is much poorer than many of us ever suspected. I think the data that Dr. Nielsen and Dr. Ehrhardt presented have been in a large part with children who have received optimal medical care, optimal psychological support, and I think the data that Dr. Soderholm presented was just the opposite. I think in our enthusiasm about maximizing growth and maximizing sexual development, we should not forget that these children are abnormal. They are chromosomally abnormal, they are developmentally abnormal. We now have some data from Dr. Elkin that intellectually they perhaps are more abnormal than we have suspected or given credit to. And I think it is going to be very important that we participate as actively as possible as pediatricians in the long-term follow-up of these children as they go into adult life, because the experience may be a lot more pessimistic than we have been led to believe.

DR. JUDITH HALL: You have taken some of my thunder. I think the real problem is that we do not know what the situation is in adults. And in studies where you pick up people at a later time, who either have not ever been treated at all, or have not been followed, we really do not know the natural history. I think it is quite clear, both from what was presented this morning and certainly from the women that we follow, that appropriate estrogenization at puberty is essential to their psychosocial development, that it is very important that they develop breasts and that they have periods. But I can also tell you from some of the older women that after 10 years of menstruating, they get kind of tired of it. And the real question then is whether estrogen is important to women between 25 and 50 in terms of avoiding other kinds of problems and in terms of their general health care maintenance. And we do not know that. In other words, we think it is, but the data are not there, so it is hard to be convinced absolutely that they should continue it. I could not agree with you more that these girls, who we are doing a wonderful job on right now, need to be followed. What we are finding is that we cannot find them as adults. We have scoured the hills looking for Turners, and if any of you know Ginna Seibert, you know she is a scourer. We have one-fourth of the adult women that we ought to have in the Seattle area. So they are not found, for whatever reasons, whether it is because they are not on estrogens and are not motivated, or because they have thought badly of themselves at the time they have learned about their situation. We do not know the natural history.

DR. EHRHARDT: I just want to underline what Dr. Rosenfeld and Dr. Hall said. I really appreciated the data by Dr. Soderholm, and I am glad it came up, because I did not want to leave you with that estrogen treatment at the right time is not important. It is not important within a well-treated group. We could not see the difference in terms of social functioning, but then when I listen to Dr. Soderholm about untreated women who still look totally undeveloped in their 20s and 30s, then of course we get back to the critical importance to do replacement therapy. Probably extreme short stature then becomes again of great importance. So you have to see both of these sets of data in perspective, and it is nice that that came up this morning.

DR. NIELSEN: A comment on Analise Söderholm's data: I am all for estrogen treatment, but I think also that some of the results you presented could be due to the contact you got with the women, I think very much it could be. We have in Denmark also contact with a number of Turner women who do not want to have the estrogen treatment. Their gynecologist says they have to have it. Otherwise they lose the calcium in their bones, and all terrible things happen. They have had very much psychological problems in this, and we have told them if they feel bothered, they can stop for a while. We have several who manage much better without estrogen, so I think it is a very complex problem we have to deal with. We are now doing a study of life expectancy in Turner syndrome, and this has shocked us quite a lot. You know, probably, the ASA study from Edinburgh on the small group. We have a larger group, because we have from the whole of Denmark a central register. However we turn it around, there is a lack of life expectancy of 12 to 15 years. We are now analyzing very carefully those women. Of course, most of them are women who have not been treated with estrogens, and we will come back with some results about this. We are doing a national study also on bone mineral content and lipoproteins in relation to estrogen treatment during life, and from there I suppose we will have some results which will tell us about what to do. But I think it is very complex and very much individual, and we have to be very careful to say it should be so.

DR. ARTHUR ROBINSON: I would like to emphasize the importance of what Dr. Nielsen said about intrauterine diagnosis. I get a tremendous number of calls from women all over this country. Thousands of them are having amniocentesis nowadays to rule out Down's syndrome and they find that they have a fetus with a sex chromosomal abnormality. I am appalled by what the physicians in this country are telling these women. And they do not do what Dr. Nielsen said, which is to give some of the positive information about these individuals. We are tremendously impressed by the difference in what is happening today and what has happened previously in these untreated women, because these parents now have an opportunity to choose whether or not they want the fetus. Those who do want the fetus and continue the pregnancy have a very positive attitude towards the kind of anticipatory guidance that Dr. Nielsen was talking about, and I think the prognosis is very different from much of what we have heard before.

DR. ANNLIS SÖDERHOLM: I would like to comment about the treatment. Turner syndrome is an endocrinologic deficiency state, and in another disease where the hormone production is not normal, you do not hesitate to give, for instance, thyroxine. Why should we discuss this thing? I think these women do not have estrogen, so why don't we give them estrogen? I know when I met these untreated women, some of them had been asked do you want treatment, but they were so shy, they did not dare to tell their doctor I want menstruation, I want breasts, because these were things that were taboo. It is a shame to talk about them. It was after a long time of contact they very carefully told me that they want to have it. And secondly, many of the women without estrogen had severe menopausal symptoms. They had hot flashes and all kinds of psychosomatic disturbances which disappeared when the estrogen replacement started.

DR. RAYMOND L. HINTZ: Dr. Nielsen, how you think patients should be screened for Turner syndrome? Obviously, you are making the diagnosis much more frequently in Denmark than perhaps we are in the North American continent. To what do you attribute your success?

DR. NIELSEN: I think I mentioned in my presentation that one should make a chromosomal examination of all with one sign of Turner syndrome and of all with a growth stature 2 standard deviations or more below mean and I think then that you will catch them all or practically all. I would like to mention this chart. It would be very nice to have early information and booklets about Turner syndrome and referral to contact groups. I think I have the addresses of all Turner contact groups around the world including the United States. So I think it is important that everybody concerned with Turner has those addresses. About the screening, we have been doing for some years a screening of all newborns, but this is within the framework of a bigger study, studying the environmental influence on pregnancy, on childbirth, and on the child. In this connection we offer chromosome examination to all parents and 95% accept it. We have now examined, I believe, 30,000. I believe this will continue as a service because everybody thinks it is extremely important so when you have a chromosome aberration you get the information, the advice, and you come back here every second year to get more information. That, of course, is too expensive all over the world, but this is the ideal way.

37

On the Adolescent and Adult Patient with Turner Syndrome

Annlis Söderholm

Social Service Center, Helsinki, Finland

INTRODUCTION

In 1972-1976 a psychiatric follow-up study of girls with Turner syndrome was carried out by Vappu Taipale at the Children's Hospital, University of Helsinki (1). She analyzed the adolescent development of 49 patients, focusing on their psychic balance, defenses, and psychosocial adjustment. The aim was to create an overall therapeutic program which would promote these girls' psychosocial maturation as effectively as possible.

At age 9-12 the healthy and intact aspects of personality remained dominant. The turning point, whereupon the development began to assume abnormal features, took place at the age of 13, when lack of pubertal development led the girls into ever-increasing isolation from agemates and withdrawal from their world. Lack of substitution therapy meant failing gender identity, the girls no longer being able to identify with their developing agemates. This resulted in life situations in which the girls could be described as having a neuter identity. The older teenager tried to defend herself against the traumatic situation occasioned by the underdevelopment by means of increasing isolation and denial of emotions. A rigidity and stolidity gradually developed which severely limited the entire capacity for emotional life.

Therapy created a relieved and favorable attitude in all age groups. Gender identity was rapidly integrated into that of a girl, even in older teenagers, whereas progress towards the gender identity of an adult woman was slow. Girls diagnosed and treated late (≥16 years) were at risk of disturbed psychological development, and their general life situation included many external risk factors associated, for example, with training and employment. Characteristic were feelings of inadequacy related to a woman, mother, or female agemate, but not to someone of the opposite sex. What the untreated girl lacked was not only puberty but also all the features of adolescent development. Without preceding pubertal development a full range psychologic adolescence is impossible.

There are many reports on children and adolescents with Turner syndrome but few on adults, and little has been known about the difference between women who are adequately treated and those who have not received any treatment at all. In 1980-1985 I studied 62 adult patients at the Children's Hospital in Helsinki (2). My aim was, among other things, to define the psychosocial problems encountered by these patients and to study the effect of hormonal replacement on previously untreated adult women.

I was able to find 22 untreated patients and 26 patients who had been diagnosed and treated late (at 15-29 years of age). These were paired with 14 young adult women followed by the Endocrine Clinic of our hospital. All the patients were interviewed and investigated, and replacement therapy was begun in 15 untreated women aged 24-45 years (mean age 32 years).

Comparison of the three groups included their social developmental history: educational and working status, living and civil status, social network and support, and sexual relationships.

The interview was semistructured and included questions about somatic, social, and psychic history. The patients given replacement therapy were seen every 4-5 months for at least 3 years, the others just once.

It was clear that lack of endocrine replacement therapy seriously endangers normal psychosocial development.

WORKING AND PROFESSIONAL STATUS

The untreated patients had a less successful working and professional status than those who received treatment. For instance, 9 of the 12 patients who were on disability pensions were untreated and had been pensioned off at a mean age of 29.5 years.

LIVING AND CIVIL STATUS

Only 3 of the 22 untreated women had been able to separate from their parents before these died. None of the untreated patients were married. Among the 26 patients diagnosed and treated late, 19 had separated from their parents for reasons of marriage, work, training, or housing. Thirteen were married.

SOCIAL SUPPORT AND SOCIAL NETWORK

Social support is the degree to which an individual's basic social needs are met by others (3). These include affection, esteem or approval, a sense of belonging, identity, and security. These needs may be met by the provision of socioemotional aid (e.g., affection, sympathy and understanding, acceptance, and esteem) or instrumental aid (e.g., advice, information, help with family and work responsibilities, financial aid). The social support system is the subset of persons in the individual's total social network upon whom she relies for socioemotional aid, instrumental aid, or both (4).

The untreated patients had fewer important social contacts than the treated patients. Nine of the 22 women reported having no friends save members of their parental home, and only 8 felt that they had good and sufficient friend relations. In the treated groups only 4 of the 40 women had no friends.

At the interview a 50-year-old patient expressed her feelings as follows:

I have always considered my lack of female development much worse than my short stature. After the age of 16 there were always some discussions in which I was unable to participate. There are some subjects you simply avoid. It is such a sore point. You feel more and more on the outside of things. You get left behind when other young people go out.

SEXUAL RELATIONSHIPS

Only one of the untreated patients had had a sexual relationship with a man. Of the 40 treated women, 22 had had sexual intercourse, the first experience between 18 and 41 years of age. Two of the untreated women stated explicitly that their sexual infantilism had made sexual relations impossible. One of these women told me:

Perhaps the fact that I am underdeveloped has meant that I don't go anywhere, I am mostly alone and I have never been with men. You just can't think of relationships with men; you don't go out looking for them either.

PSYCHIATRIC DISTURBANCES

Until recently, women with the Turner syndrome have been described as having an unusually high tolerance to stress and being emotionally inert. This was true for women with adequate hormonal replacement and psychosocial care. My study showed that this was not the case in the absence of replacement therapy. Seven of 62 women had been treated in mental hospital because of psychotic episodes or depression, and 7 had been seen by psychiatrists in outpatient clinics. Common to 12 of the 14 patients with psychic disturbances was that they were untreated at the onset of symptoms.

REPLACEMENT THERAPY FOR ADULT WOMEN

Of the 15 women whom I started on replacement therapy, one with severe psychic symptoms discontinued all medication, and one died after 2 years in a traffic accident. The other patients have now been followed for 5-7 years. None have reported any negative effects of the replacement therapy, which was started at a mean age of 32 years (24-45 years). In a letter sent 18 months after substitution was started, a 35-year-old woman wrote:

> Prior to therapy I felt like only half a woman, although I was accepted as a human being. The first menstruation was a wonderful surprise. Now even I am able to menstruate. The therapy has been something very positive in my life. I now feel like a total woman who can menstruate like other agemates.

Substitution therapy had a positive organizing effect on the patients' view of themselves as women. Without sexual characteristics and/or without experience of menstruation, these women were unable to identify completely with others of their own sex. Therapy made identification possible, even though this was quite a new experience for women who had had to repress any knowledge of the biological processes inherent in a woman's life. "Doctor, I must say I had an odd feeling, but for the first time in my life I felt like a human being," said one of the women who experienced her first menstruation at the age of 40. The first menstruation, which appeared after 5-6 months of therapy, seemed to mark a positive turning point for the patients' self-esteem as women. In addition to the symbolic meaning of menstruation, therapy meant that for the first time they could visualize having genitals—menstruation was a visible and tangible proof of having internal genitals like other women.

The rapid appearance of a positive psychological effect with hormonal replacement does not mean that therapy can easily or rapidly change learned social behaviour. For most women, the social situation is more or less the same after 6-7 years of therapy. Stepping outside the parental home is still difficult, and none of the women studied have been able to improve their working status. Three of the women have, however, established a heterosexual relationship. One is a 40-year-old woman on a disability pension whose therapy started at the age of 36. After 3 years of therapy she told me: "For me, therapy has been of immense help. I could never have believed in the beginning that it would help me so much. I don't think I had ever been able to be with men. Now I feel I'm like other women, that I've experienced those things other women experience."

REFERENCES

1. Taipale V. Adolescence in Turner's syndrome. Academic dissertation, University of Helsinki, 1979.

2. Söderholm A. Turners syndrome. En psykosocial och somatisk undersökning av 62 kvinnor. Academic dissertation, University of Helsinki, 1985.
3. Kaplan BH, Cassel JC, Gore S. Social support and health. Medical Care
   1977; XV suppl:47–58.
4. Thoits PA. Conceptual, methodological, and theoretical problems in
   studying social support as a buffer against life stress. Health Soc Behav
   1982; 23:145–159.

38

Growth Potential in Turner Syndrome

Michael Preece

Institute of Child Health, University of London, London, England

INTRODUCTION

The most consistent feature of Turner syndrome is short stature; it is also one of the most distressing. For this reason much energy is expended in the search for treatment options that may increase height, particularly if such increases are sustained into adult life. It is also important that any therapy for other aspects of the condition, such as the induction of puberty with estrogens, must not impair growth and hopefully should increase stature. For example, in the past there has been concern over the timing of the introduction of estrogen replacement as, in the doses then advocated, a hastening of epiphyseal fusion was a concomitant effect.

In considering potential mature height, it is necessary first to review historical data of adult height, then to assess methods of predicting mature height, and finally to review the various therapeutic options.

HISTORICAL GROWTH DATA

The growth of girls with Turner syndrome has already been reviewed in Chapter 12 using data from a large sample of German girls (1). In this group the mature height was estimated as 146 cm, based on 14 women in that study but supported by data from various other reports. More recently a further study amalgamated data from a variety of sources to yield an estimate of 143 cm calculated from a total of 138 women from Germany, France, Finland, and the United Kingdom (2). Considering the great variety of source data, from many different countries, these estimates are not that inconsistent.

A further problem relates to the uncertainty as to whether the adult height of women with Turner syndrome has been subject to the secular trend (3). If this were the case then the mature height of patients who are still growing today should be greater than the historical controls. Unfortunately, it is very difficult to establish this from published data as the dates of birth are not reported and the relationship between them and the date of publication is far from certain. Because of the correlation between the heights of affected women and their parents (4), it is also likely that ethnic differences will account for a greater proportion of variance than the secular trend.

PREDICTION OF ADULT HEIGHT IN TURNER SYNDROME

Further progress in the assessment of height potential in Turner syndrome is to some extent dependent on the degree of predictability of growth in the syndrome. Conventional height prediction methods (5-7) are unlikely to be helpful because they are all based on source data from normal children or those with constitutional growth delay (6). A direct extrapolation to Turner syndrome is not valid, and other approaches are necessary (8).

Figure 1 shows a growth chart which has been developed specifically for Turner syndrome using data from five European studies. Initially, four data sets were used to develop the first set of standards, and the fifth study was only used to validate the prediction of mature height (2). Subsequently, the fifth study (U.K. data) was incorporated for the final chart (published by Castlemead Publications, Ware, Hertfordshire, U.K.).

When the heights of individual girls are plotted on these charts it is clear that their growth is remarkably predictable and to a very close approximation on the final height is on the same centile as heights recorded at earlier ages. This is illustrated in Figure 2 (heights are actually plotted in terms of standard deviation scores (SDS) as these are statistically more tractable).

While the centile (or SDS) at diagnosis gives a close approximation of mature height, the prediction may be further refined using the regression equation:

$$SDS_{final} = 0.21 \ (\pm 0.07) + 1.13 \ (\pm 0.07) \cdot SDS_{initial}$$

with a residual SD of 0.30 SD units and 95% confidence limits of the order of ± 2.0 cm. In general, bone-age measurements did not improve the prediction unless there was a very substantial degree of maturational delay (2).

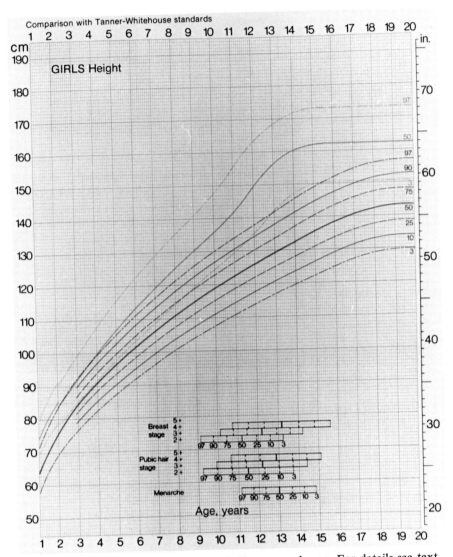

Figure 1 A growth chart for girls with Turner syndrome. For details see text.

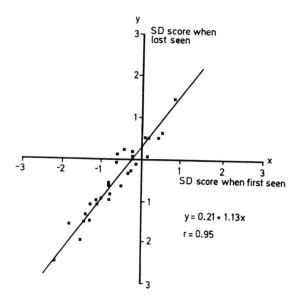

Figure 2 The relationship between height SD from the Turner standards when first measured (age 3–12) and when last seen between the ages of 19 and 24 years in 29 girls with Turner syndrome. (Reproduced from Ref. 3 with kind permission of the authors and publishers.)

EFFECTS OF HORMONE THERAPY ON GROWTH POTENTIAL

We may now assess the possibility of modifying the adult height of women with Turner syndrome by appropriate treatment during childhood. Using the method described above, we can predict the eventual mature height of a young girl with untreated Turner syndrome within an acceptable degree of precision. Long-term growth response to various treatment regimens can be compared to these predictions and an objective assessment of efficacy made. The results already presented from the U.S. multicentre study (9; Chapter 32) suggest that a number of the girls receiving growth hormone and oxandrolone are already surpassing their predicted height, which strongly suggests that a significant benefit will be achieved in due course. The magnitude of this benefit will only become clear with time. Growth hormone alone is, thus far, producing smaller increases in growth velocity but bone age advance is slower and the eventual balance between these two processes cannot be assessed until more girls are nearer to mature height. Oxandrolone alone is unlikely to increase mature height, which is in keeping with earlier studies (10).

The impact of estrogens on mature height can also be assessed to some extent. In an earlier study 29 girls were treated with ethinyl estradiol in starting doses of 10 μg daily (2). The height SDS (from the Turner syndrome standards) was -0.60 (± 0.10) SDS before treatment rising to -0.15 (± 0.09) SDS ($p <$ 0.01) one year after starting replacement. However, by maturity (between 19 and 24 years) the mean height had fallen to -0.50 (± 0.10) SDS. There was, therefore, no long-term benefit, in terms of height, but equally there was no harmful effect on height. We can therefore use estrogen in these dosages without anxiety. It may be that much lower doses may be more beneficial as has already been suggested (11). Trials of lower doses of ethinyl estradiol, both alone and in combination with growth hormone, are now in place, but results are not yet available.

In summary, we have considerable knowledge of the height potential of untreated women with Turner syndrome. Evidence is gathering that this potential may be improved by appropriate endocrine therapy, but it is too soon to assess the magnitude of these gains and thus whether they are sufficient to justify the long commitment by the patients during childhood.

REFERENCES

1. Ranke MB, Pfluger H, Rosendahl W, Stubbe P, Enders H, Bierich JR, Majewski F. Turner syndrome: Spontaneous growth in 150 cases and review of the literature. European Journal of Paediatrics 1983; 141:81-88.

2. Lyon AJ, Preece MA, and Grant DB. Growth curve for girls with Turner syndrome. Arch Dis Childhood 1985; 60:932-935.

3. Van Wieringen JC. Secular growth changes. In Falkner, F. Tanner, JM (eds.). Human Growth. New York, Plenum Press, 1986, pp. 307-331.

4. Brook CGD, Gasser T, Werder EA, and Prader A. Height correlations between parents and mature offspring in normal subjects and in subjects with Turner's and Klinefelter's and other syndromes. Annals Hum Biol 1977; 4:17-22.

5. Bayley N, and Pinneau S. Tables for predicting adult height from skeletal age. Pediatrics 1952; 40:423-441.

6. Tanner JM, Whitehouse RH, Cameron N, Marshall WA, Healy MJR, and Goldstein H. Assessment of Skeletal Maturity and Prediction of Adult Height (TW2 Method). London, Academic Press, 1983.

7. Roche AF, Wainer H, and Thissen D. Predicting adult stature for individuals. Monographs in Paediatrics. Basel, S. Karger AG, 1975.

8. Preece MA. Prediction of adult height: Methods and problems. Acta Paediatrica Scandinavica [Suppl] 1988; 347:4-10.

9. Rosenfeld RG, Hintz RL, Johanson AJ, Sherman B, and The Genentech Collaborative Group. Results from the first 2 years of a clinical trials with recombinant DNA-derived human growth hormone (somatrem) in Turner's syndrome. Acta Paediatrica Scandinavica (Suppl) 1987; 331:59-66.

10. Sybert VP. Adult height in Turner syndrome with and without androgen therapy. Pediatrics 1984; 104:365-369.

11. Ross JL, Cassorla FG, Skerda MC, Valk IM, Loriaux DL, and Gutler GB. A preliminary study of the effect of estrogen dose on growth in Turner's Syndrome. N Engl J Med 1983;309:1104-1106.

DISCUSSION

DR. MILO ZACHMAN: I have a question about when you say you think there is an artifact in the bone-age retardation when you calculate or overestimate with the bone-age-based prediction. In the Bailey-Pinot prediction, which is right, you are also based on the bone age, so why is it only in the Tanner-Whitehouse prediction? Is it because you only looked at radius, ulna, short bones, and because the artifact is more pronounced there, or is it for some other reason?

DR. MICHAEL PREECE: I do not know the answer, Milo. In the Tanner-Whitehouse prediction system it is the RUS, as you say, the radius, ulna, and the short bones of the hand that are used. In a sense that should make it better, because it is the carpus that is most unusual, or most regularly unusual in Turner syndrome. So I am as puzzled as you are. I look at the data as it comes out.

DR. JAMES TANNER: There is a difference. Whether it accounts for it, I do not quite know, but the TW system as we use it is based on chronological age modified by bone age. The Bailey-Pinot is based on bone age modified by chronological age. They are two very different things. Between the Mark 1 and Mark 2s, the Mark 1s, as you aficionados of the field will remember, had a bone age-based alternative. We thought it would be nice to do it both ways since we didn't know which was better and we put in a bone age-based alternative. When it came to the Mark 2, we had some experience, we dropped that bone age-based alternative and said, no, that is not any good. We do not want to do it that way. And I think that is the real difference.

DR. JAMES W. FRANE: I have a number of comments. One is we have taken three different methods of the Tanner-Whitehouse that have been published over the years and, relative to the Turner girls, we found all of them to mark high.

Dr. Milo Zachman is at the Universitäts-Kinderklinik, Zürich, Switzerland. Dr. Michael Preece is at the Institute of Child Health, London, England. Dr. James Tanner is at the University of Texas Health Center, Houston, Texas. Dr. James W. Frane is with Genentech, Inc., South San Francisco, California. Dr. Jaakko Perheentupa is at the University Children's Hospital, Helsinki, Finland. Dr. Barbara M. Lippe is at the University of California at Los Angeles School of Medicine, Los Angeles, California.

So in that sense we do not think any of them are applicable to untreated Turner girls. I think that the agreement between the Bailey-Pinot and the Lyon or Ranke projection, or whatever, is a matter of luck. I do not think there is anything that is scientifically based in the method there. Both Peter Compton and I have been intrigued by the difference caused by the so-called bone age adjustment to the Lyon prediction, because the way we adjust it, it does not cause a change in the average prediction. It only changes the individual predictions, especially those where the bone ages are particularly advanced or retarded. We are very interested in hearing more about how you do that. Also, I was curious as to why you would use the Lyon prediction after the child is treated, because it seems to me that by definition it would not be applicable once the child is treated.

DR. PREECE: Well the first thing, the method of modifying is simply to enter the standard score tables at the bone age rather than the chronological age. It is nothing sophisticated, it is simply that, and therefore you would expect to make a difference to the height prediction, because on average you are entering the tables at a "younger age," because of the bone age delay that was inherent in the cohort. That is why that happens. I have forgotten what the second point was.

DR. FRANE: The fact that you apply the Lyon prediction, if I understand correctly, after the child is treated. Because the norms are for untreated girls, I do not see why.

DR. PREECE: The reason for looking at that was sort of trying to allow for the change in bone maturation, which is different between the four treatment groups. If there had been the same change in bone age in all four treatment groups, then of course it would not have mattered. But because there was a difference, I felt that we had to try and allow for that in some simple way. An alternative would have been to put it in as a covariate in the analysis of variance, but in fact it comes out with essentially the same answer.

DR. FRANE: When you take your chart and you enter at the bone age rather than at the age, it seems to me that you need to adjust the chart also, because as illustrated in the Ranke paper, the average Turner girl has a bone age retardation of about 1.3 years, so it seems to me you have got to shift the norms at the same time. I do not think you can just take the old chart and enter at the bone age.

DR. PREECE: No, I think it is a naive thing to do, but it was just an exercise in looking at the effect. If the bone age delay that is seen is all due to maturational delay, which I do not think it is, but if it was all due to maturational delay, then it would be right. Given that it is probably a complex of a bit of maturational delay and a bit of dysmorphology, then of course it falls down.

DR. FRANE: I think we are going to have some more exciting discussions on this.

DR. JAAKKO PERHEENTUPA: I guess what I was going to say is just about the same. If we use a Turner syndrome-specific growth standard, why should it not be used also in Turner syndrome-specific bone age scale, because there is a systematic difference between normal and Turner?

DR. PREECE: In principle there is no reason not to. You could use the criteria of one of the bone aging systems. It could just as well be the Tanner-Whitehouse, and just restandardize on X-rays of Turner syndrome girls if we get a large enough group of them to do that. There is no reason why it should not be done.

DR. BARBARA LIPPE: I have a slightly different kind of question, but I have not been able to get the answer from anybody else, so I thought I would try you. Given the ascertainment bias that we know we have in terms of who is diagnosed as having Turner's, are the final heights of the girls normally distributed? That is, do they really fit an absolute normal Gaussian distribution?

DR. PREECE: I did not show that. Yes, they do. The numbers, if you look at the actual attained final heights, are distributed indistinguishably from a Gaussian population, but the numbers are quite small. So you cannot do very rigorous tests of the normality. And equally, height predictions by whatever method is used have a Gaussian distribution.

DR. RON G. ROSENFELD: The average bone age delay in the Genentech Collaborative Study of 1.3 years is exactly the same as that reported by Ranke for his 150 German girls, and that group of 150 girls constitutes almost half of the database for the Lyon paper. We felt that that was all the more evidence in support of the validity of using the Lyon growth curves, uncorrected, for bone age as a way of projecting final adult height for this cohort of girls.

DR. PREECE: If we are just taking an untreated group of girls, then I would absolutely agree with you, and I think to the best of our knowledge that prediction method is as good as any. The problem is what happens when you then interfere by using oxandrolone and/or growth hormone, because you cannot blithely go on not thinking that maturation is being altered differentially between the treatment groups. So you had to bring something in. That is why it was done. Otherwise, I would entirely agree with you.

39

The Long-Term Behavior of Patients with Turner Syndrome

An Update

Jennifer I. Downey and Anke A. Ehrhardt

*Columbia University College of Physicians and Surgeons,
and New York State Psychiatric Institute, New York, New York*

INTRODUCTION

The behavior of patients with Turner syndrome has been the subject of many studies. Researchers have been intrigued by different aspects of the syndrome— genetic abnormality, short stature, lack of spontaneous pubertal development, and infertility. Psychological studies are particularly important for the clinicians who follow patients with Turner syndrome and their families, since long-term endocrine management requires behavioral data, e.g., on the importance of timing of estrogen replacement therapy or, more recently, the effect of growth hormone on behavior adjustment.

We will present in this paper an update on the three areas that have been the main focus of psychoendocrine studies: (a) cognitive abilities, (b) psychosexual development, and (c) psychopathology and behavioral adjustment. We will present a longitudinal perspective rather than limit our discussion to one developmental phase, such as childhood, adolescence, or adulthood.

COGNITIVE ABILITIES

Intelligence and mental functioning in patients with Turner syndrome has been the topic of many studies. From all available evidence so far, it appears that IQ scores of persons with Turner syndrome follow the normal curve rather than clustering in the moderately or severely retarded range. Girls with Turner syndrome are not more often represented in institutions for the mentally retarded (1,2); they are also not different in overall intelligence from their unaffected siblings (3). This is in contrast to earlier reports based on clinical case examples and unrepresentative samples.

Turner syndrome is associated with a specific pattern of strengths and weaknesses in mental functioning. Many patients with this syndrome have difficulties in visual-motor coordination, motor learning (4-6), spatio-temporal processing (7), and sense of direction and perceptual stability (8). These specific difficulties appear more frequently in patients with Turner syndrome than usually observed but are not obligatory features of the clinical picture. The specific manifestations of these cognitive deficits vary in different studies depending on assessment methods and patient sample sizes, but most studies agree that Turner patients typically demonstrate a characteristic pattern of significantly lower nonverbal IQ compared to verbal IQ (9,10).

The etiology of this distinctive but variable pattern of mental abilities is poorly understood. One explanation (11) has attributed the problems of many Turner individuals with visual-motor coordination to a general developmental delay, proposing the deficiency may resolve with further brain maturation. However, a recent study from our Program of Developmental Psychoendocrinology of adult Turner women compared with constitutional short stature (CSS) women and unaffected Turner sisters (12)* found that the Turner women showed the same cognitive pattern as reported previously for children and adolescents: In comparison to the control groups, they had significantly lower scores on WAIS subtests measuring Arithmetic, Digit Span, Block Design, Object Assembly, and Digit Symbol/Coding as well as significantly lower scores on the Benton Revised Visual Retention Test, which measures ability to recall and reproduce drawings of geometric shapes. Interestingly, on a six-item self-assessment test requiring the women to rate their facility with spatial tasks relative to peers (13), the Turner women reported more difficulties on only one of the items—finding their way around a strange city. The Turner women were no different than the CSS subjects in reporting difficulty with the other five items—learning to use new equipment, assembling objects from parts, arranging things in a space-efficient manner, picturing the final result of a construction project, and interpreting charts to others.

---

*This study of psychological outcome in adult women with Turner syndrome will be referred to throughout the chapter. Twenty-three Turner women between the ages of 19 and 38 were compared with 23 women diagnosed in childhood as having constitutional short stature. In a second comparison 10 Turner women from the original 23 were compared to their normal adult sisters, so that 10 pairs were studied.

The data on cognitive abilities in Turner syndrome makes it essential that an individual patient be assessed carefully with standard psychometric testing and the results be evaluated not only as to the full-scale IQ alone, but always with special attention to the verbal IQ versus the performance IQ and to other specific aspects of mental functioning. Some Turner individuals are totally unaffected and indeed may have high spatial relations ability. Therefore, individual psychometric assessment is required in order not to make false predictions based on an average pattern that may not apply to the individual patient.

No clinician should ever counsel parents of a newborn with Turner syndrome by saying that mental retardation will probably be one of the features of the clinical picture. This information has to be corrected in textbooks since the implications of such erroneous predictions can have grave consequences if the parent believes the physician and raises the child with too low expectations, sometimes fulfilling a damaging prophesy.

PSYCHOSEXUAL DEVELOPMENT

Psychosexual development in girls with Turner syndrome does not differ from that in other girls. Despite the lack of gonadal development with the concomitant lack of exposure to fetal gonadal hormones, female gender identity and gender role behavior in childhood develop normally (14,15). Girls with Turner syndrome have been found to be interested in the same toys, games, peers, friendships, etc. as matched normal controls, with actually more pronounced interest in stereotypical feminine pursuits such as doll play. While adolescence, especially if sex hormone replacement therapy is initiated relatively late, is often a critical time and may lead to more problems in adjustment, psychosexual development remains feminine with no goals and interests different from other females.

In adulthood, Turner women typically continue to have a female gender identity and retain some of the same tendencies to more stereotypical feminine behavior. For instance, in our study of adult Turner women compared with CSS women (16), the Turner women reported more preference for female friends over male, less physical activity and athletic interest, and less open expression of anger.

When we move from gender role behavior to sexual behavior in Turner individuals, there is evidence that some women exhibit problems, though by no means universally. Nielsen and colleagues' 1977 study (11) in Denmark of 45 Turner individuals compared with 46 of their unaffected sisters found that only 42% of all patients who were over age 18 had ever been married or lived with a man compared to 80% of the sisters, and that 42% had never had sexual intercourse compared with 13% of the sisters. McCauley et al. (17) interviewed 25 adult women with Turner syndrome regarding their friendships and sexual relationships and found high rates of inexperience with social and sexual relationships with men. Five of the women had never dated at all, and nine others had never had an ongoing relationship with a man. None of these 14 women (56%) had ever had sexual intercourse. Of the 12 TUS women who had had sexual intercourse, 3 reported severe sexual dysfunction with very infrequent intercourse and/or vaginismus and dyspareunia.

In the study previously mentioned comparing adult women with Turner syndrome to women with CSS and to normal siblings, we also assessed sexual behavior (18). Age at attaining important *romantic* milestones was comparable for the earlier milestones such as first crush. But for the Turner women who had ever reached the milestones, there was increasing delay with each additional milestone until finally with age at first love, the delay was 4 years, compared to the CSS women. When we looked at age of attaining *sexual* milestones such as first holding hands, first romantic kiss, up to intercourse, we found similar patterns of comparable age at first holding hands, but 4 years delay in age when Turner women had experienced first intercourse. In addition, some of the women never reached the advanced romantic and sexual milestones. For instance, 7 Turner women had never been in love (compared to 1 CSS woman), and 10 had never had intercourse (compared to 2 CSS women).

On the other hand, Turner women were just as likely to have masturbated as the control women and to have begun to do so at about the same age. If they were currently sexually active with a partner, they were just as likely to be orgasmic with intercourse. We did not find any increased incidence of vaginismus or dyspareunia in our Turner sample, but the sexually active Turner women did report a significantly longer latency period during sexual activity before vaginal lubrication took place. The same patterns were found when the Turner women were compared to their unaffected sisters.

These findings on masturbation experience and orgasm with intercourse do not suggest that Turner women have a lower sexual drive, but the data from all three studies—Nielsen's, McCauley's, and ours—suggest that Turner women have more difficulty in establishing a sexual relationship with a partner, and even when they do, that they are more prone to have difficulties with sexual intercourse, perhaps because the regimen of estrogen replacement therapy on which they are maintained is not really adequate to establish normal vaginal lubrication with sexual arousal. On the other hand, there are always individuals who overcome any limiting factor. For instance, there was a woman in our study who was sexually active and asymptomatic with intercourse even though she had totally discontinued estrogen therapy. Endocrine factors are also clearly not the only impediment to healthy sexual adjustment for Turner women. Even when patients are on hormone replacement therapy and are very attractive and have no visible stigmata of Turner syndrome except for short stature, some of them may harbor false beliefs about their ability to perform sexually. This inhibition may act as an impediment to their seeking out experiences in which they could establish a relationship with a partner.

All of us who counsel Turner patients and their families must clearly state that there is nothing about Turner syndrome which should prevent a woman from functioning normally as a sexual partner and indicate that if symptoms develop, often this is simply a sign that the hormone replacement regimen should be reevaluated or a vaginal lubricant added.

PSYCHOPATHOLOGY AND SOCIAL FUNCTIONING

The third area of interest is psychopathology and behavioral adjustment in individuals with Turner syndrome. For the girl with Turner syndrome, risk of difficulty depends in part on how severely affected she is physically—whether she must cope with multiple birth defects or predominantly with the three cardinal features of Turner syndrome—short stature, sex hormone deficiency, and infertility. During childhood, girls with Turner syndrome usually adjust surprisingly well, though short stature may become an issue in middle childhood and may lead to behavior problems, as in other slow-growing children (19). Money and Mittenthal (20) characterized the personality style of many girls with Turner syndrome as "inertia of emotional arousal" and suggested that their compliance and lack of behavior problems during childhood may be a beneficial trait, which enables them to tolerate the adversities of their condition. The same trait was reported in other studies when girls with Turner syndrome scored low on questionnaires that measure neuroticism, spontaneity, activity, and enthusiasm (14,21).

More recent studies of girls with Turner syndrome have suggested that there is at least a subgroup of these patients who have increased behavior problems. Sonis et al. (22), in a comparison of 16 Turner girls with normal controls, observed that the Turner children had poorer attention skills, poorer peer relationships, and more immaturity. They seemed "hyperactive." McCauley et al. (23) noted in a study of 17 Turner girls ages 9–17 compared to constitutional short stature controls that the Turner girls had fewer friends, needed more structure to socialize and to complete tasks, and had more difficulty understanding social cues. They also had more behavior problems, especially in the area of social ineptitude and isolation.

During the second decade of life, at the time when peers go into spontaneous puberty, it appears that the psychological risks for girls with Turner syndrome increase markedly. The timing of induced puberty is crucial because it will determine how long they will be out of step with their peers in terms of secondary sex characteristics. It appears that having to cope with looking younger and immature in addition to being shorter than one's peers presents a significant additional risk for psychopathology. In a clinical follow-up study of 73 girls and women with Turner syndrome ranging over a wide age span, Money and Mitten-thal (20) stressed the risk of delayed pubertal development on psychological adjustment. They compared two groups of girls between the ages of 14 and 18, one treated with estrogen versus one still untreated, and found that environmental response to the immature group was very different, increasing the risk of behavior problems. Girls with immature appearance were also significantly less likely to begin dating and establishing romantic friendships.

In a prospective study in Finland (24,25) 26 girls with Turner syndrome were followed over several years during adolescence. In the older girls, estrogen replacement was given between ages 15.3 and 19.9. Psychological evaluation of patients up to age 12 confirmed earlier clinical impressions that many patients with Turner syndrome are well adjusted in childhood. However, a turning point was age 13, at which time the patient group started to fall behind in psychological maturation and often became loners or developed more severe pathology. Those patients who still were undeveloped at age 14 were often afflicted with marked anxiety, serious behavior problems, and a tendency to withdraw. The substitution therapy was found to initiate the process of adolescence and to be of emotional help to the girls.

Psychopathology can express itself in a variety of ways which are not unique to a particular disorder like Turner syndrome, yet may occur more frequently in it. An association between anorexia nervosa and Turner syndrome has been suggested, and to date at least 16 cases have been reported of the two conditions occurring together (11,26-31). However, since the incidence of anorexia nervosa in the general population is not known, it is not clear whether anorexia nervosa is genuinely increased in girls with Turner syndrome compared to its incidence in normal girls.

Assessments of psychopathology in adult Turner individuals have generally suggested that incidence of psychiatric disorder is low and probably no greater than for unaffected women. Money and Mittenthal's chart review (20) of 73 Turner patients seen at the Psychohormonal Research Unit at Johns Hopkins Hospital found seven patients with mild psychopathology, defined as "lacking the ability to meet the demands of life in a way completely acceptable to family and community" and three patients with "severe psychopathology," defined as "long-term failure to maintain a minimally acceptable everyday-life adjustment." Using the same definitions of psychopathology, Nielsen et al. (11) found no significant differences between 45 TUS individuals and their unaffected sisters: Five of the 45 TUS patients and two of the 46 sisters had psychopathological symptoms.

Our own study (32), which differed from the two described above because it included no children or adolescents, yielded similar findings. The 23 TUS women and 23 CSS controls were assessed with the SADS-L, a semistructured interview which generates a lifetime history of psychiatric disorders by Research

Diagnostic Criteria (33). Turner women and controls did not differ significantly in the number who had *ever* had a psychiatric disorder or in the number who were *currently* ill. There were indications that the CSS women actually had more vulnerability to mental disorders since they had significantly earlier ages of onset of first illness, more different disorders per subject, and a greater number of episodes of mental disorder over their lifetime. A comparison of 10 Turner women with their unaffected sisters showed no differences in any of these measures of psychopathology. On the SCL-90-R, an instrument which measures current psychiatric symptoms (34), there were no differences between the groups. On the other hand, compared to the CSS controls, Turner women had significantly lower scores on the Global Assessment Scale (35), an instrument measuring overall psychological functioning over the previous month. We felt that the Turner women achieved lower scores on the GAS because it measures positive psychological health as well as the absence of symptoms.

Thus, in adulthood, Turner individuals have been found to have no increased incidence of psychiatric disorder. Mental health, however, comprises more than psychopathology; it also includes social functioning. This is the area in which Turner women appear to be having the most difficulty. For instance, Nielsen et al. (11) reported that while Turner women had as high academic and occupational achievement as their siblings, they were less socially mature, that is, they were significantly less likely to have left their parental home, to have had sexual intercourse, or to have married. McCauley et al. (17) in their study of 30 Turner women between the ages of 21 and 48 years, found that while the women reported in general adequate relationships with friends, they had limited social and sexual experience with men and, as mentioned above, when they were sexually active, a high incidence of sexual dysfunction. A subgroup of subjects reported considerable depression and difficulties with self-esteem.

Our own study of Turner women supports this picture of some impairment in social functioning in Turner adults. Compared to the short-stature women, TUS women were significantly less likely to have a heterosexual partner, whether spouse or boyfriend, and to have ever had heterosexual experience in the past. They also reported having fewer friends and placing less reliance on their closest friend. Finally, despite comparable verbal IQs—one of the best predictors of educational attainment—the Turner women had lower educational and occupational attainment than did the CSS women.

The available studies to date suggest that most Turner girls do well in childhood, with a minority suffering from hyperactivity and/or social immaturity. In adolescence, with the delay in puberty and the increased importance of height comparable to peers, psychological risk increases. In adulthood, although problems have less of a crisis-like presentation and although psychiatric disorders are not increased, achieving a mature level of psychosocial functioning remains a difficulty for a significant number of Turner individuals.

An important clinical implication of this is that professionals who are consulted about Turner individuals need to be aware that the problems these patients have do not tend to be of the acting-out kind which are most likely to distress family members, school personnel, and employers. Rather, these patients, when having difficulty, tend to become socially withdrawn and isolated, and their lack of attention-getting behavior and complaint may lead to oversight that any help is needed. Thus, professionals who counsel Turner patients and their families need to ask about social functioning with an awareness of what is age-appropriate so that intervention can be made if a Turner individual is beginning to withdraw from her peer group or if social awkardness is becoming a problem.

SUMMARY AND IMPLICATIONS FOR CLINICAL MANAGEMENT

Turner syndrome is a clinical syndrome with widely varying presentations. Affected individuals may have multiple physical abnormalities and health problems or be totally normal in appearance and health except for short stature, lack of spontaneous puberty, and infertility. Cognitive abilities also vary greatly. While it is now clear that mental retardation does not occur more frequently in Turner syndrome, the fact remains that a Turner individual may have cognitive deficits which make certain tasks such as space-form tasks difficult, or she may be totally unaffected. Thus, one of our patients needed to be accompanied to our office in order to find it, while another, obviously without any space-form difficulty, possessed a private pilot's license. Gender-role behavior is typically very feminine, and tomboyish behavior is unusual but would surely not be abnormal. Turner women as a group do not have more mental disorders than do unaffected women, but individuals may still suffer from such conditions as depressive disorders and anorexia nervosa. Social and sexual functioning may be impaired or may be not only adequate, but extraordinary.

For this reason, we feel that a balanced approach to the Turner patient and her family is essential. It is valuable to be aware of what kind of difficulties are most likely to occur and what developmental stages such as adolescence can be particularly troublesome. On the other hand, we should not assume without evidence that a particular problem will occur since predicting problems where none exist can be stigmatizing and as harmful as not seeing them when they are there. Professionals who combine an up-to-date knowledge of Turner syndrome with a careful investigative approach to the individual patient and give appropriate counseling and individualized guidance are in a position to be of enormous help to Turner individuals and their families.

REFERENCES

1. Ferguson-Smith MA. Karyotype-phenotype correlations in gonadal dysgenesis and their bearing on the pathogenesis of malformations. J Med Genetics 1965; 2:142-155.
2. Palmer CG, and Reichman A. Chromosomal and clinical findings in 110 females with Turner syndrome. Human Genetics 1976; 35:35-49.
3. Garron DC. Intelligence among persons with Turner's syndrome. Behavior Genetics 1977; 7:105-127.
4. Shaffer JW. A specific cognitive deficit in gonadal aplasia (Turner's syndrome). J Psychol 1962; 18:403-406.
5. Money J. Cytogenetic and psychosexual incongruities with a note on space form blindness. Am J Psychiatry 1963; 119:820-827.
6. Alexander D, Ehrhardt AA, and Money J. Defective figure drawing, geometric and human, in Turner's syndrome. J Nervous and Mental Dis 1966; 152:161-167.
7. Silbert A, Wolff PH, and Lilienthal J. Spatial and temporal processing in patients with Turner's syndrome. Behavior Genetics 1977; 7:11-21.
8. Waber DP. Neuropsychological aspects of Turner's syndrome. Devel Med and Child Neurol 1979; 21:58-70.
9. Thielgard A. Cognitive style and gender role. Danish Med Bull 1972; 19: 276-282.
10. Money J, and Granoff D. IQ and the somatic stigmata of Turner's syndrome. J Mental Deficiency 1965; 70:69-77.
11. Nielsen J, Nyborg H, and Dahl G. *Turner's Syndrome*. Risskov, Denmark, Acta Jutlandica, 1977.
12. Downey J, Elkin E, Ehrhardt AA, Gruen R, Bell JJ, and Morishima A. Cognitive ability and educational and career attainment in women with Turner syndrome (submitted).
13. Lunneborg PW. Sex differences in self-assessed, everyday spatial abilities. Percep Motor Skills 1982; 55:200-202.
14. Shaffer JW. Masculinity, femininity and other personality traits in gonadal aplasia (Turner's syndrome). In H. Biegel (Ed.), *Advances in sex research*. New York, Hoeber, 1963, pp. 219-232.
15. Ehrhardt AA, Greenberg N, and Money J. Female gender identity and absence of fetal gonadal hormones: Turner's syndrome. Johns Hopkins Med J 1970; 126:237-248.
16. Downey J, Ehrhardt AA, Morishima A, Bell J, and Gruen R. Gender role development in two clinical syndromes: Turner syndrome versus constitutional short stature. J Am Acad Child and Adult Psychiatry, 1987; 26(4):566-573.
17. McCauley E, Sybert VP, and Ehrhardt AA. Psychosocial adjustment of adult women with Turner syndrome. Clin Genetics 1986; 29:284-290.
18. Downey J, Ehrhardt AA, Gruen R, Bell JJ, and Morishima A. Sexual behavior in Turner syndrome (in preparation).

19. Meyer-Bahlburg HFL. Psychosocial management of short stature. In D Shaffer, AA Ehrhardt, and LL Greenhill (Eds.). *Clinical guide to child psychiatry*. New York, Free Press, 1985, pp. 110–144.

20. Money J, and Mittenthal S. Lack of personality pathology in Turner's syndrome: Relation to cytogenetics, hormones, and physique. Behavior Genetics 1970; 1:43–56.

21. Baekgaard W, and Nyborg H. Neuroticism and extraversion in Turner's syndrome. J Abnormal Psychol 1978; 87:583–586.

22. Sonis WA, Levine-Ross J, Blue J, Cutler GB, Loriaux PL, and Klein RP. Hyperactivity and Turner's syndrome. Paper presented at American Academy of Child Psychiatry Meetings, San Francisco, 1983.

23. McCauley E, Ito J, and Kay T. Psychosocial functioning in girls with Turner's syndrome and short stature: Social skills, behavior problems, and self-concept. J Amer Acad Child Psychiatry 1986; 25:105–112.

24. Perheentupa J, Lenko HL, Nevalainen I, Niittymaki M, Söderholm A, and Taipale V. Hormonal treatment of Turner's syndrome. Acta Paediatrica Scandinavica 1975; 256:24–25.

25. Taipale V. *Adolescence in Turner's Syndrome*. Helsinki, Finland, University of Helsinki, 1979.

26. Liston EH, and Shershow LW. Concurrence of anorexia nervosa and gonadal dysgenesis: A critical review with practical considerations. Arch Gen Psychiatry 1973; 29:834–836.

 7. Kron L, Katz JL, Gorzynski G, and Weiner H. Anorexia nervosa and gonadal dysgenesis: Further evidence of a relationship. Arch Gen Psychiatry 1977; 34:332–335.

28. Darby PL, Garfinkel PE, Vale JM, Kirwan PJ, and Brown GM. Anorexia nervosa and 'Turner syndrome': Cause or coincidence? Psychol Med 1981; 11:141–145.

29. Taipale V, Niittymaki M, and Nevalainen I. Turner's syndrome and anorexia nervosa symptoms. Acta Paedopsychiatrica 1982; 48:231–238.

30. Dongherty GG, Rockwell WJK, Sutton G, and Ellinwood EH. Anorexia nervosa in treated gonadal dysgenesis: Case report and review. J Clin Psychiatry 1983; 44:219–221.

31. Larocca FEF. Concurrence of Turner's syndrome, anorexia nervosa, and mood disorders: Case report. J Clin Psychiatry 1985; 46:296–297.

32. Downey J et al. Psychopathology and social functioning in women with Turner syndrome. J. Nerv and Mental Disease 1989; 177(4):191–201.

33. Spitzer RL, and Endicott J. *Schedule for affective disorders and schizophrenia: Life-time version*. New York, New York Psychiatric Institute, 1979.

34. Derogatis LR. *SCL-90-R: Administration, scoring, and procedures manual*. Towson, MD, Clinical Psychometric Research, 1983.

35. Endicott J, Spitzer RL, Fleiss JL, and Cohen J. The global assessment scale: A procedure for measuring overall severity of psychiatric disturbance. Arch Gen Psychiatry 1976; 33:766–771.

DISCUSSION

DR. RAYMOND HINTZ: What was the range of heights of these girls? The average was 142, but was the range?

UNIDENTIFIED: The average height listed was 4'8" (±2.5 inches), and two standard deviations would have taken it up to a little bit over 5 feet.

DR. JUDITH G. HALL: We have recently observed a physical finding that may well be related to psychological function. Michael Hayden, my colleague, has done PET scan studies on five women with Turner syndrome. There is a panel of neurologic and normal patients who can be used as controls for the PET scan. On PET scan, you can actually see visualization of areas of the brain and quantitate by doing slices at various areas and then measuring the amount of uptake in those areas.

In the Turner women there was significantly lower uptake in the occipital and the parietal area, where there is decreased utilization of glucose in the Turner women. That does not mean that the structure is abnormal. It means that those areas are less active under the test situation.

I think the reason this is important is that it gives us a structural area to either monitor or follow, and perhaps we have to think about what is different in those areas—imprinting, estrogen, or other things. All of these women had been on estrogen, three of them were on estrogen at the time of this study. There were no differences between those women who were presently on estrogen and those who were not.

I cannot interpret the data any more than that at this point, but I think it gives us some sense that there may be something related to the visual area of brain in Turner women and may give us a basis for some of the things that we observe in them.

DR. HINTZ: Who served as controls for the normals?

DR. HALL: There is a panel of patients of 100 women and 100 men. The closest ones in age, socioeconomic background, and family history were chosen.

DR. HINTZ: But is there a variance in size?

DR. HALL: No. If you look among the normal panel, being short does not make any difference.

Dr. Raymond Hintz is at the Stanford University School of Medicine, Stanford, California. Dr. Judith G. Hall is at the University of British Columbia, Vancouver, British Columbia, Canada.

40

The Management of the Adult with Turner Syndrome
The Natural History of Turner Syndrome

Judith G. Hall

University of British Columbia, Vancouver, British Columbia, Canada

Turner syndrome is a multisystem disorder. The type and frequency of various congenital anomalies are fairly well defined in newborns and young girls with Turner syndrome. However, the natural history and medical complications in adult women are much less well described, and there is even less information on their appropriate management.

Over a decade ago, Virginia Sybert and I started a clinic for adult women with Turner syndrome in Seattle, Washington in order to try to define the natural history in adults with Turner syndrome (1). The clinic population as well as a review of the available medical literature allowed us to recognize a number of specific problems seen in adult women with Turner syndrome. These are outlined here. Most medical complications of adult women did not seem to relate to a particular karyotype.

There is still a great deal to be learned about the natural history of adults with Turner syndrome. This paper includes a flowchart to alert the clinician caring for patients with Turner syndrome to the medical complications of various ages and outlines suggestions for regular screening. Each of these medical complications appear to be relatively rare in individuals with Turner syndrome, and certainly no one individual will have all of the complications. However, many problems do have an increased incidence (albeit hard to establish exactly how high) and therefore bear watching.

GYNECOLOGIC AND OBSTETRIC COMPLICATIONS

Most patients with Turner syndrome have gonadal dysgenesis, but occasionally a woman will have spontaneous menses and, rarely, even become pregnant without medical assistance (2). Early menopause occurs in most women with Turner syndrome who have spontaneous menses. Although the pelvis is somewhat android in configuration, an increased need for cesarean section does not occur.

There is an increased incidence of chromosome abnormalities in the children of fertile Turner syndrome women (3). The exact risk is not clear, but it definitely appears to be above the background 0.5% risk for a chromosome anomaly in non-Turner women. Therefore, prenatal diagnosis to rule out a chromosomal anomaly is appropriately offered to pregnant women with Turner syndrome. In most cases, replacement hormonal therapy should be provided from the age appropriate for puberty induction until an age similar to menopause in other women. Usually hormonal replacement therapy is discontinued between ages 45 and 50 years.

GENITOURINARY TRACT

Approximately 60% of women with Turner syndrome have some type of structural or positional renal tract anomaly compared to 10% of non-Turner women (4,5). These abnormalities rarely result in renal malfunction. However, it would appear that those women with structural renal tract anomalies have an increased risk of silent urinary tract infections and silent hydronephrosis. Thus, it would appear to be appropriate to screen for renal and collecting system anomalies and to monitor those women with abnormalities for urinary tract infections during adult life.

Women with Turner syndrome with 46,XY/45,X karyotype are at increased risk for gonadoblastomas and malignant degeneration of Wolfian tract remnants. Ideally, these would have been surgically removed in childhood (6), but if they have not been, they should be removed as soon as possible after the karyotypic abnormality is recognized.

ENDOCRINE DISTURBANCES

Patients with Turner syndrome have an increased incidence of autoimmune endocrine disease including hypothyroidism and possibly diabetes mellitus. There is an increased incidence of thyroid antibodies (as many as 60% of Turner syndrome women compared to 20% of non-Turner women) (7,8), but hyperthyroidism is rarely seen (about 1%). Symptomatic autoimmune hypothyroidism is seen in about 30% of adult Turner syndrome women. It is appropriate to monitor regularly for autoimmune thyroid disease by determining the presence of autoantibodies or elevated TSH. It appears that women with iso-chromosome X do have a higher risk for acute Hashimoto's thyroiditis and Graves' disease (9).

There is an increased incidence of glucose tolerance abnormalities in women with Turner syndrome (between 30 and 60% have impaired serum glucose response to an oral glucose load) (10) but they rarely develop frank diabetes. For this, regular screening of urine rather than a GTT may be the appropriate way to screen for functional diabetes in Turner syndrome.

Obesity is a common complication of Turner syndrome (11). Forty percent of affected adult women have a significant problem controlling their weight. This is complicated by the presence of peripheral edema. Early dietary counseling and careful caloric maintenance at a young age are important preventive measures. Unfortunately, hypertension is often associated with the obesity of Turner syndrome and provides a second reason for controlling weight gain.

ORTHOPEDIC AND SKELETAL ABNORMALITIES

There are a large number of skeletal changes seen in Turner syndrome that prove helpful in suspecting the diagnosis. These include short fourth metacarpal, cubitus valgus, midface hypoplasia, Madelung's deformity, increasing angulation of the carpal bones, pes cavus, irregular tibial metaphyses with a mushroom projection of the medial surface of the proximal tibial metaphyses, Schmorl's nodes of the vertebrae and android configuration of the pelvis (12,13).

Scoliosis requiring therapy is a fairly frequent finding in Turner syndrome (about 10%) and particularly needs to be watched for during induction of puberty (14).

Congenital dislocation of the hips is also seen with increased frequency (about 15%) and is associated with degenerative arthritis of the hips in older women.

Osteoporosis is said to have an increased frequency in Turner syndrome, however, it may well be that translucency, trabecular bone patterns, and decreased mineral content of the bone appear to look like osteoporisis but do not predispose to fractures (15). These changes do not appear to improve very much with estrogen therapy, nor does it appear that women with the Turner syndrome are at increased risk for osteoporotic fracture in old age.

CRANIOFACIAL INVOLVEMENT AND COMPLICATIONS

Women with the Turner syndrome tend to have a high palate and mildly nasal speech. They frequently have had chronic and recurrent otitis media as children

(16), and many adults (at least one sixth) have hearing loss (including both conductive and neurosensory).

Half of individuals with the Turner syndrome have opthalmologic problems including ptosis, amblyopia, cataracts, nystagmus, color blindness, or strabismus (present in one third of all Turner syndrome women).

Because of the high palate and small jaw, malocclusion and crowding of teeth is frequent (17,18). If orthodontic work has not been performed, adults with Turner syndrome may have a cosmetic problem. An increased incidence of sinusitis and mastoiditis has also been reported.

Because of the high palate, shortened tracheal length, and short neck, it has been suggested that anesthetizing patients with Turner syndrome may be a problem (19), but complications have not been reported.

CARDIOVASCULAR COMPLICATIONS

Lymphedema is present in about half of the individuals with Turner syndrome at birth, and although it may subside, it can be a problem throughout life. Peripheral lymphedema can be treated with support hose, diuretics, and salt restriction, but frequently lymphedema is aggravated by the menstrual cycle. This may occasionally take the form of a chyloris collection of fluid in the thorax or abdomen and occasionally as fluid and protein loss in the GI tract (20).

Structural abnormalities of the heart were described earlier. All types of heart defects are seen, although postductal coarctation of the aorta is most typical. Approximately half of affected individuals have some structural cardiac anomaly, but it is usually corrected by adulthood if symptomatic. However, a surprisingly large number of women with Turner syndrome (as many as one third) have bicuspid aortic valves (21); thus echocardiographic evaluation is appropriate. Prophylactic antibiotic use with dental work or surgery may be indicated.

Aneurysm with dissection of the aorta has been described (21) but would appear to be very rare in the absence of hypertension, bicuspid aortic valve, or coarctation. When any of these risk factors are present, screening cardiac and aortic echocardiography should be performed every few years.

Hypertension is a frequent complication of Turner syndrome, even without either coarctation of the aorta or renal abnormalities (23). Approximately 30% of Turner women have blood pressures of 140/90 or higher. The hypertension seems to be particularly related to obesity, some forms of estrogens, and fluid retention. When these factors are corrected or controlled, most Turner women have normal blood pressures. Regular monitoring of blood pressure is mandatory.

SKIN ABNORMALITIES

Prominent ears and webbing of the neck occasionally requires cosmetic surgical correction. It is important to be aware that keloid formation is frequent in Turner syndrome, so care should be used at the time of any surgical procedure, including ear piercing (24).

Patients with Turner syndrome have an increased number of nevi, and these should be removed if they are in an area where they will be rubbed (1). Atrophic skin, alopecia, hirsutism, and increased wrinkling are seen in older women with Turner syndrome and may be related to relative estrogen deficiency.

GI DISEASE

Bleeding of the bowel from hemangiomas is seen with increased frequency in Turner syndrome at all ages, although it seems to respond to estrogen therapy (25,26). In addition, inflammatory bowel disease (27) and anorexia nervosa (28) are seen more frequently than expected. Treatment is as with any other patient.

LIFETIME MANAGEMENT

The management of each of the abnormalities in individuals with Turner syndrome is usually not different from that in the general population. However, monitoring for these abnormalities and complications is appropriate in all individuals with Turner syndrome. Table 1 is an attempt to outline age-related concerns. After the age of 25, it makes sense for the individual with Turner syndrome to establish a regular yearly checkup with an internist who knows to monitor for these particular problems.

The actual frequency of various problems is not yet clearly defined. The recognition of these and other potential problems in adult women with Turner syndrome is important for better long-term management and for an understanding of the pathogenetic processes that occur in the absence of a second normal X chromosome.

The lay support group, The Turner's Syndrome Society, York University, ASB 006, 4700 Keele St., Downsview Ontario, M3J 1P3, Canada can be very helpful to individuals and families.

Table 1 Medical Care Flowchart

	Newborn or when diagnosed	Childhood	Adolescent	Adult
Gonadal dysgenesis	Karyotype to establish diagnosis. If 46XY remove gonads by 5 years of age. Gonadotrophins before age 5 to determine if functional gonadal tissue present	Fertility counseling and reassurance about options available for various ways to have children discussed with girl	Gonadotrophins prior to hormone replacement if not evaluated at earlier age. Hormone replacement with yearly pelvic examination. Endometrial biopsy if abnormal bleeding	Usually hormone replacement until mid-40s. If fertile, offer prenatal diagnosis with all pregnancies
GU	Renal ultrasound to look for renal structural anomalies. If structural anomalies, yearly urine to screen for occult UTI	If structural anomalies, yearly urine to screen for occult UTI	If structural anomalies, yearly urine to screen for occult UTI	If structural anomalies, yearly urine to screen for occult UTI
Growth	Plot growth on growth curve yearly	Plot growth curve yearly. Check yearly for thyroid antibodies and/or TSH. Watch for obesity. Develop good dietary habits to avoid overweight	Plot growth curve yearly. Initiate hormone replacement to maximize growth. Watch for obesity	Check yearly for thyroid antibodies and/or TSH. Watch for obesity
Skeletal	R/O dislocated hips knee problems	Watch for scoliosis. Examine wrists for Madelung. Watch knees for tibial problems	Watch for scoliosis. Examine wrists for Madelung. Examine knees for tibial problems	

Craniofacial	Feeding problem with high palate, use cleft palate nipple Otitis frequent Check ears with colds Treat aggressively	Otitis frequent— Check ears with colds Treat aggressively Crowded jaw— may need orthodontic work Start planning and evaluating by 6 years Prominent ears—may need cosmetic repair (beware of potential for keloid formation)		Otitis frequent Check with colds Treat aggressively Crowded jaw— may need orthodontic work
Cardiovascular	Observe for lymphedema and treat symptomatically (support hose, diuretics, salt restriction)* R/O coarctation—US study Treat as needed R/O bicuspid valve—US study Use prophylactic antibiotics if present	R/O Hypertension— check yearly Treat as necessary Try weight reduction for treatment	Watch for fluid retention and recurrence of edema As start hormone replacement treat symptomatically Check yearly for hypertension and aortic root size	Observe for lymphedema and treat symptomatically (support hose, diuretics, salt restriction) Check yearly for hypertension and aortic root size

Table 1 (Continued)

	Newborn or when diagnosed	Childhood	Adolescent	Adult
Skin	If web neck prominent, consider repair—beware of potential for keloid formation	Multiple nevi appear—Remove if in areas where rub, (beware of potential for keloid formation) Toenails may rub against shoes Treat with V-wedge resection If considering ear-piercing, be aware of potential for keloids	If considering ear piercing or surgery be aware of potential for keloids Consider removal of nevi if rubbing	Consider removal of nevi if rubbing Beware of keloids with any surgery
Central nervous system		Screen for spatial abilities If problem discuss with schools to arrange help Psychosocial anticipatory counselling	Psychologic support opportunity to discuss either with other Turner girls, family or with psychologist	
Other	Check stool guaiac for GI bleeding in infancy and childhood	Check urine every 1–2 years for diabetes	Be aware of increased risk for anorexia nervosa, inflammatory bowel disease and psychiatric illness Check urine every 1–2 years for diabetes	Check urine every 1–2 years for diabetes

*Ultrasound

REFERENCES

1. Hall JG, Sybert VP, Williamson RA, Fisher NL, Reed SD. Turner's syndrome. West J Med 1982; 137:32–44.
2. King CR, Magenis E, Bennett S. Pregnancy and the Turner syndrome. Obstet Gynecol 1978; 52:617–624.
3. Taysi K. Brief clinical report: Del(X) (q26) in a phenotypically normal woman and her daughter who has trisomy 21. Am J Med Genet 1983; 14:367–372.
4. Egli F, Stalder G. Malformations of kidney and urinary tract in common chromosomal aberrations. Hum Genet 1973; 18:1–15.
5. Rahal F, Young Rb, Mamunes P. Gonadal dysgenesis associated with a multicystic kidney. Am J Dis Child 1973; 126:505–506.
6. Knudtzon J, Aarskos D. 45,X/46, XY mosaicism. A clinical review and report of ten cases. Eur J Pediatr 1987; 146:266–271.
7. Gruneiro de Papendieck L, Iorcansky S, Coco R, Rivarola MA, Bergada C. High incidence of thyroid disturbances in 49 children with Turner syndrome. J Pediatr 1987; 111:258–261.
8. Germain EL, Plotnick LP. Age-related anti-thyroid antibodies and thyroid abnormalities in Turner syndrome. Acta Paediatr Scan 1986; 75:750–755.
9. Sparkes RS, Motulsky AG. The Turner syndrome with isochromosome X and Hashimoto's thyroiditis. Ann Intern Med 1967; 67:132–144.
10. Polychronakos C, Letarte J, Collu R. Carbohydrate intolerance in children and adolescents with Turner syndrome. J Pediatr 1980; 96:1009–1014.
11. Delsado JA, Trahms CM, Sybert VP. Measurement of body fat in Turner syndrome. Clin Genet 1986; 29:291–297.
12. Leszczynki S, Kosowica J. Radiological changes in the skeletal system in Turner's syndrome—Review of 102 cases. Prog Radiol 1965; 1:510–517.
13. Finby N, Archibald RM. Skeletal abnormalities associated with gonadal dysgenesis. Am J Radiol 1965; 93:354–361.
14. Crawford JD. Management of children with Turner's syndrome. In: Papadatos CJ, Bartsocas CS, eds. The Management of Genetic Disorders. New York, Alan R Liss, 1979, pp. 97–109.
15. Park E. Cortical bone measurements in Turner's syndrome. Am J Phys Anthropol 1977; 46:455–462.
16. Szpunar J, Rybak M. Middle ear disease in Turner's syndrome. Arch Otolaryng 1968; 87:34–40.
17. Filipsson R, Lindsten J, Almquist S. Time of eruption of the permanent teeth, cephalometric and tooth measurement and sulphation factor activity in 45 patients with Turner's syndrome with different types of X chromosome aberrations. Acta Endocrinol 1965; 48:91–113.
18. Lammi S. Occlusal morphology in 45,X females. J Craniofac Genet Dev Biol 1986; 6:351–355.
19. Divekar VM, Kothari MD, Kamdar BM. Anaesthesia in Turner's syndrome. Can Anaesth Soc J 1983; 30:417–418.

20. Triesman J, Collins FS. Adult Turner syndrome associated with chylous ascites and vascular anomalies. Clin Genet 1987;31:218-223.
21. Miller MJ, Geffner ME, Lippe BM, Itami RM, Kaplan SA, DiSessa TG, Isabel-Jones JB, Friedman WF. Echocardiography reveals a high incidence of bicuspid aortic valve in Turner's syndrome. J Pediatr 1983;102:47-50.
22. Lie JT. Aortic dissection in Turner's syndrome. Am Heart J 1982; 103: 1077-1080.
23. Virdis R, Cantu MC, Ghizoni L, Ammenti A, Nori G, Volta C, Cravidi C, Vanelli M, Balestrazzi P, Bernasconi S. Blood pressure behaviour and control in Turner syndrome. Clin Exp Hypertens 1986;8:787-791.
24. Haddad HM, Wilkins. Congenital anomalies associated with gonadal aplasia: Review of 55 cases. Pediatrics 1959;23:885-902.
25. Burge DM, Middleton AW, Kamath R, Fasher BJ. Intestinal hemorrhage in Turner's syndrome. Arch Dis Child 1981; 56:557-558.
26. O'Hare JP, Hamilton M, Davies JD, Corrall RJ, Mountford R. Oestrogen deficiency and bleeding from large bowel telangiectasia in Turner's syndrome. J R Soc Med 1986; 79:746-747.
27. Arulanantham K, Kramer MS, Gryboski JD. The association of inflammatory bowel disease and X chromosomal abnormality. Pediatrics 1980; 66: 63-66.
28. Dougherty GG, Rockwell WJK, Sutton G, Ellinwood EH. Anorexia nervosa in treated gonadal dysgenesis: Case report and review. J Clin Psychiatry 1983;44:219-221.

DISCUSSION

DR. JUDSON VAN WYCK: I used to think that the wandering blood theory (Bonneville) was kind of nuts, but now that we are diagnosing patients in utero through amniocentesis at a very early age and the suggestion that the accumulations of lymphedema may play an etiologic role in some of the things that distort the body image the grossest, I am asking the questions whether, when this diagnosis is made early on in gestation, imaging techniques should be promptly instituted and what can be done with the more aggressive intrauterine attacks on problems such as this, because this may be one frontier where we can really make a huge difference if we understood this part of their pathophysiology.

Dr. Judson Van Wyck is at the University of North Carolina at Chapel Hill, Chapel Hill, North Carolina. Dr. Judith G. Hall is at the University of British Columbia, Vancouver, British Columbia, Canada. Dr. Arthur Robinson is at the University of Colorado Health Science Center, and the National Jewish Center, Denver, Colorado. Dr. Michael Preece is at the Institute of Child Health, London, England.

DR. JUDITH G. HALL: My impression, and I would ask Dr. Robinson to comment as well, is that those fetuses that show severe edema are destined to die. In other words, those who are picked up with hydrops such that you can actually see it on ultrasound will usually go ahead and terminate spontaneously in the second trimester. When you look at those fetuses that are picked up by karyotype of either chorionic villi or cells from amniocentesis, what you see is no edema at that stage. I suspect that the damage has already been done by the time we are recognizing that fetus in utero. What you might like to try is something to open up their lymphatics or decrease intravascular volume.

DR. ARTHUR ROBINSON: I think you are absolutely right and we are very excited now about the possibility of looking at this chromosomal commitment idea, that perhaps the parental origin of the X chromosome and its degree of methylation may be very important in telling you how seriously affected the fetus is.

DR. MICHAEL PREECE: I have a couple of minor points which I suppose are, broadly speaking, immunological. I would like to add to the observation of somatotroph antibodies that we have reported in one case some 8 or 9 years ago. We have seen a second case subsequently. These go often with the multiple endocrine immunological abnormalities, but with very specific antibodies to the somatotroph and which result in associated growth hormone secretory abnormalities. So it is a worthwhile diagnosis to make.

DR. HALL: Would you suggest that they should be screened for then by the endocrinologist, or is this something that you think occurs in adulthood?

DR. PREECE: Well, I think it depends a little bit on whether growth hormone becomes a more or less routine treatment for Turner syndrome when this becomes an irrelevance. If not, then it has to be borne in mind, because one of our patients had growth hormone deficiency related to this. I would also be interested in other people's reactions to our very clear impression of an excessive incidence of juvenile rheumatoid arthritis in our Turner syndrome population.

DR. HALL: Well, as I suggested, we have seen degenerative arthritis in the adults. I am not aware of JRA being reported, and I guess the real question is what the incidence is and whether it is related in some way to the immunologic background of these girls.

DR. PREECE: In our own patient population, which I suppose is about 120 patients currently, we have had 4 juvenile rheumatoids, so it is a real excess, and this is indistinguishable from ordinary juvenile rheumatoids to my understanding.

DR. HALL: And what are the HLA types, or has that been looked at?

DR. PREECE: I cannot tell you offhand.

DR. MARGARET MC GILLIVRAY: We don't have any in the 141 that I am currently following, so it may be related to something else in the population.

DR. PREECE: True.

DR. JOHANNES NIELSEN: Turner girls and Turner women are not patients and we should try not to make them patients. I am a little afraid that they should be screened for all that has been mentioned here. They will certainly become patients and they will manage more poorly, I think, than if we leave them untouched. Of course, we should be aware of the most serious things, but should not screen them for everything and not let this out to general practitioners or whoever might do this. Another thing is, and you mentioned it also, I believe your group is a select group and we certainly do not find these frequencies in more unselected groups in Denmark, where many have never been in the hands of any physicians except that the diagnosis was made probably in screening programs or by chance. So I think also we should be aware of publications on selected groups belonging to different clinics. When you talk about frequency of abnormalities, you have to have unselected groups, but of course you do not have it, and you just cannot get it.

DR. HALL: I believe in the importance of Turner support groups, and I was waiting until the end of the conference to see if anybody was going to mention the North American Turner's Support group. There is one based in Toronto which is very active and has some very good literature. It is my impression that the support groups are not used much, and they are so helpful to a family when a diagnosis is first made and to a girl to meet and talk with somebody else with Turner syndrome. But I think then what happens is those groups learn that there are medical complications and the families want to know what to screen for. My hope would be not to upset people, but rather to say these are the things to screen for. Let your doctor take care of it and that is it.

41

Turner Syndrome in Adult Women
Two Illustrative Cases

Andrew R. Hoffman

Stanford University School of Medicine, Stanford, California

Although the incidence of Turner syndrome has been estimated to be as high as ~1 in 1000 women, relatively few of these patients are seen by internists or adult endocrinologists. The population of adult women with Turner syndrome can be divided into three distinct groups: 1. those patients who had been diagnosed, evaluated and treated as children; 2. individuals who received the diagnosis of Turner syndrome but never received treatment or evaluation for multisystem abnormalities; and 3. patients in whom the diagnosis is made only in adult life, if it is made at all. Since the first group of patients have been carefully evaluated over a period of years, it is more likely that they will enter into a continuing health care system as adults. While some patients will escape from specialized care, most of the serious congenital anomolies should have been diagnosed during childhood. Patients in the latter two groups, however, have not received adequate care. The challenge to internists and gynecologists, therefore, is to find these individuals, to evaluate them extensively, and to be willing to reevaluate patients who currently carry the diagnosis of Turner syndrome.

The importance of careful, life-long medical evaluation was recently emphasized by a prospective epidemiologic study of individuals with Turner syndrome who survived infancy in the United Kingdom (1). One hundred and fifty-six patients with Turner syndrome were followed for an average of 17 years. While the expected mortality in this group of women was estimated to be 3.6 deaths, 15 of the Turner patients died. Even when the 16 patients with congenital

507

cardiac anomalies were removed from the evaluation, the mortality in the Turner population was increased threefold. The investigators estimated that life expectancy in Turner syndrome is reduced by 11 years at age 20, by 10 years at age 40, and, by 8 years at age 60. The reasons for the increased mortality are not known, but patients with Turner syndrome have an increased incidence of glucose intolerance (2) and hypertension (3), two conditions associated with substantial cardiovascular morbidity.

Two patients recently seen at Stanford University Hospital clearly illustrate some of the special problems in the diagnosis and care of adults with Turner syndrome:

CASE 1

A 36-year-old Chinese woman was admitted with a dissecting aneurysm of the aortic arch and transient left hemiparesis. Surgical repair was achieved with graft replacement of the ascending aorta and part of the aortic arch. Turner syndrome had been diagnosed by buccal smear at age 18 when the patient presented with primary amenorrhea to a physician in Taiwan. Estrogen replacement was attempted with birth control pills, but no further evaluation was performed. The patient had been followed for hypertension in the United States, but did not volunteer information concerning the diagnosis of Turner syndrome. On physical examination, she was short (149 cm) and prepubertal. The karyotype was 45X;46,X, pseudodicentic Y (q21.2) mosaicism. Because of the presence of Y chromosome material, she underwent laparotomy and removal of two streak gonads; no tumor was found.

A recent study has demonstrated that there is an 8.8% incidence of aortic root dilatation by echocardiography in patients with Turner syndrome. Risk factors for aortic dissection in this population include coarctation of the aorta, bicuspid aortic valve, and systemic hypertension. On pathologic examination, cystic medial necrosis is often observed (4).

The finding of any Y chromosomal material in a patient with gonadal dysgenesis mandates gonadectomy because of the high risk of gonadal malignancy. In a review of the literature from 1953 to 1983, 140 cases of neoplasia in dysgenetic gonads had been reported (5). A Y chromosome or a fragment of it were present in 90.7% of the cases. Bilateral tumors were discovered in 38.4% of the patients, underlining the importance of bilateral gonadectomy. While 53.1% of the tumors were gonadoblastomas, neoplasms that are virtually always benign, 19.6% of the patients harbored dysgerminomas. Moreover, dysgerminomatous elements were found in conjunction with gonadoblastoma in an additional 17.5% of cases. Other neoplasms included choriocarcinoma, embryonal cell carcinoma, Sertoli cell tumor, and interstitiallike carcinoma. Many adult patients with Turner syndrome were diagnosed in childhood by buccal smear, a method that will not detect the presence of a Y chromosome. Therefore, it is important to discover how patients who carry the diagnosis of Turner syndrome were previously evaluated and to obtain a karyotype on each patient who had been diagnosed by buccal smear to determine if Y chromosomal material is present. When ordering karyotypes in adult patients, it must be recalled that aneuploidy is frequently seen in individuals over age 40, and that a 45,XO mosaic karyotype is not uncommon in older, normal women (6).

CASE 2

A 33-year-old Hispanic woman was referred to the Endocrine Service for evaluation of osteoporosis and secondary amenorrhea. Menarche occurred at age 11, and the patient experienced normal menses from age 12 to 15. By age 16, she had menstrual periods every 2-4 months. Behcet's syndrome was diagnosed in her late teens, and she has received intermittent glucocorticoid therapy ever since. Oligoamenorrhea and infertility persisted until age 31; there have been no subsequent menstrual periods. The menstrual irregularities were attributed to her severe chronic illness, and no evaluation had been initiated. The patient was short (148 cm) but bore no other stigmata of Turner syndrome. Serum FSH was in the menopausal range at 54 mIU/ml, and the karyotype was 46,X, del (X)(q21).

This patient demonstrates the importance of evaluating longstanding menstrual abnormalities, even in patients with debilitating diseases. In premature ovarian failure, Turner syndrome or mosaicism should be considered, since normal menstrual cycles and even fertility are occasionally seen in women with gonadal dysgenesis (7). Osteoporosis may occur as a consequence of hypoestrogenemia secondary to chronic amenorrhea or oligoamenorrhea. While there is currently no published data to indicate that osteoporosis is a significant problem in patients with Turner syndrome, it would be important to study a population of these women to determine the role of long-term estrogen therapy in the preservation of their bone mass. Moreover, since estrogen therapy has been shown to be beneficial in decreasing cardiovascular mortality in postmenopausal women (8), sex hormone replacement therapy should be offered to all adult women with Turner syndrome.

In summary, women with Turner syndrome must not be allowed to disappear from the health care system once they graduate from pediatric care. Frequent monitoring of the cardiovascular system is necessary, since these patients are at risk for diseases of the aortic valve, the aorta, and the coronary arteries. Thus, patients should be vigorously screened for hypertension and glucose intolerance and be cautioned to avoid obesity, a common condition in this syndrome. Estrogen replacement therapy, with progesterone-induced cycling, should also be discussed with each patient. Finally, Hashimoto's thyroiditis is common in

Turner syndrome, and, therefore, thyroid function tests should be obtained on all adult patients.

ACKNOWLEDGMENT

Supported in part by a grant from the National Institutes of Health (AG 01312).

REFERENCES

1. Price WH, Clayton JF, Collyer S, DeMey R, Wilson J. Mortality ratios, life expectancy, and causes of death in patients with Turner's syndrome. J Epidemiol Commun Health 1986; 40:97–102.
2. Polychronakos C, Letarte J, Collu R, Ducharme JR. Carbohydrate intolerance in children and adolescents with Turner syndrome. J Pediatrics 1980; 96:1009–1014.
3. Hall JG, Sybert VP, Williamson RA, Fisher NL, Reed SD. Turner's syndrome. West J Med 1982; 137:32–44.
4. Lin AE, Lippe BM, Geffner ME, Gomes A, Lois JF, Barton CW, Rosenthal A, Friedman WF. Aortic dilatation, dissection, and rupture in patients with Turner syndrome. J Pediatr 1986; 100:820–826.
5. Troche V, Hernandez E. Neoplasia arising in dysgenetic gonads. Obstet Gynecol Survey 1986; 41:74–79.
6. Court-Brown WM. Human Population Cytogenetics. North-Holland, Amsterdam, 1967.
7. Reyes FI, Koh KS, Faiman C. Fertility in women with gonadal dysgenesis. Am J Obstet Gynecol 1976; 126:668–670.
8. Stampfer MJ, Willett WC, Colditz GA, Rosner B, Speizer FE, Hennekens CH. A prospective study of postmenopausal estrogen therapy and coronary heart disease. N Engl J Med 1985; 313:1044–1049.

Summary of Part V

Intellectual and Psychosocial Development in Turner Syndrome

Raymond L. Hintz

Stanford University School of Medicine, Stanford, California

The scientific advances in the field of genetics and Turner syndrome reviewed in this symposium are of limited importance unless they can be translated into benefit for the girls who have Turner syndrome. To a large extent, the success of our treatment must be judged ultimately by the patient's feelings of self-worth and her ability to function in society. The papers in this section examine what is now known about the intellectual and psychosocial development and outcome of patients with Turner syndrome. Using this base of information, more rational and comprehensive therapeutic approaches to Turner syndrome should be developed.

Chapter 39 details long-term studies in patients who have Turner syndrome. These studies show that the gender-role behavior in Turner syndrome is basically normal compared either to their siblings or to normal short controls. Their sexuality demonstrates a delaying of heterosexual behavior, with significantly later ages of having boyfriends, "going steady," love, and intercourse. On the other hand, measures of psychopathology are either the same or actually decreased when compared to controls. The intellectual function of the patients with Turner syndrome is within the range of normal as a group, but shows a decreased ability to reproduce figures when compared to either the sibling or the short female control groups. The assessment of social functioning shows a decrease in educational level, occupational level, and a lower proportion who were married or had a steady significant other. Interestingly, there was no correlation

found between the height of Turner syndrome patients and any of these outcome parameters. The authors emphasize that women with Turner syndrome
have a wide range of abilities and problems, just like 46,XX women, and it is
crucial to individualize the approach to each patient.

Dr. Johannes Nielsen (Chapter 36) reviewed the Danish experience with 115
girls with Turner syndrome found among 460,000 girls born between 1955 and
1966. They represent 85% of all the patients in this age range. The overall
picture of school performance in this group is normal, with some increased difficulties in mathematics. In addition, they have excellent records of obtaining and
keeping employment as adults. Dr. Nielsen stressed the importance of early
diagnosis and the provision of complete information to both parents and patients. In addition, he clearly feels that contact groups for Turner syndrome patients are crucial both for the education of the patients with Turner syndrome
and for the education of the public. One of the problems brought up by Dr.
Nielsen is that the prenatal diagnosis of Turner syndrome is being made with
increasing frequency, and in Denmark the vast majority of them are aborted.
In Dr. Nielsen's view, this is inappropriate, and clearly demonstrates the need for
increased education of both physicians and the public about Turner syndrome.

Dr. Soderholm (Chapter 37) shared her experience dealing with untreated
adults with Turner syndrome. In her experience, treatment with estrogens makes
a marked difference in the outlook and psyche of adults with Turner syndrome.

Dr. Michael Preece reviewed the present knowledge about the growth patterns
of Turner syndrome and the various ways of predicting adult height. There is a
remarkable stability in the Z scores (height standard deviation from the mean)
in girls with Turner syndrome. This allows a reasonable prediction of adult
height in girls with Turner syndrome using only their height at a given age and is
at least as good as any prediction of adult height using any of the bone age
methods.

Dr. Judith Hall emphasized the need for a comprehensive approach to girls
with Turner syndrome, and the value of continuing follow-up of adults with
this syndrome. These women are subject to a variety of increased risks of
medical problems associated with Turner syndrome, and their life expectancy is
clearly decreased. Continued comprehensive care by physicians aware of Turner
syndrome and its potential complications is a necessity.

The overall picture that emerges from these contributions is that much more
needs to be done in research, in education, in psychological counseling, and in
medical follow-up to ensure that each one of these girls achieves her own best
human potential.

Index

About the Editors

RON G. ROSENFELD is Professor of Pediatrics at Stanford University School of Medicine, Stanford, California. The coauthor of one book and author or coauthor of more than 150 scientific papers, Dr. Rosenfeld is the recipient of the Ross Award for Research from the Society for Pediatric Research. He is a Fellow of the American Academy of Pediatrics and member of the Endocrine Society, Lawson Wilkins Pediatric Endocrine Society, Society for Pediatric Research, American Federation for Clinical Research, American Diabetes Association, Alpha Omega Alpha, and Phi Beta Kappa. Dr. Rosenfeld received the B.A. degree (1968) from Columbia University, New York, New York, and M.D. degree (1973) from Stanford University School of Medicine, Stanford, California.

MELVIN M. GRUMBACH is Edward B. Shaw Professor of Pediatrics, Emeritus Chairman, Department of Pediatrics, and Acting Director of the Laboratory of Molecular Endocrinology at the University of California, San Francisco. He also serves as Attending Physician at the Medical Center of the University of California, San Francisco, and San Francisco General Hospital. Among his awards are the Borden Award of the American Academy of Pediatrics and the Williams Award of the Endocrine Society. The author or coauthor of more than 280 scientific articles and monographs, Dr. Grumbach has been an invited speaker at numerous conferences and symposia throughout the world. He is past president of the Endocrine Society and the Lawson Wilkins Pediatric Endocrine Society, a Fellow of the American Academy of Pediatrics, American Association for the Advancement of Science, and New York Academy of Sciences, and member of the Institute of Medicine, National Academy of Sciences; American Pediatric Society; Society of Pediatric Research; American Association of Physicians; American Society for Clinical Investigation; Endocrine Society; Alpha Omega Alpha; and Sigma Xi, among other prestigious societies. Dr. Grumbach received the M.D. degree (1948) from Columbia University College of Physicians & Surgeons, New York, New York.